W9-BMQ-394

CLINICIAN'S POCKET DRUG REFERENCE 2007

EDITORS

Leonard G. Gomella, MD, FACS
Steven A. Haist, MD, MS, FACP
Aimee G. Adams, PharmD
Kelly M. Smith, PharmD

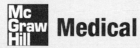

McGraw Hill Medical

New York   Chicago   San Francisco   Lisbon
London   Madrid   Mexico City   Milan   New Delhi
San Juan   Seoul   Singapore   Sydney   Toronto

The McGraw·Hill Companies

Clinician's Pocket Drug Reference 2007

Copyright © 2007 by Leonard G. Gomella. Published by The McGraw-Hill Companies, Inc. All rights reserved. Printed in Canada. Except as permitted under the United States Copyright Act of 1976, no part of this publication may be reproduced or distributed in any form or by any means, or stored in a data base or retrieval system, without the prior written permission of the publisher.

1 2 3 4 5 6 7 8 9 0   TRAFTRA   0 9 8 7 6

ISBN-13: 978-0-07-147768-0
ISBN-10: 0-07-147768-3
ISSN: 1540-6725

The book was set in Times Roman by Pine Tree Composition, Inc.
The editors were Jim Shanahan and Harriet Lebowitz.
The senior production supervisor was Sherri Souffrance.
Project management was provided by Pine Tree Composition, Inc.
Transcontinental Gagne was printer and binder.

This book is printed on acid-free paper.

International Edition ISBN-13: 978-0-07-128656-5; ISBN-10: 0-07-128656-X
Copyright © 2007. Exclusive rights by The McGraw-Hill Companies, Inc., for manufacture and export. This book cannot be reexported from the country to which it is consigned by McGraw-Hill. The International Edition is not available in North America.

CONTENTS

CONSULTING EDITORS

Vincenzo Berghella, MD
Professor, Department of Obstetrics
and Gynecology
Director, Division of Maternal-Fetal
Medicine
Thomas Jefferson University
Philadelphia, Pennsylvania

Tricia L. Gomella, MD
Part-Time Clinical Assistant
Professor of Pediatrics
Johns Hopkins University School
of Medicine
Baltimore, Maryland

Alan T. Lefor, MD, MPH, FACS
Director, Division of Surgical
Oncology
Director, Surgical Education and
Academic Affairs
Department of Surgery
Cedars-Sinai Medical Center
Los Angeles, California;
Associate Professor of Clinical
Surgery,
Department of Surgery,
University of California, Los
Angeles
Los Angeles, California

Nick A. Pavona, MD
Professor, Department of Surgery,
Division of Urology
Benjamin Franklin University
Medical Center
Chadds Ford, Pennsylvania

Carol Beck, PhD
Assistant Dean, Jefferson College of
Graduate Studies
Assistant Professor, Department
of Pharmacology & Experimental
Therapeutics
Thomas Jefferson University
Philadelphia, Pennsylvania

CONTRIBUTORS

Kazumi Morita, PharmD
Infectious Disease Pharmacy
Specialty Resident
University of Kentucky Medical
Center
Lexington, Kentucky

Molly Kent, PharmD
Pharmacy Practice Resident
University of Kentucky Medical
Center
Lexington, Kentucky

Amanda M. Ball, PharmD
Pharmacy Practice Resident
University of Kentucky Medical
Center
Lexington, Kentucky

April D. Miller, PharmD
Pharmacy Practice Resident
University of Kentucky Medical
Center
Lexington, Kentucky

Stella Papadopoulos, PharmD
Critical Care Pharmacy Specialty
Resident
University of Kentucky Medical
Center
Lexington, Kentucky

Peter N. Johnson, PharmD
Pediatrics Pharmacy Specialty
Resident
University of Kentucky Medical
Center
Lexington, Kentucky

Felix Yam, PharmD
Primary Care Pharmacy Specialty
Resident
University of Kentucky Medical
Center
Lexington, Kentucky

PREFACE

We are pleased to present the sixth edition of the *Clinician's Pocket Drug Reference*. This book is based on the drug presentation style used since 1983 in the *Clinician's Pocket Reference*, popularly known as the Scut Monkey Book.

Our goal is to identify the most frequently used and clinically important medications based on input from our readers and editorial board. The book includes over 1000 generic medications and is designed to represent a cross section of those used in medical practices across the country.

The style of drug presentation includes key "must-know" facts of commonly used medications, essential information for both the student and practicing physician. The inclusion of common uses of medications rather than just the official labeled indications are based on the uses of the medication supported by publications and community standards of care. All uses have been reviewed by our editorial board.

It is essential that students and residents in training learn more than the name and dose of the medications they prescribe. Certain common side effects and significant contraindications are associated with most prescription medications. Although health-care providers should ideally be completely familiar with the entire package insert of any medication prescribed, such a requirement is unreasonable. References such as the *Physician's Desk Reference* and the drug manufacturer's Web site make package inserts readily available for many medications, but may not highlight clinically significant facts or provide key data for generic drugs and those available over the counter.

The limitations of difficult-to-read package inserts were acknowledged by the Food and Drug Administration in early 2001, when it noted that physicians do not have time to read the many pages of small print in the typical package insert. In the future, package inserts will likely be redesigned to ensure that important drug interactions, contraindications, and common side effects are highlighted for easier practitioner reference. The editorial board has analyzed the information on both brand and generic medications and has made this key prescribing information available in this pocket-sized book. Information in this book is meant for use by health-care professionals who are familiar with these commonly prescribed medications.

This 2007 edition has been completely reviewed and updated by our editorial board. Over 30 new drugs have been added, and changes in other medications based on FDA actions have been incorporated. New to this edition is a section on commonly used vitamin combinations.

We express special thanks to our spouses and families for their long-term support of this book and the entire Scut Monkey project. The contributions of the members of the editorial board are deeply appreciated. The assistance of Denise Tropea and the team at McGraw-Hill, are also to be thanked.

Your comments and suggestions are always welcome and encouraged because improvements to this and all our books would be impossible without the interest and feedback of our readers. We hope this book will help you learn some of the key elements in prescribing medications and allow you to care for your patients in the best way possible.

Leonard G. Gomella, MD, FACS
Philadelphia, PA
Leonard.Gomella@jefferson.edu

Steven A. Haist, MD, MS, FACP
Lexington, KY
sahaist@uky.edu

Aimee G. Adams, PharmD
Lexington, KY
argelh1@email.uky.edu

Kelly M. Smith, PharmD
Lexington, KY
ksmit1@email.uky.edu

MEDICATION KEY

MEDICATIONS ARE LISTED BY PRESCRIBING CLASS, AND THE INDI-
VIDUAL MEDICATIONS ARE THEN LISTED IN ALPHABETICAL ORDER
BY GENERIC NAME. SOME OF THE MORE COMMONLY RECOGNIZED
TRADE NAMES ARE LISTED FOR EACH MEDICATION (IN PARENTHESES
AFTER THE GENERIC NAME).

> **Generic Drug Name (Selected Common Brand Names)
> [Controlled Substance]** WARNING: Summarized version of the
> "Black Box" precautions deemed necessary by the FDA. These are sig-
> nificant precautions and contraindications concerning the individual med-
> ication. **Uses:** This includes both FDA-labeled indications bracketed by *
> and other "off label" uses of the medication. Because many medications
> are used to treat various conditions based on the medical literature and
> not listed in their package insert, we list common uses of the medication
> rather than the official "labeled indications" (FDA approved) based on
> input from our editorial board **Action:** How the drug works. This infor-
> mation is helpful in comparing classes of drugs and understanding side
> effects and contraindications **Spectrum:** Specifies activity against se-
> lected microbes **Dose:** *Adults.* Where no specific pediatric dose is given,
> the implication is that this drug is not commonly used or indicated in that
> age group. At the end of the dosing line, important dosing modifications
> may be noted (ie, take with food, avoid antacids, etc) **Caution:** [preg-
> nancy/fetal risk categories, breast-feeding (as noted below)] cautions
> concerning the use of the drug in specific settings **Contra:** Contraindica-
> tions **Disp:** Common dosing forms **SE:** Common or significant side ef-
> fects **Notes:** Other key information about the drug.

CONTROLLED SUBSTANCE CLASSIFICATION

Medications under the control of the US Drug Enforcement Agency (Schedule I–V
controlled substances) are indicated by the symbol [C]. Most medications are "uncontrolled" and do not require a DEA prescriber number on the prescription. The
following is a general description for the schedules of DEA controlled substances:

Schedule (C-I) I: All nonresearch use forbidden (eg, heroin, LSD, mescaline).

Schedule (C-II) II: High addictive potential; medical use accepted. No telephone call-in prescriptions; no refills. Some states require special prescription form (eg, cocaine, morphine, methadone).

Schedule (C-III) III: Low to moderate risk of physical dependence, high risk of psychologic dependence; prescription must be rewritten after 6 months or five refills (eg, acetaminophen plus codeine).

Schedule (C-IV) IV: Limited potential for dependence; prescription rules same as for schedule III (eg, benzodiazepines, propoxyphene).

Schedule (C-V) V: Very limited abuse potential; prescribing regulations often same as for uncontrolled medications; some states have additional restrictions.

FDA FETAL RISK CATEGORIES

Category A: Adequate studies in pregnant women have not demonstrated a risk to the fetus in the first trimester of pregnancy; there is no evidence of risk in the last two trimesters.

Category B: Animal studies have not demonstrated a risk to the fetus, but no adequate studies have been done in pregnant women.

or

Animal studies have shown an adverse effect, but adequate studies in pregnant women have not demonstrated a risk to the fetus during the first trimester of pregnancy, and there is no evidence of risk in the last two trimesters.

Category C: Animal studies have shown an adverse effect on the fetus, but no adequate studies have been done in humans. The benefits from the use of the drug in pregnant women may be acceptable despite its potential risks.

or

No animal reproduction studies and no adequate studies in humans have been done.

Category D: There is evidence of human fetal risk, but the potential benefits from the use of the drug in pregnant women may be acceptable despite its potential risks.

Category X: Studies in animals or humans or adverse reaction reports, or both, have demonstrated fetal abnormalities. The risk of use in pregnant women clearly outweighs any possible benefit.

Category ?: No data available (not a formal FDA classification; included to provide complete data set).

BREAST-FEEDING

No formally recognized classification exists for drugs and breast-feeding. This shorthand was developed for the *Clinician's Pocket Drug Reference*.

+	Compatible with breast-feeding
M	Monitor patient or use with caution
±	Excreted, or likely excreted, with unknown effects or at unknown concentrations
?/–	Unknown excretion, but effects likely to be of concern
–	Contraindicated in breast-feeding
?	No data available

ABBREVIATIONS

AB: Antibody

ABMT: autologous bone marrow transplantation

ACE: angiotensin-converting enzyme

ACLS: advanced cardiac life support

ACS: acute coronary syndrome, American Cancer Society, American College of Surgeons

ADH: antidiuretic hormone

ADHD: attention-deficit hyperactivity disorder

ADR: adverse drug reaction

AF: atrial fibrillation

ALL: acute lymphocytic leukemia

ALT: alanine aminotransferase

AMI: acute myocardial infarction

AML: acute myelogenous leukemia

amp: ampule

ANC: absolute neutrophil count

aPTT: activated partial thromboplastin time

APAP: acetaminophen [*N*-acetyl-*p*-aminophenol]

ARB: angiotensin II receptor blocker

ARDS: adult respiratory distress syndrome

ASA: aspirin (acetylsalicylic acid)

AUC: area under the curve

AV: atrioventricular

AVM: arteriovenous malformation

BCL: B-cell lymphoma

BM: bone marrow; bowel movement

BMT: bone marrow transplantation

BOO: bladder outlet obstruction

BSA: body surface area

BUN: blood urea nitrogen

Ca: calcium

CA: cancer

CAD: coronary artery disease

CAP: cancer of the prostate

CBC: complete blood count

CCB: calcium channel blocker

CF: cystic fibrosis

CHF: congestive heart failure

CLL: chronic lymphocytic leukemia

CML: chronic myelogenous leukemia

CMV: cytomegalovirus

Contra: contraindicated

COPD: chronic obstructive pulmonary disease

CP: chest pain

CPP: central precocious puberty

CR: controlled release

CrCl: creatinine clearance

CRF: chronic renal failure

CV: cardiovascular

CVA: cerebrovascular accident, costovertebral angle

CVH: common variable hypergammaglobulinemia

D: diarrhea

D_5LR: 5% dextrose in lactated Ringer's solution

D_5NS: 5% dextrose in normal saline

D$_5$W: 5% dextrose in water

D/C: discontinue

DI: diabetes insipidus

Disp: dispensed as, how the drug is supplied

DKA: diabetic ketoacidosis

dL: deciliter

DM: diabetes mellitus

DMARD (Disease-modifying antirheumatic drug) drugs defined in randomized trials to decrease erosions and joint space narrowing in rheumatoid arthritis (eg, D-penicillamine, methotrexate, azathioprine)

DN: diabetic nephropathy

dppr: dropper

DOT: directly observed therapy

DVT: deep venous thrombosis

Dz: disease

EC: enteric-coated

ECC: emergency cardiac care

ECG: electrocardiogram

ED: erectile dysfunction

ELISA: enzyme-linked immunosorbent assay

EMIT: enzyme-multiplied immunoassay text

EPS: extrapyramidal symptoms (tardive dyskinesia, tremors and rigidity, restlessness [akathisia], muscle contractions [dystonia], changes in breathing and heart rate)

ER: extended release

ESRD: end-stage renal disease

ET: endotracheal

EtOH: ethanol

FSH: follicle-stimulating hormone

5-FU: fluorouracil

Fxn: function

G-CSF: granulocyte colony-stimulating factor

gen: generation

GERD: gastroesophageal reflux disease

GF: growth factor

GFR: glomerular filtration rate

GI: gastrointestinal

GIST: Gastrointestinal stromal tumor

GM-CSF: granulocyte-macrophage colony-stimulating factor

GnRH: gonadotropin-releasing hormone

gt, gtt: drop, drops (*gutta*)

HA: headache

HCL: hairy cell leukemia

Hct: hematocrit

HCTZ: hydrochlorothiazide

HD: hemodialysis

Hgb: hemoglobin

HIT: heparin-induced thrombocytopenia

HIV: human immunodeficiency virus

HMG-CoA: hydroxymethylglutaryl coenzyme A

hs: at bedtime (*hora somni*)

HSV: herpes simplex virus

5-HT: 5-hydroxytryptamine

HTN: hypertension

Hx: history of

IBD: irritable bowel disease

IBS: irritable bowel syndrome

ICP: intracranial pressure

IFIS: Intraoperative Floppy Iris Syndrome

Ig: immunoglobulin

IM: intramuscular

Inf: Infusion

Infxn: infection

Inh: inhalation

INH: isoniazid

INR: international normalized ratio

Insuff: insufficiency

intravag: intravaginal

IOP: intraocular pressure
ISA: intrinsic sympathomimetic activity
IT: intrathecal
ITP: idiopathic thrombocytopenic purpura
IV: intravenous
K: potassium
LDL: low-density lipoprotein
LFT: liver function test
LH: luteinizing hormone
LHRH: luteinizing hormone-releasing hormone
LMW: low molecular weight
LVD: left ventricular dysfunction
LVSD: left ventricular systolic dysfunction
MAC: *Mycobacterium avium* complex
MAO/MAOI: monoamine oxidase/inhibitor
mEq: milliequivalent
MI: myocardial infarction, mitral insufficiency
mL: milliliter
MoAb: monoclonal antibody
MRSA: methicillin-resistant *Staphylococcus aureus*
MS: multiple sclerosis
MSSA: methicillin-sensitive *Staphylococcus aureus*
MTT: monotetrazolium
MTX: methotrexate
MyG: myasthenia gravis
N: nausea
NA: narrow angle
NAG: narrow angle glaucoma
ng: nanogram
NG: nasogastric
NHL: non-Hodgkin's lymphoma
NIDDM: non-insulin-dependent diabetes mellitus

nl: normal
NO: nitric oxide
NPO: nothing by mouth (*nil per os*)
NRTI: nucleoside reverse transcriptase inhibitor
NS: normal saline
NSAID: nonsteroidal antiinflammatory drug
NSCLC: non-small-cell lung cancer
N/V: nausea and vomiting
N/V/D: nausea, vomiting, diarrhea
OAB: overactive bladder
OCP: oral contraceptive pill
OD: overdose
ODT: orally disintegrating tablets
OK: recommended
OTC: over the counter
PAT: paroxysmal atrial tachycardia
pc: after eating (*post cibum*)
PCN: penicillin
PCP: *Pneumocystis jiroveci* (formerly *carinii*) pneumonia
PCWP: pulmonary capillary wedge pressure
PDE5: phosphodiesterase type 5
PDGF: platelet-derived growth factor
PE: pulmonary embolus, physical examination, pleural effusion
PFT: pulmonary function test
pg: picogram
PID: pelvic inflammatory disease
plt: platelet
PMDD: premenstrual dysphoric disorder
PO: by mouth (*per os*)
PPD: purified protein derivative
PR: by rectum
PRG: pregnancy
PRN: as often as needed (*pro re nata*)
PSVT: paroxysmal supraventricular tachycardia
pt: patient

PT: prothrombin time
PTCA: percutaneous transluminal
   coronary angioplasty
PTH: parathyroid hormone
PTT: partial thromboplastin time
PUD: peptic ulcer disease
PVC: premature ventricular
   contraction
PWP: pulmonary wedge pressure
Px: prevention
q: every (*quaque*)
q_h: every _ hours
qd: every day
qh: every hour
qhs: every hour of sleep (before
   bedtime)
qid: four times a day (*quater in die*)
qod: every other day
RA: rheumatoid arthritis
RCC: renal cell carcinoma
RDA: recommended dietary
   allowance
RDS: respiratory distress syndrome
resp: respiratory
RSV: respiratory syncytial virus
RT: reverse transcriptase
RTA: renal tubular acidosis
Rx: prescription or therapy
Rxn: reaction
SCr: serum creatinine
SDV: Single Dose Vial
SIADH: syndrome of inappropriate
   antidiuretic hormone
SL: sublingual
SLE: systemic lupus erythematosus
Sol/soln: solution
SPAG: small particle aerosol
   generator
Sp: species
SQ: subcutaneous
SR: sustained release

SSRI: selective serotonin reuptake
   inhibitor
SSS: sick sinus syndrome
S/Sys: signs & symptoms
stat: immediately (*statim*)
supl: supplement
supp: suppository
SVT: supraventricular tachycardia
Sx: symptom
Sz: seizure
tab/tabs: tablet/tablets
TB: tuberculosis
TCA: tricyclic antidepressant
TTS: transdermal therapeutic system
TFT: thyroid function test
TIA: transient ischemic attack
tid: three times a day (*ter in die*)
TMP: trimethoprim
TMP—SMX: trimethoprim—
   sulfamethoxazole
tox: toxicity
TPA: tissue plasminogen activator
tri: trimester
TTP: thrombotic thrombocytopenic
   purpura
Tx: treatment
uln: upper limits of normal
URI: upper respiratory infection
UTI: urinary tract infection
Vag: vaginal
VF: ventricular fibrillation
VRE: vancomycin-resistant
   Enterococcus
VT: ventricular tachycardia
WHI: Women's Health Initiative
WNL: within normal limits
WPW: Wolff—Parkinson—White
   syndrome
XR: extended release
ZE: Zollinger—Ellison (syndrome)

CLASSIFICATION (Generic and common brand names)

ALLERGY

Antihistamines

Azelastine (Astelin, Optivar)
Cetirizine (Zyrtec, Zyrtec D)
Chlorpheniramine (Chlor-Trimeton)

Clemastine Fumarate (Tavist)
Cyproheptadine (Periactin)
Desloratadine (Clarinex)
Diphenhydramine (Benadryl)

Fexofenadine (Allegra)
Hydroxyzine (Atarax, Vistaril)
Loratadine (Claritin, Alavert)

Miscellaneous Antiallergy Agents

Budesonide (Rhinocort, Pulmicort)

Cromolyn Sodium (Intal, NasalCrom, Opticrom)

Montelukast (Singulair)

ANTIDOTES

Acetylcysteine (Acetadote, Mucomyst)
Amifostine (Ethyol)
Charcoal (SuperChar, Actidose, Liqui-Char Activated)
Deferasirox (Exjade)

Dexrazoxane (Zinecard)
Digoxin Immune Fab (Digibind)
Flumazenil (Romazicon)
Ipecac Syrup (OTC Syrup)
Mesna (Mesnex)

Naloxone (Narcan)
Physostigmine (Antilirium)
Succimer (Chemet)

ANTIMICROBIAL AGENTS

Antibiotics

AMINOGLYCOSIDES
Amikacin (Amikin)
Gentamicin (Garamycin, G-Mycitin)

Neomycin
Streptomycin

Tobramycin (Nebcin)

CARBAPENEMS

Ertapenem (Invanz)

Imipenem-Cilastatin (Primaxin)

Meropenem (Merrem)

CEPHALOSPORINS, FIRST GENERATION

Cefadroxil (Duricef, Ultracef)

Cefazolin (Ancef, Kefzol)

Cephalexin (Keflex, Keftab)

Cephradine (Velosef)

CEPHALOSPORINS, SECOND GENERATION

Cefaclor (Ceclor)
Cefmetazole (Zefazone)
Cefonicid (Monocid)
Cefotetan (Cefotan)

Cefoxitin (Mefoxin)
Cefprozil (Cefzil)

Cefuroxime (Ceftin [oral], Zinacef [parenteral])
Loracarbef (Lorabid)

CEPHALOSPORINS, THIRD GENERATION

Cefdinir (Omnicef)
Cefditoren (Spectracef)
Cefixime (Suprax)
Cefoperazone (Cefobid)
Cefotaxime (Claforan)

Cefpodoxime (Vantin)
Ceftazidime (Fortaz, Ceptaz, Tazidime, Tazicef)
Ceftibuten (Cedax)

Ceftizoxime (Cefizox)
Ceftriaxone (Rocephin)

CEPHALOSPORINS, FOURTH GENERATION

Cefepime (Maxipime)

FLUOROQUINOLONES

Ciprofloxacin (Cipro)
Gatifloxacin (Tequin)
Gemifloxacin (Factive)
Levofloxacin (Levaquin, Quixin Ophthalmic)

Lomefloxacin (Maxaquin)
Moxifloxacin (Avelox)
Norfloxacin (Noroxin, Chibroxin Ophthalmic)

Ofloxacin (Floxin, Ocuflox Ophthalmic)

MACROLIDES

Azithromycin (Zithromax)
Clarithromycin (Biaxin)

Dirithromycin (Dynabac)
Erythromycin (E-Mycin, E.E.S., Ery-Tab)

Erythromycin & Sulfisoxazole (Eryzole, Pediazole)

KETOLIDE

Telithromycin (Ketek)

PENICILLINS

Amoxicillin (Amoxil, Polymox)
Amoxicillin & Clavulanic Acid (Augmentin)
Ampicillin (Amcill, Omnipen)
Ampicillin-Sulbactam (Unasyn)
Dicloxacillin (Dynapen, Dycill)

Nafcillin (Nallpen)
Oxacillin (Bactocill, Prostaphlin)
Penicillin G, Aqueous (Potassium or Sodium) (Pfizerpen, Pentids)
Penicillin G Benzathine (Bicillin)

Penicillin G Procaine (Wycillin)
Penicillin V (Pen-Vee K, Veetids)
Piperacillin (Pipracil)
Piperacillin-Tazobactam (Zosyn)
Ticarcillin (Ticar)
Ticarcillin/Potassium Clavulanate (Timentin)

TETRACYCLINES

Doxycycline (Vibramycin)

Tetracycline (Achromycin V, Sumycin)

Tigecycline (Tygacil)

Miscellaneous Antibiotic Agents

Aztreonam (Azactam)
Clindamycin (Cleocin, Cleocin-T)
Fosfomycin (Monurol)
Linezolid (Zyvox)
Metronidazole (Flagyl, MetroGel)

Quinupristin-Dalfopristin (Synercid)
Rifaximin (Xifaxan)
Trimethoprim-Sulfamethoxazole [Co-Trimoxazole] (Bactrim, Septra)

Vancomycin (Vancocin, Vancoled)

Antifungals

Amphotericin B (Fungizone)
Amphotericin B Cholesteryl (Amphotec)
Amphotericin B Lipid Complex (Abelcet)
Amphotericin B Liposomal (AmBisome)

Anidulafungin (Eraxis)
Caspofungin (Cancidas)
Clotrimazole (Lotrimin, Mycelex)
Clotrimazole & Betamethasone (Lotrisone)
Econazole (Spectazole)
Fluconazole (Diflucan)
Itraconazole (Sporanox)

Ketoconazole (Nizoral)
Miconazole (Monistat)
Nystatin (Mycostatin)
Oxiconazole (Oxistat)
Sertaconazole (Ertaczo)
Terbinafine (Lamisil)
Triamcinolone & Nystatin (Mycolog-II)
Voriconazole (VFEND)

Antimycobacterials

Dapsone (Avlosulfon)
Ethambutol (Myambutol)
Isoniazid (INH)

Pyrazinamide
Rifabutin (Mycobutin)
Rifampin (Rifadin)

Rifapentine (Priftin)
Streptomycin

Antiprotozoals

Nitazoxanide (Alinia)   Tinidazole (Tindamax)

Antiretrovirals

Abacavir (Ziagen)
Amprenavir (Agenerase)
Delavirdine (Rescriptor)
Didanosine [ddI] (Videx)
Efavirenz (Sustiva)
Efavirenz 600
    mg/emtricitabine 200
    mg/tenofovir
    disoproxil fumarate
    300 mg (Atripla)
Fosamprenavir (Lexiva)
Indinavir (Crixivan)
Lamivudine (Epivir,
    Epivir-HBV)
Lopinavir/Ritonavir
    (Kaletra)
Nelfinavir (Viracept)
Nevirapine (Viramune)
Ritonavir (Norvir)
Saquinavir (Fortovase)
Stavudine (Zerit)
Tenofovir (Viread)
Tenofovir/Emtricitabine
    (Truvada)
Zalcitabine (Hivid)
Zidovudine (Retrovir)
Zidovudine &
    Lamivudine
    (Combivir)

Antivirals

Acyclovir (Zovirax)
Adefovir (Hepsera)
Amantadine
    (Symmetrel)
Atazanavir (Reyataz)
Cidofovir (Vistide)
Emtricitabine (Emtriva)
Enfuvirtide (Fuzeon)
Famciclovir (Famvir)
Foscarnet (Foscavir)
Ganciclovir (Cytovene,
    Vitrasert)
Interferon Alfa-2b &
    Ribavirin Combo
    (Rebetron)
Oseltamivir (Tamiflu)
Palivizumab (Synagis)
Peg Interferon Alfa 2a
    (Peg Intron)
Penciclovir (Denavir)
Ribavirin (Virazole)
Rimantadine
    (Flumadine)
Valacyclovir (Valtrex)
Valganciclovir (Valcyte)
Zanamivir (Relenza)

Miscellaneous Antimicrobial Agents

Atovaquone (Mepron)
Atovaquone/Proguanil
    (Malarone)
Daptomycin (Cubicin)
Pentamidine (Pentam
    300, NebuPent)
Trimetrexate (Neutrexin)

ANTINEOPLASTIC AGENTS

Alkylating Agents

Altretamine (Hexalen)
Busulfan (Myleran,
    Busulfex)
Carboplatin (Paraplatin)
Cisplatin (Platinol)
Oxaliplatin (Eloxatin)
Procarbazine (Matulane)
Triethylenetriphosphami
de (Thio-Tepa)

NITROGEN MUSTARDS

Chlorambucil (Leukeran)

Cyclophosphamide (Cytoxan, Neosar)

Ifosfamide (Ifex, Holoxan)

Mechlorethamine (Mustargen)

Melphalan [L-PAM] (Alkeran)

NITROSOUREAS

Carmustine [BCNU] (BiCNU, Gliadel)

Streptozocin (Zanosar)

Antibiotics

Bleomycin Sulfate (Blenoxane)

Dactinomycin (Cosmegen)

Daunorubicin (Daunomycin, Cerubidine)

Doxorubicin (Adriamycin, Rubex)

Epirubicin (Ellence)

Idarubicin (Idamycin)

Mitomycin (Mutamycin)

Antimetabolites

Clofarabine (Clolar)

Cytarabine [ARA-C] (Cytosar-U)

Cytarabine Liposome (DepoCyt)

Floxuridine (FUDR)

Fludarabine Phosphate (Flamp, Fludara)

Fluorouracil [5-FU] (Adrucil)

Gemcitabine (Gemzar)

Mercaptopurine [6-MP] (Purinethol)

Methotrexate (Folex, Rheumatrex)

Nelarabine (Arranon)

Pemetrexed (Alimta)

6-Thioguanine [6-TG]

Hormones

Anastrozole (Arimidex)

Bicalutamide (Casodex)

Estramustine Phosphate (Estracyt, Emcyt)

Exemestane (Aromasin)

Fluoxymesterone (Halotestin)

Flutamide (Eulexin)

Fulvestrant (Faslodex)

Goserelin (Zoladex)

Leuprolide (Lupron, Viadur, Eligard)

Levamisole (Ergamisol)

Megestrol Acetate (Megace)

Nilutamide (Nilandron)

Tamoxifen

Triptorelin (Trelstar Depot, Trelstar LA)

Mitotic Inhibitors

Etoposide [VP-16] (VePesid)

Vinblastine (Velban, Velbe)

Vincristine (Oncovin, Vincasar PFS)

Vinorelbine (Navelbine)

Monoclonal Antibodies

Cetuximab (Erbitux)   Erlotinib (Tarceva)   Trastuzumab (Herceptin)

Miscellaneous Antineoplastic Agents

Aldesleukin [Interleukin-2, IL-2] (Proleukin)
Aminoglutethimide (Cytadren)
L-Asparaginase (Elspar, Oncaspar)
BCG [Bacillus Calmette-Guérin] (TheraCys, Tice BCG)
Bevacizumab (Avastin)
Bortezomib (Velcade)
Cladribine (Leustatin)
Dacarbazine (DTIC)

Docetaxel (Taxotere)
Gefitinib (Iressa)
Gemtuzumab Ozogamicin (Mylotarg)
Hydroxyurea (Hydrea, Droxia)
Imatinib (Gleevec)
Irinotecan (Camptosar)
Letrozole (Femara)
Leucovorin (Wellcovorin)
Mitoxantrone (Novantrone)

Paclitaxel (Taxol, Abraxane)
Pemetrexed (Alimta)
Rasburicase (Elitek)
Sorafenib (Nexavar)
Sunitinib (Sutent)
Thalidomide (Thalomid)
Topotecan (Hycamtin)
Tretinoin, Topical [Retinoic Acid] (Retin-A, Avita, Renova)

CARDIOVASCULAR (CV) AGENTS

Aldosterone Antagonist

Eplerenone (Inspra)

Alpha$_1$-Adrenergic Blockers

Doxazosin (Cardura)   Prazosin (Minipress)   Terazosin (Hytrin)

Angiotensin-Converting Enzyme (ACE) Inhibitors

Benazepril (Lotensin)
Captopril (Capoten)
Enalapril (Vasotec)
Fosinopril (Monopril)

Lisinopril (Prinivil, Zestril)
Moexipril (Univasc)
Perindopril Erbumine (Aceon)

Quinapril (Accupril)
Ramipril (Altace)
Trandolapril (Mavik)

Angiotensin II Receptor Antagonists

Candesartan (Atacand)
Eprosartan (Teveten)

Irbesartan (Avapro)
Losartan (Cozaar)

Telmisartan (Micardis)
Valsartan (Diovan)

Antiarrhythmic Agents

Adenosine (Adenocard)
Amiodarone (Cordarone, Pacerone)
Atropine
Digoxin (Lanoxin, Lanoxicaps)
Disopyramide (Norpace, NAPAmide)

Dofetilide (Tikosyn)
Esmolol (Brevibloc)
Flecainide (Tambocor)
Ibutilide (Corvert)
Lidocaine (Anestacon Topical, Xylocaine)
Mexiletine (Mexitil)

Procainamide (Pronestyl, Procan)
Propafenone (Rythmol)
Quinidine (Quinidex, Quinaglute)
Sotalol (Betapace, Betapace AF)

Beta-Adrenergic Blockers

Acebutolol (Sectral)
Atenolol (Tenormin)
Atenolol & Chlorthalidone (Tenoretic)
Betaxolol (Kerlone)
Bisoprolol (Zebeta)

Carteolol (Cartrol, Ocupress Ophthalmic)
Carvedilol (Coreg)
Labetalol (Trandate, Normodyne)
Metoprolol (Lopressor, Toprol XL)

Nadolol (Corgard)
Penbutolol (Levatol)
Pindolol (Visken)
Propranolol (Inderal)
Timolol (Blocadren)

Calcium Channel Antagonists

Amlodipine (Norvasc)
Diltiazem (Cardizem, Cartia XT, Dilacor, Diltia XT, Tiamate, Tiazac)
Felodipine (Plendil)

Isradipine (DynaCirc)
Nicardipine (Cardene)
Nifedipine (Procardia, Procardia XL, Adalat, Adalat CC)
Nimodipine (Nimotop)

Nisoldipine (Sular)
Verapamil (Calan, Isoptin)

Centrally Acting Antihypertensive Agents

Clonidine (Catapres)
Methyldopa (Aldomet)

Diuretics

Acetazolamide (Diamox)
Amiloride (Midamor)
Bumetanide (Bumex)
Chlorothiazide (Diuril)
Chlorthalidone (Hygroton)

Furosemide (Lasix)
Hydrochlorothiazide (HydroDIURIL, Esidrix)
Hydrochlorothiazide & Amiloride (Moduretic)

Hydrochlorothiazide & Spironolactone (Aldactazide)
Hydrochlorothiazide & Triamterene (Dyazide, Maxzide)

Indapamide (Lozol)   Spironolactone   Torsemide (Demadex)
Mannitol   (Aldactone)   Triamterene (Dyrenium)
Metolazone (Mykrox,
  Zaroxolyn)

Inotropic/Pressor Agents

Digoxin (Lanoxin,   Epinephrine (Adrenalin,   Nesiritide (Natrecor)
  Lanoxicaps)   Sus-Phrine, EpiPen)   Norepinephrine
Dobutamine (Dobutrex)   Inamrinone (Inocor)   (Levophed)
Dopamine (Intropin)   Isoproterenol (Isuprel)   Phenylephrine (Neo-
                              Milrinone (Primacor)   Synephrine)

Lipid-Lowering Agents

Atorvastatin (Lipitor)   Fenofibrate (TriCor)   Pravastatin (Pravachol)
Cholestyramine   Fluvastatin (Lescol)   Rosuvastatin (Crestor)
  (Questran, LoCholest)   Gemfibrozil (Lopid)   Simvastatin (Zocor)
Colesevelam (WelChol)   Lovastatin (Mevacor,
Colestipol (Colestid)   Altocor)
Ezetimibe (Zetia)   Niacin (Niaspan)

Lipid-Lowering/Antihypertensive Combos

Amlodipine/Atorvastatin
  (Caduet)

Vasodilators

Alprostadil   Isosorbide Dinitrate   Bid Ointment, Nitro-
  [Prostaglandin E₁]   (Isordil, Sorbitrate,   Bid IV, Nitrodisc,
  (Prostin VR)   Dilatrate-SR)   Transderm-Nitro)
Epoprostenol (Flolan)   Isosorbide Mononitrate   Nitroprusside (Nipride,
Fenoldopam (Corlopam)   (Ismo, Imdur)   Nitropress)
Hydralazine (Apresoline)   Minoxidil (Loniten,   Tolazoline (Priscoline)
Iloprost (Ventavis)   Rogaine)   Treprostinil Sodium
                              Nitroglycerin (Nitrostat,   (Remodulin)
                                Nitrolingual, Nitro-

Miscellaneous Cardiovascular Agents

Conivaptan (Vaprisol)   Ranolazine (Ranexa)

CENTRAL NERVOUS SYSTEM AGENTS

Antianxiety Agents

Alprazolam (Xanax)
Buspirone (BuSpar)
Chlordiazepoxide
   (Librium, Mitran,
   Libritabs)
Clorazepate (Tranxene)

Diazepam (Valium)
Doxepin (Sinequan,
   Adapin)
Hydroxyzine (Atarax,
   Vistaril)
Lorazepam (Ativan)

Meprobamate (Equanil,
   Miltown)
Oxazepam (Serax)

Anticonvulsants

Carbamazepine (Tegretol)
Clonazepam (Klonopin)
Diazepam (Valium)
Ethosuximide (Zarontin)
Fosphenytoin (Cerebyx)
Gabapentin (Neurontin)

Lamotrigine (Lamictal)
Levetiracetam (Keppra)
Lorazepam (Ativan)
Oxcarbazepine (Trileptal)
Pentobarbital (Nembutal)
Phenobarbital

Phenytoin (Dilantin)
Tiagabine (Gabitril)
Topiramate (Topamax)
Valproic Acid
   (Depakene, Depakote)
Zonisamide (Zonegran)

Antidepressants

Amitriptyline (Elavil)
Bupropion (Wellbutrin,
   Zyban)
Citalopram (Celexa)
Desipramine
   (Norpramin)
Doxepin (Sinequan,
   Adapin)
Duloxetine (Cymbalta)

Escitalopram (Lexapro)
Fluoxetine (Prozac,
   Sarafem)
Fluvoxamine (Luvox)
Imipramine (Tofranil)
Mirtazapine (Remeron)
Nefazodone
Nortriptyline (Aventyl,
   Pamelor)

Paroxetine (Paxil)
Phenelzine (Nardil)
Selegiline transdermal
   (Emsam)
Sertraline (Zoloft)
Trazodone (Desyrel)
Venlafaxine (Effexor)

Antiparkinson Agents

Amantadine (Symmetrel)
Apomorphine (Apokyn)
Benztropine (Cogentin)
Bromocriptine (Parlodel)
Carbidopa/Levodopa
   (Sinemet)

Entacapone (Comtan)
Pergolide (Permax)
Pramipexole (Mirapex)
Rasagiline mesylate
   (Azilect)
Ropinirole (Requip)

Selegiline (Eldepryl)
Tolcapone (Tasmar)
Trihexyphenidyl
   (Artane)

Antipsychotics

Aripiprazole (Abilify)
Chlorpromazine
   (Thorazine)

Clozapine (Clozaril)
Fluphenazine (Prolixin,
   Permitil)

Haloperidol (Haldol)
Lithium Carbonate
   (Eskalith, Lithobid)

Molindone (Moban)
Olanzapine (Zyprexa)
Perphenazine (Trilafon)
Prochlorperazine
(Compazine)

Quetiapine (Seroquel)
Risperidone (Risperdal)
Thioridazine (Mellaril)
Thiothixene (Navane)

Trifluoperazine
(Stelazine)
Ziprasidone (Geodon)

Sedative Hypnotics

Chloral Hydrate
(Aquachloral,
Supprettes)
Diphenhydramine
(Benadryl)
Estazolam (ProSom)
Eszopiclone (Lunesta)

Flurazepam (Dalmane)
Hydroxyzine (Atarax,
Vistaril)
Midazolam (Versed)
Pentobarbital
(Nembutal)
Phenobarbital

Propofol (Diprivan)
Quazepam (Doral)
Secobarbital (Seconal)
Temazepam (Restoril)
Triazolam (Halcion)
Zaleplon (Sonata)
Zolpidem (Ambien)

Miscellaneous CNS Agents

Atomoxetine (Strattera)
Galantamine (Reminyl)
Interferon beta 1a
(Rebif)
Memantine (Namenda)

Methylphenidate, Oral
(Concerta, Ritalin,
Ritalin-SR others)
Methylphenidate,
Transdermal
(Daytrana)

Natalizumab (Tysabri)
Nimodipine (Nimotop)
Rivastigmine (Exelon)
Sodium Oxybate (Xyrem)
Tacrine (Cognex)

DERMATOLOGIC AGENTS

Acitretin (Soriatane)
Acyclovir (Zovirax)
Alefacept (Amevive)
Anthralin (Anthra-Derm)
Amphotericin B
(Fungizone)
Bacitracin, Topical
(Baciguent)
Bacitracin & Polymyxin
B, Topical (Polysporin)
Bacitracin, Neomycin, &
Polymyxin B, Topical
(Neosporin Ointment)
Bacitracin, Neomycin,
Polymyxin B, &
Hydrocortisone,
Topical (Cortisporin)

Bacitracin, Neomycin,
Polymyxin B, &
Lidocaine, Topical
(Clomycin)
Calcipotriene (Dovonex)
Capsaicin (Capsin,
Zostrix)
Ciclopirox (Loprox)
Ciprofloxacin (Cipro)
Clindamycin (Cleocin)
Clotrimazole &
Betamethasone
(Lotrisone)
Dibucaine (Nupercainal)
Doxepin, Topical
(Zonalon)
Econazole (Spectazole)

Efalizumab (Raptiva)
Erythromycin, Topical
(A/T/S, Eryderm,
Erycette, T-Stat)
Finasteride (Proscar,
Propecia)
Gentamicin, Topical
(Garamycin, G-
Mycitin)
Haloprogin (Halotex)
Imiquimod Cream, 5%
(Aldara)
Isotretinoin [13-cis
Retinoic acid]
(Accutane,
Amnesteem, Claravis,
Sotret)

Ketoconazole (Nizoral)
Lactic Acid & Ammonium Hydroxide [Ammonium Lactate] (Lac-Hydrin)
Lindane (Kwell)
Metronidazole (Flagyl, MetroGel)
Miconazole (Monistat)
Minoxidil (Loniten, Rogaine)
Mupirocin (Bactroban)
Naftifine (Naftin)
Neomycin Sulfate (Myciguent)
Nystatin (Mycostatin)

Oxiconazole (Oxistat)
Penciclovir (Denavir)
Permethrin (Nix, Elimite)
Pimecrolimus (Elidel)
Podophyllin (Podocon-25, Condylox Gel 0.5%, Condylox)
Pramoxine (Anusol Ointment, ProctoFoam-NS)
Pramoxine & Hydrocortisone (Enzone, ProctoFoam-HC)
Selenium Sulfide (Exsel Shampoo, Selsun Blue

Shampoo, Selsun Shampoo)
Silver Sulfadiazine (Silvadene)
Steroids, Topical (Table 5, page 217)
Tacrolimus (Prograf, Protopic)
Tazarotene (Tazorac)
Terbinafine (Lamisil)
Tolnaftate (Tinactin)
Tretinoin, Topical [Retinoic Acid] (Retin-A, Avita, Renova)

DIETARY SUPPLEMENTS

Calcium Acetate (Calphron, Phos-Ex, PhosLo)
Calcium Glubionate (Neo-Calglucon)
Calcium Salts [Chloride, Gluconate, Gluceptate]
Cholecalciferol [Vitamin D_3] (Delta D)
Cyanocobalamin [Vitamin B_{12}]
Ferric Gluconate Complex (Ferrlecit)

Ferrous Gluconate (Fergon)
Ferrous Sulfate
Fish Oil (Omacor, OTC)
Folic Acid
Iron Dextran (DexFerrum, INFeD)
Iron Sucrose (Venofer)
Magnesium Oxide (Mag-Ox 400)
Magnesium Sulfate
Multivitamins (Table 15, page 233)

Phytonadione [Vitamin K] (Aqua-MEPHYTON)
Potassium Supplements (Kaon, Kaochlor, K-Lor, Slow-K, Micro K, Klorvess)
Pyridoxine [Vitamin B_6]
Sodium Bicarbonate [$NaHCO_3$]
Thiamine [Vitamin B_1]

EAR (OTIC) AGENTS

Acetic Acid & Aluminum Acetate (Otic Domeboro)
Benzocaine & Antipyrine (Auralgan)
Ciprofloxacin, Otic (Cipro HC Otic)
Neomycin, Colistin, & Hydrocortisone

(Cortisporin-TC Otic Drops)
Neomycin, Colistin, Hydrocortisone, & Thonzonium (Cortisporin-TC Otic Suspension)

Polymyxin B & Hydrocortisone (Otobiotic Otic)
Sulfacetamide & Prednisolone (Blephamide)
Triethanolamine (Cerumenex)

ENDOCRINE SYSTEM AGENTS

Antidiabetic Agents

Acarbose (Precose)
Chlorpropamide
   (Diabinese)
Glimepiride (Amaryl)
Glipizide (Glucotrol)
Glyburide (DiaBeta,
   Micronase, Glynase)
Glyburide/Metformin
   (Glucovance)

Insulins, Systemic
   (Table 6)
Insulin Human
   Inhalation Powder
   (Exubera)
Metformin (Glucophage)
Miglitol (Glyset)
Nateglinide (Starlix)
Pioglitazone (Actos)

Pioglitazone/Metformin
   (ActoPlus Met)
Repaglinide (Prandin)
Rosiglitazone (Avandia)
Tolazamide (Tolinase)
Tolbutamide (Orinase)

Hormone & Synthetic Substitutes

Calcitonin (Cibacalcin,
   Miacalcin)
Calcitriol (Rocaltrol,
   Calcisex)
Cortisone Systemic,
   Topical
Desmopressin (DDAVP,
   Stimate)
Dexamethasone
   (Decadron)

Fludrocortisone Acetate
   (Florinef)
Glucagon
Hydrocortisone Topical
   & Systemic (Cortef,
   Solu-Cortef)
Methylprednisolone
   (Solu-Medrol)
Prednisolone
Prednisone

Testosterone (AndroGel,
   Androderm, Striant,
   Testim, Testoderm)
Vasopressin [Antidiuretic
   Hormone, ADH]
   (Pitressin)

Hypercalcemia/Osteoporosis Agents

Etidronate Disodium
   (Didronel)

Gallium Nitrate (Ganite)
Ibandronate (Boniva)

Pamidronate (Aredia)
Zoledronic acid (Zometa)

Obesity

Sibutramine (Meridia)

Osteoporosis Agents

Alendronate (Fosamax)
Raloxifene (Evista)

Risedronate (Actonel)
Teriparatide (Forteo)

Zoledronic Acid
   (Zometa)

Thyroid/Antithyroid

Levothyroxine
(Synthroid, Levoxyl)
Liothyronine (Cytomel)
Methimazole (Tapazole)

Potassium iodide [Lugol
Solution] (SSKI,
Thyro-Block)

Propylthiouracil [PTU]

Miscellaneous Endocrine Agents

Cinacalcet (Sensipar)

Demeclocycline
(Declomycin)

Diazoxide (Hyperstat,
Proglycem)

EYE (OPHTHALMIC) AGENTS

Glaucoma Agents

Acetazolamide (Diamox)
Apraclonidine (Iopidine)
Betaxolol, Ophthalmic
(Betopic)
Brimonidine (Alphagan)
Brinzolamide (Azopt)
Carteolol (Cartrol,
Ocupress Ophthalmic)
Ciprofloxacin,
Ophthalmic (Ciloxan)
Cyclosporine,
Ophthalmic (Restasis)
Dipivefrin (Propine)
Dorzolamide (Trusopt)

Dorzolamide & Timolol
(Cosopt)
Echothiophate Iodine
(Phospholine
Ophthalmic)
Epinastine (Elestat)
Gatifloxacin Ophthalmic
(Zymar Ophthalmic)
Latanoprost (Xalatan)
Levobunolol (A-K Beta,
Betagan)
Levocabastine (Livostin)
Levofloxacin (Levaquin,
Quixin & Iquix
Ophthalmic)

Lodoxamide (Alomide)
Moxifloxacin (Vigamox)
Neomycin, Polymyxin,
& Hydrocortisone
(Cortisporin
Ophthalmic & Otic)
Norfloxacin (Chibroxin)
Ofloxacin (Ocuflox
Ophthalmic)
Rimexolone (Vexol
Ophthalmic)
Timolol, Ophthalmic
(Timoptic)
Trifluridine, Ophthalmic
(Viroptic)

Ophthalmic Antibiotics

Bacitracin, Ophthalmic
(AK-Tracin
Ophthalmic)
Bacitracin & Polymyxin
B, Ophthalmic (AK
Poly Bac Ophthalmic,

Polysporin
Ophthalmic)
Bacitracin, Neomycin, &
Polymyxin B
Spore Ophthalmic,
Neosporin
Ophthalmic)

Bacitracin, Neomycin,
Polymyxin B, &
Hydrocortisone,
Ophthalmic (AK
Spore HC Ophthalmic,
Cortisporin
Ophthalmic)

Ciprofloxacin, Ophthalmic (Ciloxan)
Erythromycin, Ophthalmic (Ilotycin Ophthalmic)
Gentamicin, Ophthalmic (Garamycin, Genoptic, Gentacidin, Gentak)
Neomycin & Dexamethasone (AK-Neo-Dex Ophthalmic, NeoDecadron Ophthalmic)
Neomycin, Polymyxin B, & Dexamethasone (Maxitrol)
Neomycin, Polymyxin B, & Prednisolone (Poly-Pred Ophthalmic)
Ofloxacin (Floxin, Ocuflox Ophthalmic)
Silver Nitrate (Dey-Drop)
Sulfacetamide (Bleph-10, Cetamide, Sodium Sulamyd)
Sulfacetamide & Prednisolone (Blephamide)
Tobramycin, Ophthalmic (AKTob, Tobrex)
Tobramycin & Dexamethasone (TobraDex)
Trifluridine (Viroptic)

Miscellaneous Ophthalmic Agents

Artificial Tears (Tears Naturale)
Cromolyn Sodium (Opticrom)
Cyclopentolate (Cyclogyl)
Cyclopentolate with phenylephrine (Cyclomydril)
Cyclosporine Ophthalmic (Restasis)
Dexamethasone, Ophthalmic (AK-Dex Ophthalmic, Decadron Ophthalmic)
Emedastine (Emadine)
Ketorolac, Ophthalmic (Acular, Aculair LS, Aculair PF)
Ketotifen (Zaditor)
Lodoxamide (Alomide)
Naphazoline & Antazoline (Albalon-A Ophthalmic)
Naphazoline & Pheniramine Acetate (Naphcon A)
Nepafenac (Nevanac)
Olopatadine (Patanol)
Pemirolast (Alomast)
Rimexolone (Vexol Ophthalmic)
Scopolamine ophthalmic

GASTROINTESTINAL AGENTS

Antacids

Alginic Acid (Gaviscon)
Aluminum Hydroxide (Amphojel, ALternaGEL)
Aluminum Hydroxide with Magnesium Carbonate (Gaviscon)
Aluminum Hydroxide with Magnesium Hydroxide (Maalox)
Aluminum Hydroxide with Magnesium Hydroxide & Simethicone (Mylanta, Mylanta II, Maalox Plus)
Aluminum Hydroxide with Magnesium Trisilicate (Gaviscon, Gaviscon-2)
Calcium Carbonate (Tums, Alka-Mints)
Magaldrate (Riopan, Lowsium)
Simethicone (Mylicon)

Antidiarrheals

Bismuth Subsalicylate
(Pepto-Bismol)
Diphenoxylate with
Atropine (Lomotil)

Kaolin-Pectin (Kaodene,
Kao-Spen, Kapectolin,
Parepectolin)
Lactobacillus (Lactinex
Granules)

Loperamide (Imodium)
Octreotide (Sandostatin,
Sandostatin LAR)
Paregoric [Camphorated
Tincture of Opium]

Antiemetics

Aprepitant (Emend)
Chlorpromazine
(Thorazine)
Dimenhydrinate
(Dramamine)
Dolasetron (Anzemet)
Dronabinol (Marinol)
Droperidol (Inapsine)
Granisetron (Kytril)

Meclizine (Antivert)
Metoclopramide (Reglan,
Clopra, Octamide)
Nabilone (Cesamet)
Ondansetron (Zofran)
Palonosetron (Aloxi)
Prochlorperazine
(Compazine)

Promethazine
(Phenergan)
Scopolamine (Scopace)
Thiethylperazine
(Torecan)
Trimethobenzamide
(Tigan)

Antiulcer Agents

Cimetidine (Tagamet)
Esomeprazole (Nexium)
Famotidine (Pepcid)
Lansoprazole (Prevacid)

Nizatidine (Axid)
Omeprazole (Prilosec,
Zegerid)
Pantoprazole (Protonix)

Rabeprazole (AcipHex)
Ranitidine Hydrochloride
(Zantac)
Sucralfate (Carafate)

Cathartics/Laxatives

Bisacodyl (Dulcolax)
Docusate Calcium
(Surfak)
Docusate Potassium
(Dialose)
Docusate Sodium (Doss,
Colace)
Glycerin Suppository

Lactulose (Constulose,
Generlac, Chronulac,
Cephulac, Enulose)
Magnesium Citrate
Magnesium Hydroxide
(Milk of Magnesia)
Mineral Oil

Polyethylene Glycol
Electrolyte Solution
(GoLYTELY, CoLyte)
Psyllium (Metamucil,
Serutan, Effer-Syllium)
Sodium Phosphate
(Visicol)
Sorbitol

Enzymes

Pancreatin (Pancrease,
Cotazym, Creon,
Ultrase)

Miscellaneous GI Agents

Alosetron (Lotronex)
Balsalazide (Colazal)
Dexpanthenol (Ilopan-Choline Oral, Ilopan)
Dibucaine (Nupercainal)
Dicyclomine (Bentyl)
Hydrocortisone, Rectal (Anusol-HC Suppository, Cortifoam Rectal, Proctocort)
Hyoscyamine (Anaspaz, Cystospaz, Levsin)
Hyoscyamine, Atropine, Scopolamine, &

Phenobarbital (Donnatal)
Infliximab (Remicade)
Lubiprostone (Amitiza)
Mesalamine (Rowasa, Asacol, Pentasa)
Metoclopramide (Reglan, Clopra, Octamide)
Misoprostol (Cytotec)
Olsalazine (Dipentum)
Pramoxine (Anusol Ointment, ProctoFoam-NS)

Pramoxine with Hydrocortisone (Enzone, ProctoFoam-HC)
Propantheline (Pro-Banthine)
Sulfasalazine (Azulfidine)
Tegaserod Maleate (Zelnorm)
Vasopressin (Pitressin)

HEMATOLOGIC AGENTS

Anticoagulants

Ardeparin (Normiflo)
Argatroban (Acova)
Bivalirudin (Angiomax)
Dalteparin (Fragmin)

Enoxaparin (Lovenox)
Fondaparinux (Arixtra)
Heparin
Lepirudin (Refludan)

Protamine
Tinzaparin (Innohep)
Warfarin (Coumadin)

Antiplatelet Agents

Abciximab (ReoPro)
Aspirin (Bayer, Ecotrin, St. Joseph's)
Clopidogrel (Plavix)

Dipyridamole (Persantine)
Dipyridamole & Aspirin (Aggrenox)

Eptifibatide (Integrilin)
Reteplase (Retavase)
Ticlopidine (Ticlid)
Tirofiban (Aggrastat)

Antithrombotic Agents

Alteplase, Recombinant [tPA] (Activase)
Aminocaproic Acid (Amicar)
Anistreplase (Eminase)

Aprotinin (Trasylol)
Danaparoid (Organan)
Dextran 40 (Rheomacrodex)
Reteplase (Retavase)

Streptokinase (Streptase, Kabikinase)
Tenecteplase (TNKase)
Urokinase (Abbokinase)

Hematopoietic Stimulants

Darbepoetin Alfa
(Aranesp)
Epoetin Alfa
[Erythropoietin, EPO]
(Epogen, Procrit)

Filgrastim [G-CSF]
(Neupogen)
Oprelvekin (Neumega)
Pegfilgrastim (Neulasta)

Sargramostim [GM-CSF] (Leukine)

Volume Expanders

Albumin (Albuminar,
Buminate, Albutein)

Dextran 40
(Rheomacrodex)
Hetastarch (Hespan)

Plasma Protein Fraction
(Plasmanate)

Miscellaneous Hematologic Agents

Antihemophilic Factor
VIII (Monoclate)
Decitabine (Dacogen)

Desmopressin (DDAVP,
Stimate)

Lenalidomide
(Revlimid)
Pentoxifylline (Trental)

IMMUNE SYSTEM AGENTS

Immunomodulators

Abatacept (Orencia)
Adalimumab (Humira)
Anakinra (Kineret)
Etanercept (Enbrel)
Interferon Alfa (Roferon
A, Intron A)

Interferon Alfacon-1
(Infergen)
Interferon Beta-1b
(Betaseron)
Interferon Gamma-1b
(ActImmune)

Mycophenolic Acid
(Myfortic)
Natalizumab (Tysabri)
Peg Interferon Alfa-2b
(PEG-Intron)

Immunosuppressive Agents

Azathioprine (Imuran)
Basiliximab (Simulect)
Cyclosporine
(Sandimmune, NeORL)
Daclizumab (Zenapax)
Lymphocyte Immune
Globulin

[Antithymocyte
Globulin, ATG]
(Atgam)
Muromonab-CD3
(Orthoclone OKT3)
Mycophenolate Mofetil
(CellCept)

Sirolimus (Rapamune)
Steroids, Systemic
(Table 4, page 216)
Tacrolimus (Prograf,
Protopic)

Vaccines/Serums/Toxoids

Cytomegalovirus
Immune Globulin
[CMV-IG IV]
(CytoGam)

Diphtheria, Tetanus
Toxoids, & Acellular
Pertussis Adsorbed,
Hepatitis B

(recombinant), &
Inactivated Poliovirus
Vaccine (IPV)
Combined (Pediarix)

Haemophilus B Conjugate Vaccine (ActHIB, HibTITER, PedvaxHIB, Prohibit)

Hepatitis A Vaccine (Havrix, Vaqta)

Hepatitis A (Inactivated) & Hepatitis B Recombinant Vaccine (Twinrix)

Hepatitis B Immune Globulin (HyperHep, H-BIG)

Hepatitis B Vaccine (Engerix-B, Recombivax HB)

Human Papillomavirus (Types 6, 11, 16, 18)

Recombinant Vaccine (Gardasil)

Immune Globulin, IV (Gamimune N, Sandoglobulin, Gammar IV)

Influenza Vaccine (Fluzone, FluShield, Fluvirin)

Influenza Virus Vaccine Live, Intranasal (FluMist)

Measles, Mumps, Rubella, and Varicella Virus Vaccine Live (Proquad)

Meningococcal Polysaccharide Vaccine (Menomune)

Pneumococcal 7-Valent Conjugate Vaccine (Prevnar)

Pneumococcal Vaccine, Polyvalent (Pneumovax-23)

Rotavirus vaccine, live, oral, pentavalent (RotaTeq)

Tetanus Immune Globulin

Tetanus Toxoid

Varicella Virus Vaccine (Varivax)

Zoster vaccine, live (Zostavax)

MUSCULOSKELETAL AGENTS

Antigout Agents

Allopurinol (Zyloprim, Lopurin, Aloprim)

Colchicine

Probenecid (Benemid)

Sulfinpyrazone (Anturane)

Muscle Relaxants

Baclofen (Lioresal)

Carisoprodol (Soma)

Chlorzoxazone (Paraflex, Parafon Forte DSC)

Cyclobenzaprine (Flexeril)

Dantrolene (Dantrium)

Diazepam (Valium)

Metaxalone (Skelaxin)

Methocarbamol (Robaxin)

Orphenadrine (Norflex)

Neuromuscular Blockers

Atracurium (Tracrium)

Pancuronium (Pavulon)

Rocuronium (Zemuron)

Succinylcholine (Anectine, Quelicin, Sucostrin)

Vecuronium (Norcuron)

Miscellaneous Musculoskeletal Agents

Edrophonium (Tensilon)

Leflunomide (Arava)

Methotrexate (Folex, Rheumatrex)

OB/GYN AGENTS

Contraceptives

Estradiol Cypionate &
Medroxyprogesterone
Acetate (Lunelle)
Etonogestrel/Ethinyl
Estradiol (NuvaRing)
Levonorgestrel Implant
(Norplant)

Medroxyprogesterone
(Provera, Depo-
Provera)
Norgestrel (Ovrette)
Oral Contraceptives,
Monophasic (Table 7,
page 221)

Oral Contraceptives,
Multiphasic (Table 7,
page 223)
Oral Contraceptives,
Progestin Only (Table
7, page 224)

Emergency Contraceptives

Ethinyl Estradiol, &
Levonorgestrel
(Preven)

Levonorgestrel (Plan B)

Estrogen Supplementation Agents

Esterified Estrogens
(Estratab, Menest)
Esterified Estrogens with
Methyltestosterone
(Estratest)
Estradiol (Estrace)
Estradiol, Transdermal
(Estraderm, Climara,
Vivelle)
Estrogen, Conjugated
(Premarin)

Estrogen, Conjugated-
Synthetic (Cenestin)
Estrogen, Conjugated
with
Medroxyprogesterone
(Prempro, Premphase)
Estrogen, Conjugated
with
Methylprogesterone
(Premarin with
Methylprogesterone)

Estrogen, Conjugated
with
Methyltestosterone
(Premarin with
Methyltestosterone)
Ethinyl Estradiol
(Estinyl, Feminone)
Norethindrone
Acetate/Ethinyl
Estradiol (FemHRT)

Vaginal Preparations

Amino-Cerv pH 5.5
Cream

Miconazole (Monistat)
Nystatin (Mycostatin)

Terconazole (Terazol 7)
Tioconazole (Vagistat)

Miscellaneous Ob/Gyn Agents

Dinoprostone (Cervidil
Vaginal Insert,
Prepidil Vaginal Gel)
Gonadorelin (Lutrepulse)
Leuprolide (Lupron)
Lutropin Alfa (Luveris)

Magnesium Sulfate
Medroxyprogesterone
(Provera, Depo-
Provera)
Methylergonovine
(Methergine)

Mifepristone [RU 486]
(Mifeprex)
Oxytocin (Pitocin)
Terbutaline (Brethine,
Bricanyl)

PAIN MEDICATIONS

Local Anesthetics (Table 3, page 215)

Benzocaine & Antipyrine (Auralgan)
Bupivacaine (Marcaine)
Capsaicin (Capsin, Zostrix)
Cocaine
Dibucaine (Nupercainal)
Lidocaine (Anestacon Topical, Xylocaine)
Lidocaine & Prilocaine (EMLA, LMX)
Pramoxine (Anusol Ointment, ProctoFoam-NS)

Migraine Headache Medications

Acetaminophen with Butalbital w/wo Caffeine (Fioricet, Medigesic, Repan, Sedapap-10, Two-Dyne, Triapin, Axocet, Phrenilin Forte)
Almotriptan (Axert)
Aspirin & Butalbital Compound (Fiorinal)
Aspirin with Butalbital, Caffeine, & Codeine (Fiorinal with Codeine)
Eletriptan (Relpax)
Frovatriptan (Frova)
Naratriptan (Amerge)
Serotonin 5-HT$_1$ Receptor Agonists (See Table 11, page 228)
Sumatriptan (Imitrex)
Zolmitriptan (Zomig)

Narcotic Analgesics

Acetaminophen with Codeine (Tylenol No. 3, 4)
Alfentanil (Alfenta)
Aspirin with Codeine (Empirin No. 2, 3, 4)
Buprenorphine (Buprenex)
Butorphanol (Stadol)
Codeine
Dezocine (Dalgan)
Fentanyl (Sublimaze)
Fentanyl, Transdermal (Duragesic)
Fentanyl, Transmucosal (Actiq System)
Hydrocodone & Acetaminophen (Lorcet, Vicodin)
Hydrocodone & Aspirin (Lortab ASA)
Hydrocodone & Ibuprofen (Vicoprofen)
Hydromorphone (Dilaudid)
Levorphanol (Levo-Dromoran)
Meperidine (Demerol)
Methadone (Dolophine)
Morphine (Avinza XR, Duramorph, Infumorph, MS Contin, Kadian SR, Oramorph SR, Palladone, Roxanol)
Morphine, Liposomal (DepoDur)
Nalbuphine (Nubain)
Oxycodone (OxyContin, OxyIR, Roxicodone)
Oxycodone & Acetaminophen (Percocet, Tylox)
Oxycodone & Aspirin (Percodan, Percodan-Demi)
Oxymorphone (Numorphan)
Pentazocine (Talwin)
Propoxyphene (Darvon)
Propoxyphene & Acetaminophen (Darvocet)
Propoxyphene & Aspirin (Darvon Compound-65, Darvon-N with Aspirin)

Nonnarcotic Analgesics

Acetaminophen [APAP] (Tylenol)

Aspirin (Bayer, Ecotrin, St. Joseph's)
Tramadol (Ultram)

Tramadol/Acetaminophen (Ultracet)

Nonsteroidal Antiinflammatory Agents

Celecoxib (Celebrex)
Diclofenac (Cataflam, Voltaren)
Diflunisal (Dolobid)
Etodolac (Lodine)
Fenoprofen (Nalfon)
Flurbiprofen (Ansaid)

Ibuprofen (Motrin, Rufen, Advil)
Indomethacin (Indocin)
Ketoprofen (Orudis, Oruvail)
Ketorolac (Toradol)
Meloxicam (Mobic)
Nabumetone (Relafen)

Naproxen (Aleve, Naprosyn, Anaprox)
Oxaprozin (Daypro)
Piroxicam (Feldene)
Sulindac (Clinoril)
Tolmetin (Tolectin)
Valdecoxib (Bextra)

Miscellaneous Pain Medications

Amitriptyline (Eluvil)
Imipramine (Tofranil)

Pregabalin (Lyrica)
Tramadol (Ultram)

Ziconotide (Prialt)

RESPIRATORY AGENTS

Antitussives, Decongestants, & Expectorants

Acetylcysteine (Acetadote, Mucomyst)
Benzonatate (Tessalon Perles)
Codeine
Dextromethorphan (Mediquell, Benylin DM, PediaCare 1)
Guaifenesin (Robitussin)
Guaifenesin & Codeine (Robitussin AC, Brontex)

Guaifenesin & Dextromethorphan
Hydrocodone & Guaifenesin (Hycotuss Expectorant)
Hydrocodone & Homatropine (Hycodan, Hydromet)
Hydrocodone & Pseudoephedrine (Detussin, Histussin-D)
Hydrocodone, Chlorpheniramine,

Phenylephrine, Acetaminophen, & Caffeine (Hycomine)
Potassium Iodide (SSKI, Thyro Block)
Pseudoephedrine (Sudafed, Novafed, Afrinol)

Bronchodilators

Albuterol (Proventil, Ventolin, Volmax)

Albuterol & Ipratropium (Combivent)

Aminophylline
Bitolterol (Tornalate)

Ephedrine

Epinephrine (Adrenalin, Sus-Phrine, EpiPen)

Formoterol (Foradil Aerolizer)

Isoproterenol (Isuprel)

Levalbuterol (Xopenex)

Metaproterenol (Alupent, Metaprel)

Pirbuterol (Maxair)

Salmeterol (Serevent)

Terbutaline (Brethine, Bricanyl)

Theophylline (Theo24, TheoChron)

Respiratory Inhalants

Acetylcysteine (Acetadote, Mucomyst)

Beclomethasone (Beconase, Vancenase Nasal Inhaler)

Beclomethasone (QVAR)

Beractant (Survanta)

Budesonide (Rhinocort, Pulmicort)

Calfactant (Infasurf)

Cromolyn Sodium (Intal, Nasalcrom, Opticrom)

Dexamethasone, Nasal (Dexacort Phosphate Turbinaire)

Flunisolide (AeroBid, Nasarel)

Fluticasone, Oral, Nasal (Flonase, Flovent)

Fluticasone Propionate & Salmeterol Xinafoate (Advair Diskus)

Ipratropium (Atrovent)

Nedocromil (Tilade)

Tiotropium (Spiriva)

Triamcinolone (Azmacort)

Miscellaneous Respiratory Agents

Alpha₁-Protease Inhibitor (Prolastin)

Dornase Alfa (Pulmozyme)

Montelukast (Singulair)

Omalizumab (Xolair)

Zafirlukast (Accolate)

Zileuton (Zyflo)

URINARY/GENITOURINARY AGENTS

Alprostadil, Intracavernosal (Caverject, Edex)

Alprostadil, Urethral Suppository (Muse)

Ammonium Aluminum Sulfate [Alum]

Belladonna & Opium Suppositories (B & O Supprettes)

Bethanechol (Urecholine, Duvoid)

Darifenacin (Enablex)

Dimethyl Sulfoxide [DMSO] (Rimso 50)

Flavoxate (Urispas)

Hyoscyamine (Anaspaz, Cystospaz, Levsin)

Methenamine (Hiprex, Urex)

Neomycin-Polymyxin Bladder Irrigant [Neosporin GU Irrigant]

Nitrofurantoin (Macrodantin, Furadantin, Macrobid)

Oxybutynin (Ditropan, Ditropan XL)

Oxybutynin Transdermal System (Oxytrol)

Pentosan Polysulfate (Elmiron)

Phenazopyridine (Pyridium)

Potassium Citrate (Urocit-K)

Potassium Citrate & Citric Acid (Polycitra-K)

Sildenafil (Viagra)

Solifenacin (VESIcare)
Sodium Citrate/Citric acid (Bicitra)
Tadalafil (Cialis)

Tolterodine (Detrol, Detrol LA)
Trimethoprim (Trimpex, Proloprim)

Trospium Chloride (Sanctura)
Vardenafil (Levitra)

Benign Prostatic Hyperplasia Medications

Alfuzosin (Uroxatral)
Doxazosin (Cardura, Cardura XL)

Dutasteride (Avodart)
Finasteride (Proscar, Propecia)

Tamsulosin (Flomax)
Terazosin (Hytrin)

WOUND CARE

Becaplermin (Regranex Gel)

Silver Nitrate (Dey-Drop)

MISCELLANEOUS THERAPEUTIC AGENTS

Acamprosate (Campral)
Alglucosidase alfa (Myozyme)
Cilostazol (Pletal)
Drotrecogin Alfa (Xigris)
Megestrol Acetate (Megace)
Mecasermin (Increlex)
Lanthanum Carbonate (Fosrenol)

Naltrexone (ReVia)
Nicotine Gum (Nicorette)
Nicotine Nasal Spray (Nicotrol NS)
Nicotine Transdermal (Habitrol, Nicoderm, Nicotrol)
Orlistat (Xenical)
Palifermin (Kepivance)

Potassium Iodide [Lugol Solution] (SSKI, Thyro-Block)
Sevelamer (Renagel)
Sodium Polystyrene Sulfonate (Kayexalate)
Talc (Sterile Talc Powder)
Varenicline (Chantix)

NATURAL AND HERBAL AGENTS

Black Cohosh
Chamomile
Cranberry (*Vaccinium macrocarpon*)
Dong Quai (*Angelica polymorpha, sinensis*)
Echinacea (*Echinacea purpurea*)
Ephedra/MaHuang
Evening Primrose Oil
Fish Oil
Garlic (*Allium sativum*)

Ginger (*Zingiber officinale*)
Ginkgo Biloba
Ginseng
Glucosamine Sulfate (chitosamine) & Chondroitin Sulfate
Kava Kava (Kava Kava Root Extract, *Piper methysticum*)
Melatonin

Milk Thistle (*Silybum marianum*)
Saw Palmetto (*Serenoa repens*)
St. John's Wort (*Hypericum perforatum*)
Valerian (*Valeriana officinalis*)
Yohimbine (*Pausinystalia yohimbe*)

GENERIC DRUG DATA

Abacavir (Ziagen) **WARNING:** Allergy (fever, rash, fatigue, GI, resp) reported; stop drug immediately & do not rechallenge; lactic acidosis & hepatomegaly/steatosis reported **Uses:** *HIV Infxn* **Action:** Nucleoside RT inhibitor **Dose:** *Adults.* 300 mg PO bid or 600 mg PO daily **Peds.** 8 mg/kg bid **Caution:** [C,] CDC recommends HIV-infected mothers not breast-feed (risk of infant transmission) **Disp:** Tabs 300 mg; soln 20 mg/mL **SE:** See Warning, ↑ LFTs, fat redistribution **Notes:** Numerous drug interactions

Abatacept (Orencia) **Uses:*** Mod/severe RA w/inadequate response to one or more DMARDs **Action:** Selective costimulation modulator, ↓ T-cell activation **Dose:** Initial 500 mg (<60 kg), 750 mg(60–100 kg); 1 gm (>100kg) IV over 30 min; repeat at 2 and 4 wk, then every 4 wk **Caution:** [C; ?/-] COPD; h/o recurrent, localized, chronic, or predisposition to Infxn **Contra:** w/TNF antagonists (↑ Infxn) **Disp:** Powder for IV: 250 mg/15 mL **SE:** HA, URI, N, nasopharyngitis, Infxn, malignancy, infusion Rxns (dizziness, HA, HTN), hypersensitivity, COPD exacerbations, cough, rhonchi, dyspnea **Notes:** Screen for TB prior to use; do not give w/ live vaccines w/ or w/in 3 mo discontinuing abatacept

Abciximab (ReoPro) **Uses:** *Prevent acute ischemic complications in PTCA,* MI **Action:** ↓ plt aggregation (glycoprotein IIb/IIIa inhibitor) **Dose:** Unstable angina w/ PCI: 0.25 mg/kg bolus followed by 10 mcg/min cont inf × 18–24 h, stopping 1 h after PCI; PCI: 0.25 mg/kg bolus 10–60 min pre PTCA, then 0.125 mcg/kg/min (max = 10 mcg/min) cont inf for 12 h **Caution:** [C, ?/-] **Contra:** Active or recent (w/in 6 wk) internal hemorrhage, CVA w/in 2 y or CVA w/ significant neurologic deficit, bleeding diathesis or PO anticoagulants w/in 7 d (unless PT <1.2 × control), thrombocytopenia (<100,000 cells/mcL), recent trauma or major surgery (w/in 6 wk), CNS tumor, AVM, aneurysm, severe uncontrolled HTN, vasculitis, use of dextran prior to or during PTCA, allergy to murine proteins **Disp:** Inj 2 mg/mL **SE:** Allergic Rxns, bleeding, thrombocytopenia possible **Notes:** Use w/ heparin

Acamprosate (Campral) **Uses:** *Maint abstinence from EtOH* **Action:** ↓ Glutamatergic transmission; modulates neuronal hyperexcitability; related to GABA **Dose:** 666 mg PO tid; CrCl 30–50 mL/min: 333 mg PO tid **Caution:** [C; ?/-] **Contra:** CrCl <30 mL/min **Disp:** Tabs 333 mg EC (enteric coated) **SE:** N/D, depression, anxiety, insomnia **Notes:** Does not eliminate EtOH withdrawal Sx; continue even if relapse occurs

Acarbose (Precose) **Uses:** *Type 2 DM* **Action:** α-Glucosidase inhibitor; delays digestion of carbohydrates to ↓ glucose **Dose:** 25–100 mg PO tid (w/ 1st bite each meal) **Caution:** [B, ?] Avoid if CrCl <25 mL/min; can affect digoxin levels **Contra:** IBD, cirrhosis **Disp:** Tabs 25, 50, 100 mg **SE:** Abdominal pain, D, flatulence, ↑ LFTs **Notes:** OK w/ sulfonylureas; LFTs q3mo for 1st y

Acebutolol (Sectral) **Uses:** *HTN, arrhythmias* angina **Action:** Blocks β-adrenergic receptors, β₁, & ISA **Dose:** HTN: 200–800 μg/d; arrhythmia: 400–1200 mg/day in divided doses ↓ if CrCl <50 mL/min **Caution:** [B, D in 2nd & 3rd tri, +] Can exacerbate ischemic heart Dz, do not D/C abruptly **Contra:** 2nd-, 3rd-degree heart block **Disp:** Caps 200, 400 mg **SE:** Fatigue, HA, dizziness, bradycardia

Acetaminophen [APAP, N-acetyl-p-aminophenol] (Tylenol, other generic) [OTC] **Uses:** *Mild–moderate pain, HA, fever* **Action:** Nonnarcotic analgesic; ↓ CNS synthesis of prostaglandins & hypothalamic heat-regulating center **Dose:** *Adults.* 650 mg PO or PR q4–6h or 1000 mg PO q6h; max 4 g/24 h. *Peds.* *<12 y.* 10–15 mg/kg/dose PO or PR q4–6h; max 2.6 g/24 h. Quick dosing Table 1. Administer q6h if CrCl 10–50 mL/min & q8h if CrCl <10 mL/min **Caution:** [B, +] Hepatotoxic in elderly & w/ EtOH use w/ >4 g/day; alcoholic liver Dz **Contra:** G6PD deficiency **Disp:** Tabs meltaway/dissolving 160; Tabs 325, 500, 650 mg; chew tabs 80, 160 mg; liq 100 mg/mL, 120/2.5 mL, 120 mg/5 mL, 160 mg/5 mL, 167 mg/5 mL, 325 mg/5 mL, 500 mg/15 mL; 80 mg/0.8 mL supp 80, 120, 125, 325, 650 mg **SE:** OD hepatotox at 10 g; 15 g is potentially lethal; Rx w/ N-acetylcysteine **Notes:** No antiinflammatory or plt-inhibiting action; avoid EtOH

Acetaminophen + Butalbital ± Caffeine (Fioricet, Medigesic, Repan, Sedapap-10, Two-Dyne, Triapin, Axocet, Phrenilin Forte) [C-III] **Uses:** *Tension HA,* mild pain **Action:** Nonnarcotic analgesic w/ barbiturate **Dose:** 1–2 tabs or caps PO q4/6h PRN; ↓ in renal/hepatic impair; 4 g/24 h APAP max **Caution:** [C, D, +] Alcoholic liver Dz **Contra:** G6PD deficiency **Disp:** Caps Dolgic Plus butalbital 50 mg, caffeine 40 mg, APAP 750 mg; Caps *Medigesic, Repan, Two-Dyne:* butalbital 50 mg, caffeine 40 mg, + APAP 325 mg; Caps *Axocet, Phrenilin Forte:* butalbital 50 mg + APAP 650 mg; Caps: Esgic-Plus, Zebutal: butalbital 50 mg, caffeine 40 mg, APAP 500 mg; Liq. Dolgic LQ: butalbital 50 mg, caffeine 40 mg, APAP 325 mg/15mL; Tabs *Medigesic, Fioricet, Repan:* butalbital 50 mg, caffeine 40 mg, APAP 325 mg; Phrenilin: butalbital 50 mg + APAP 325 mg; *Sedapap-10:* butalbital 50 mg + APAP 650 mg **SE:** Drowsiness, dizziness, "hangover" effect **Notes:** Butalbital habit-forming; avoid EtOH

Acetaminophen + Codeine (Tylenol No. 3, No. 4) [C-III, C-V] **Uses:** *Mild–moderate pain (No. 3); moderate–severe pain (No. 4)* **Action:** Combined APAP & narcotic analgesic **Dose:** *Adults.* 1–2 tabs q3–4h PRN (max dose APAP = 4 g/d). *Peds.* APAP 10–15 mg/kg/dose; codeine 0.5–1 mg/kg dose q4–6h (guide: 3–6 y, 5 mL/dose; 7–12 y, 10 mL/dose); ↓ in renal/hepatic impair **Caution:** [C, +] Alcoholic liver Dz **Contra:** G6PD deficiency **Disp:** Tabs 300 mg APAP + codeine; caps 325 mg APAP + codeine; susp (C-V) APAP 120 mg + codeine 12 mg/5 mL **SE:** Drowsiness, dizziness, N/V **Notes:** Codeine in No. 3 = 30 mg, No. 4 = 60 mg

Acetazolamide (Diamox) Uses: *Diuresis, glaucoma, prevent high-altitude sickness, refractory epilepsy* **Action:** Carbonic anhydrase inhibitor; ↓ renal excretion of hydrogen & ↑ renal excretion of Na⁺, K⁺, HCO₃⁻, & H₂O **Dose:** *Adults. Diuretic:* 250–375 mg IV or PO q24h. *Glaucoma:* 250–1000 mg PO q24h in ÷ doses. *Epilepsy:* 8–30 mg/kg/d PO in ÷ doses. *Altitude sickness:* 250 mg PO q8–12h or SR 500 mg PO q12–24h start 24–48 h before & 48 h after highest ascent. *Peds.* Epilepsy: 8–30 mg/kg/24 h PO in ÷ doses; max 1 g/d. *Diuretic:* 5 mg/kg/24 h PO or IV. *Alkalinization of urine:* 5 mg/kg/dose PO bid–tid. *Glaucoma:* 5–15 mg/kg/24 h PO in ÷ doses; max 1 g/d; adjust in renal impair; avoid if CrCl <10 mL/min **Caution:** [C, +] **Contra:** Renal/hepatic failure, sulfa allergy **Disp:** Tabs 125, 250 mg, ER caps 500 mg; inj 500 mg/vial, powder for reconstitution **SE:** Malaise, metallic taste, drowsiness, photosensitivity, hyperglycemia **Notes:** Follow Na⁺ & K⁺; watch for metabolic acidosis; SR forms not for epilepsy

Acetic Acid & Aluminum Acetate (Otic Domeboro) Uses: *Otitis externa* **Action:** Antiinfective **Dose:** 4–6 gtt in ear(s) q2–3h **Caution:** [C, ?] **Contra:** Perforated tympanic membranes **Disp:** 2% otic soln **SE:** Local irritation

Acetylcysteine (Acetadote, Mucomyst) Uses: *Mucolytic, antidote to APAP hepatotox * adjuvant Rx for chronic bronchopulmonary Dzs & CF* **Action:** Splits disulfide linkages between mucoprotein complexes; protects liver by restoring glutathione in APAP OD **Dose:** *Adults & Peds.* Nebulizer: 3–5 mL of 20% soln diluted w/ equal vol of H₂O or NS tid–qid. *Antidote:* PO or NG: 140 mg/kg load, then 70 mg/kg q4h for 17 doses. (Dilute 1:3 in carbonated beverage or orange juice) *Acetadote:* load 150 mg/kg over 15 min, then 50 mg/kg over 4 h, then 100 mg/kg over 16 h **Caution:** [C, ?] **Disp:** Soln inhaled and oral 10%, 20%; Acetadote IV soln 20% **SE:** Bronchospasm (inhal), N/V, drowsiness; anaphylactoid Rxns w/ IV **Notes:** Activated charcoal adsorbs acetylcysteine if given PO for APAP ingestion; start Rx for APAP overdose w/in 6–8 h

Acitretin (Soriatane) WARNING: Must not be used by females who are pregnant or intend to become pregnant during therapy or for up to 3 y following D/C of therapy; EtOH must not be ingested during therapy or for 2 mo following cessation of therapy; do not donate blood for 3 y following cessation Uses: *Severe psoriasis*; other keratinization disorders (lichen planus, etc) **Action:** Retinoid-like activity **Dose:** 25–50 mg/d PO, w/ main meal; ↑ if no response by 4 wk to 75 mg/d **Caution:** [X, –] Renal/hepatic impair; in women of reproductive potential **Contra:** See Warning **Disp:** Caps 10, 25 mg **SE:** Cheilitis, skin peeling, alopecia, pruritus, rash, arthralgia, GI upset, photosensitivity, thrombocytosis, hypertriglyceridemia **Notes:** Follow LFTs and lipids; response often takes 2–3 mo; pt agreement/informed consent prior to use

Acyclovir (Zovirax) Uses: *Herpes simplex & zoster Infxns* **Action:** Interferes w/ viral DNA synthesis **Dose:** *Adults. PO:* Initial genital herpes: 200 mg PO q4h while awake, 5 caps/d × 10 d or 400 mg PO tid × 7–10 d. *Chronic suppression:* 400 mg PO bid. *Intermittent Rx:* As for initial Rx, except treat for 5 d, or

800 mg PO bid, at prodrome. *Herpes zoster:* 800 mg PO 5×/d for 7–10 d. *IV:* 5–10 mg/kg/dose IV q8h. *Topical: Initial herpes genitalis:* Apply q3h (6×/d) for 7 d. **Peds.** 5–10 mg/kg/dose IV or PO q8h or 750 mg/m²/24 h ÷ q8h. *Chickenpox:* 20 mg/kg/dose PO qid; ↓ w/CrCl <50 mL/min **Caution:** [B, +] **Disp:** Caps 400 mg; tabs 400, 800 mg; susp 200 mg/5 mL; inj 500 mg/vial; 1000, injection soln 25 mg/mL, 50 mg/mL oint 5% and cream 5% **SE:** Dizziness, lethargy, confusion, rash, inflammation at IV site **Notes:** PO better than topical for herpes genitalis

Adalimumab (Humira)
WARNING: Cases of TB have been observed; check TB skin test prior to use; Hepatitis B reactivation has also occurred **Uses:** *Moderate–severe RA w/ an inadequate response to one or more DMARDs* **Action:** TNF-α inhibitor **Dose:** 40 mg SQ qowk; may ↑ 40 mg qwk if not on MTX **Caution:** [B, ?/–] Serious Infxns & sepsis reported **Disp:** Prefilled 0.8 mL (40 mg) syringe **SE:** Inj site Rxns, serious Infxns, neurologic events, malignancies **Notes:** Refrigerate prefilled syringe, rotate inj sites, OK w/ other DMARDs

Adefovir (Hepsera)
WARNING: Acute exacerbations of hepatitis may occur following d/c therapy (monitor LFTs); chronic use may lead to nephrotox especially w/ underlying renal impair (monitor renal Fxn); HIV resistance may emerge; lactic acidosis & severe hepatomegaly w/ steatosis reported alone or in combo w/ other antiretrovirals **Uses:** *Chronic active hepatitis B virus* **Action:** Nucleotide analog **Dose:** CrCl >50 mL/min: 10 mg PO qd; CrCl 20–49 mL/min: 10 mg PO q48h; CrCl 10–19 mL/min: 10 mg PO q72h; HD: 10 mg PO q7d postdialysis; adjust w/ CrCl <50 mL/min **Caution:** [C, –] **Disp:** Tabs 10 mg **SE:** Asthenia, HA, abdominal pain; see Warning

Adenosine (Adenocard)
Uses: *PSVT;* including associated w/ WPW **Action:** Class IV antiarrhythmic; slows AV node conduction **Dose:** *Adults.* 6 mg IV bolus; may repeat in 1–2 min; max 12 mg IV. *Peds.* 0.05 mg/kg IV bolus; may repeat q1–2 min to 0.25 mg/kg max **Caution:** [C, ?] **Contra:** 2nd- or 3rd-degree AV block or SSS (w/o pacemaker); recent MI or cerebral hemorrhage **Disp:** Inj 3 mg/mL **SE:** Facial flushing, HA, dyspnea, chest pressure, ↓ BP **Notes:** Doses >12 mg not OK; can cause momentary asystole when administered; caffeine, theophylline antagonize effects

Albumin (Albuminar, Buminate, Albutein)
Uses: *Plasma volume expansion for shock* (eg, burns, hemorrhage) **Action:** Maint of plasma colloid oncotic pressure **Dose:** *Adults.* Initial 25 g IV; subsequent dose based on response; 250 g/48h max. *Peds.* 0.5–1 g/kg/dose; inf at 0.05–0.1 g/min **Caution:** [C, ?] Severe anemia; cardiac, renal, or hepatic insuff due to added protein load & possible hypervolemia **Contra:** Cardiac failure **Disp:** Soln 5%, 25% **SE:** Chills, fever, CHF, tachycardia, ↓ BP, hypervolemia **Notes:** Contains 130–160 mEq Na⁺/L; may precipitate pulmonary edema

Albuterol (Proventil, Ventolin, Volmax)
Uses: *Asthma; prevent exercise-induced bronchospasm* **Action:** β-Adrenergic sympathomimetic bron-

chodilator; relaxes bronchial smooth muscle **Dose:** *Adults.* Inhaler: 2 inhal q4–6h PRN; 1 Rotacap inhaled q4–6h. PO: 2–4 mg PO tid–qid. Neb: 1.25–5 mg (0.25–1 mL of 0.5% soln in 2–3 mL of NS) tid–qid. *Peds.* Inhaler: 2 inhal q4–6h. *PO:* 0.1–0.2 mg/kg/dose PO; max 2–4 mg PO tid; *Neb:* 0.05 mg/kg (max 2.5 mg) in 2–3 mL of NS tid–qid **Caution:** [C, +] **Disp:** Tabs 2, 4 mg; XR tabs 4, 8 mg; syrup 2 mg/5 mL; 90 mcg/dose met-dose inhaler; soln for neb 0.083, 0.5% **SE:** Palpitations, tachycardia, nervousness, GI upset

Albuterol & Ipratropium (Combivent) Uses: *COPD* Action:
Combo of β-adrenergic bronchodilator & quaternary anticholinergic **Dose:** 2 inhal qid; neb 3 mL q 6 h **Caution:** [C, +] **Contra:** Peanut/soybean allergy **Disp:** Met-dose inhaler, 18 mcg ipratropium/103 mcg albuterol/puff; nebulization soln (DuoNeb) Ipratropium 0.5 mg Albuterol 2.5 mg/3 mL **SE:** Palpitations, tachycardia, nervousness, GI upset, dizziness, blurred vision

Aldesleukin [IL-2] (Proleukin) WARNING: Use restricted to pts w/ nl
pulmonary & cardiac Fxn **Uses:** *Metastatic RCC, melanoma* **Action:** Acts via IL-2 receptor; numerous immunomodulatory effects **Dose:** 600,000 IU/kg q8h × 14 doses (FDA-approved dose/schedule for RCC). Multiple cont inf & alternate schedules (including "high dose" using 24×10^6 IU/m^2 IV q8h on days 1–5 & 12–16) **Caution:** [C, ?/–] **Contra:** Organ allografts **Disp:** Powder for reconstitution 22×10^6 IU, when reconstituted 18 million int units/ mL = 1.1 mg/mL **SE:** Flulike syndrome (malaise, fever, chills), N/V/D, ↑ bilirubin; capillary leak syndrome w/ ↓ BP, pulmonary edema, fluid retention, & weight gain; renal & mild hematologic tox (anemia, thrombocytopenia, leukopenia) & secondary eosinophilia; cardiac tox (ischemia, atrial arrhythmias); neurologic tox (CNS depression, somnolence, rarely coma, delirium). Pruritic rashes, urticaria, & erythroderma common. **Notes:** Cont inf ↓ risk severe ↓ BP & fluid retention

Alefacept (Amevive) WARNING: Must monitor CD4 before each dose;
w/hold if <250; D/C if <250 × 1 month **Uses:** *Moderate/severe chronic plaque psoriasis* **Action:** Fusion protein inhibitor **Dose:** 7.5 mg IV or 15 mg IM once wk × 12 wk **Caution:** [B, ?/–] PRG registry; associated w/ serious Infxn **Contra:** Lymphopenia, HIV **Disp:** 7.5-, 15-mg vials **SE:** Pharyngitis, myalgia, inj site Rxn, malignancy **Notes:** IV or IM different formulations; may repeat course 12 wk later if CD4 OK

Alendronate (Fosamax, Fosamax Plus D) Uses: *Rx & prevention
of osteoporosis, Rx of steroid-induced osteoporosis & Paget Dz* **Action:** ↓ nl & abnormal bone resorption **Dose:** Osteoporosis: Rx: 10 mg/d PO or 70 mg qwk; Fosamax plus D 1 tab qwk. *Steroid-induced osteoporosis:* Rx: 5 mg/d PO. *Prevention:* 5 mg/d PO or 35 mg qwk. *Paget Dz:* 40 mg/d PO **Caution:** [C, ?] Not OK if CrCl <35 mL/min, w/NSAID use **Contra:** Esophageal anomalies, inability to sit/stand upright for 30 min, ↓ Ca^{2+} **Disp:** Tabs 5, 10, 35, 40, 70 mg, soln 70 mg/75mL, Fosamax plus D Alendronate 70 mg and cholecalciferol 2800 int units **SE:** GI disturbances, HA, pain, jaw osteonecrosis (w/dental procedures, chemo) **Notes:** Take 1st

thing in AM w/ H$_2$O (8 oz) >30 min before 1st food/beverage of the day. Do not lie down for 30 min after. Ca^{2+} & vitamin D supl necessary for regular tab

Alfentanil (Alfenta) [C-II] Uses: *Adjunct in the maint of anesthesia; analgesia* Action: Short-acting narcotic analgesic Dose: *Adults & Peds >12 y.* 3–75 mcg/kg mcg/kg (IBW) IV inf; total depends on duration of procedure Caution: [C, +/–] ↑ ICP, resp depression Disp: Inj 500 mcg/mL SE: Bradycardia, ↓ BP arrhythmias, peripheral vasodilation, ↑ ICP, drowsiness, resp depression

Alfuzosin (Uroxatral) WARNING: May prolong QTc interval Uses: *BPH* Action: α-Blocker Dose: 10 mg PO daily immediately after the same meal Caution: [B, –] Contra: W/ CYP3A4 inhibitors; moderate–severe hepatic impair Disp: Tabs 10 mg SE: Postural ↓ BP, dizziness, HA, fatigue Notes: XR tablet—do not cut or crush; fewest reports of ejaculatory disorders compared w/ other drugs in class

Alginic Acid + Aluminum Hydroxide & Magnesium Trisilicate (Gaviscon) [OTC] Uses: *Heartburn*; pain from hiatal hernia Action: Protective layer blocks gastric acid Dose: 2–4 tabs or 15–30 mL PO qid followed by H$_2$O; Caution: [B, –] Avoid in renal impair or Na$^+$-restricted diet Disp: Tabs, susp SE: D, constipation

Alglucosidase alfa (Myozyme) WARNING: Life-threatening anaphylactic Rxns have occurred w/infusion; appropriate medical support measures should be immediately available Uses: *Rx Pompe DZ* Action: Recombinant acid alpha-glucosidase; degrades glycogen in lysosomes Dose: 20 mg/kg IV q 2 wks over 4 h (see labeling for details) Caution: [B,?/-] Illness at time of inf may ↑ inf Rxns Disp: Powder 50 mg/vial SE: Hypersensitivity, fever, rash, D,V, gastroenteritis, pneumonia, URI, cough, respiratory distress, inf Rxns, cardiorespiratory failure, cardiac arrhythmia w/general anesthesia

Allopurinol (Zyloprim, Lopurin, Aloprim) Uses: *Gout, hyperuricemia of malignancy, uric acid urolithiasis* Action: Xanthine oxidase inhibitor; ↓ uric acid production Dose: *Adults.* PO: Initial 100 mg/d; usual 300 mg/d; max 800 mg/d. IV: 200–400 mg/m^2/d (max 600 mg/24 h); (after meal w/ plenty of fluid). *Peds.* Only for hyperuricemia of malignancy if <10 y: 10 mg/kg/24 h PO or 200 mg/m^2/d IV ÷ q6–8h (max 600 mg/24 h); ↓ in renal impair Caution: [C, M] Disp: Tabs 100, 300 mg; inj 500 mg/30 mL (Aloprim) SE: Skin rash, N/V, renal impair, angioedema Notes: Aggravates acute gout; begin after acute attack resolves; IV dose of 6 mg/mL final conc as single daily inf or ÷ 6-, 8-, or 12-h intervals

Almotriptan (Axert) See Table 11

Alosetron (Lotronex) WARNING: Serious GI side effects, some fatal, including ischemic colitis reported. May be prescribed only through participation in the prescribing program for Lotronex Uses: *Severe diarrhea-predominant IBS in women who fail conventional therapy* Action: Selective 5-HT$_3$ receptor antagonist Dose: *Adults.* 1 mg PO qd × 4 wk; titrate to 1 mg bid max; D/C after 4 wk at max dose if Sxs not controlled **Caution:** [B, ?/–] **Contra:** Hx chronic/severe constipation, GI obstruction, strictures, toxic megacolon, GI perforation, adhesions, ischemic colitis, Crohn Dz, ulcerative colitis, diverticulitis, thrombophlebitis, or hypercoagulable state. **Disp:** Tabs 0.5, 1 mg **SE:** Constipation, abdominal pain, nausea **Notes:** D/C immediately if constipation or Sxs of ischemic colitis develop; pt must sign informed consent prior to use "patient-physician agreement"

Alpha$_1$-Protease Inhibitor (Prolastin) Uses: *α_1-Antitrypsin deficiency*; panacinar emphysema **Action:** Replace human α_1-protease inhibitor **Dose:** 60 mg/kg IV once/wk **Caution:** [C, ?] **Contra:** Selective IgA deficiencies w/ known IgA antibodies **Disp:** Inj 500 mg/20 mL, 1000 mg/40 mL powder for inj **SE:** Fever, dizziness, flulike Sxs, allergic Rxns

Alprazolam (Xanax, Niravam) [C-IV] Uses: *Anxiety & panic disorders,* anxiety w/ depression **Action:** Benzodiazepine; antianxiety agent **Dose:** Anxiety: Initial, 0.25–0.5 mg tid; $\uparrow$ to a max of 4 mg/d in ÷ doses. Panic: Initial, 0.5 mg tid; may gradually $\uparrow$ to response; $\downarrow$ in elderly, debilitated, & hepatic impair **Caution:** [D, –] **Contra:** NA glaucoma, concomitant itra/ketoconazole **Disp:** Tabs 0.25, 0.5, 1, 2 mg; Xanax XR 0.5, 1, 2, 3 mg; Niravam (orally disintegrating tabs) 0.25, 0.5, 1, 2 mg; soln 1 mg/mL **SE:** Drowsiness, fatigue, irritability, memory impair, sexual dysfunction **Notes:** Avoid abrupt D/C after prolonged use

Alprostadil [Prostaglandin E$_1$] (Prostin VR) Uses: *Conditions where blood flow must be maintained in ductus arteriosus* sustain pulmonary/systemic circulation until surgery (eg, pulmonary atresia/stenosis, tricuspid atresia, transposition, etc.) **Action:** Vasodilator, plt inhibitor; ductus arteriosus (very sensitive) **Dose:** 0.05 mcg/kg/min IV; $\downarrow$ to lowest that maintains response **Caution:** [X, –] **Contra:** Neonatal resp distress syndrome **Disp:** Inj 500 mcg/mL **SE:** Cutaneous vasodilation, Sz-like activity, jitteriness, $\uparrow$ temp, $\downarrow$ Ca^{2+}, apnea, thrombocytopenia, $\downarrow$ BP; may cause apnea **Notes:** Keep intubation kit at bedside

Alprostadil, Intracavernosal (Caverject, Edex) Uses: *Erectile dysfunction* **Action:** Relaxes smooth muscles, dilates cavernosal arteries, $\uparrow$ lacunar spaces and blood entrapment **Dose:** 2.5–60 mcg intracavernosal; titrate at physician's office **Caution:** [X, –] **Contra:** Predisposition to priapism (eg, sickle cell); penile deformities/implants; men in whom sexual activity is inadvisable **Disp:** *Caverject:* 5, 10, 20, 40 mcg vials ± diluent syringes. *Caverject Impulse:* Self-contained syringe (29 gauge) 10 & 20 mcg. Edex: 10, 20, 40 mcg cartridges **SE:** Local pain w/ injection **Notes:** Counsel about priapism, penile fibrosis, & hematoma risks, titrate w/Obs

Alprostadil, Urethral Suppository (Muse) Uses: *Erectile dysfunction* **Action:** Urethral mucosal absorption; vasodilator, smooth muscle relaxant of corpus cavernosa **Dose:** 125–1000 mcg system 5–10 min prior to sexual activity; titrate at physician's office **Caution:** [X, –] **Contra:** Predisposition to priapism (eg, sickle cell) penile deformities/implants; men in whom sexual activity is inadvisable **Disp:** 125, 250, 500, 1000 mcg w/ a transurethral delivery system **SE:**

↓ BP, dizziness, syncope, penile/testicular pain, urethral burning/bleeding, priapism **Notes:** Supervision, titrate w/Obs

Alteplase, Recombinant [tPA] (Activase) **Uses:** *AMI, PE, acute ischemic stroke, & CV cath occlusion* **Action:** Thrombolytic; binds to fibrin in the thrombus, initiates fibrinolysis **Dose:** *AMI & PE:* 100 mg IV over 3 h (10 mg over 2 min, then 50 mg over 1 h, then 40 mg over 2 h). Stroke: 0.9 mg/kg (max 90 mg) inf over 60 min. *Cath occlusion:* 10–29 kg 1 mg/mL; ≥ 30 kg 2 mg/mL **Caution:** [C, ?] **Contra:** Active internal bleeding; uncontrolled HTN (systolic BP = >185 mm Hg/diastolic = >110 mm Hg); recent (w/in 3 mo) CVA, GI bleed, trauma, surgery; prolonged external cardiac massage; intracranial neoplasm, suspected aortic dissection, AVM/aneurysm/subarachnoid hemorrhage, bleeding/hemostatic defects, Sz at the time of stroke **Disp:** Powder for inj 2, 50, 100 mg **SE:** Bleeding, bruising (eg, venipuncture sites), ↓ BP **Notes:** Give heparin to prevent reocclusion; in AMI, doses of >150 mg associated w/ intracranial bleeding

Altretamine (Hexalen) **Uses:** *Epithelial ovarian CA* **Action:** Unknown; cytotoxic agent, unknown alkylating agent; ↓ nucleotide incorporation into DNA/RNA **Dose:** 260 mg/m²/d in 4 ÷ doses for 14–21 d of a 28-d Rx cycle; dose ↑ to 150 mg/m²/d for 14 d in multiagent regimens (per protocols); after meals and at bedtime **Caution:** [D, ?/–]. **Contra:** Preexisting BM depression or neurologic tox **Disp:** Caps 50 mg **SE:** V/D, cramps; neurologic (peripheral neuropathy, CNS depression); minimally myelosuppressive

Aluminum Hydroxide (Amphojel, AlternaGEL) [OTC] **Uses:** *Relief of heartburn, upset or sour stomach, or acid indigestion*; supl to Rx of hyperphosphatemia **Action:** Neutralizes gastric acid; binds PO_4^{-2} **Dose:** *Adults.* 10–30 mL or 300–1200 mg PO q4–6h. *Peds.* 5–15 mL PO q4–6h or 50–150 mg/kg/24 h PO ÷ q4–6h (hyperphosphatemia) **Caution:** [C, ?] **Disp:** Tabs 300, 600 mg; susp 320, 600 mg/5 mL **SE:** constipation **Notes:** OK in renal failure

Aluminum Hydroxide + Magnesium Carbonate (Gaviscon Extra Strength, Liquid) [OTC] **Uses:** *Relief of heartburn, acid indigestion* **Action:** Neutralizes gastric acid **Dose:** *Adults.* 15–30 mL PO pc & hs. *Peds.* 5–15 mL PO qid or PRN; avoid in renal impair **Caution:** ↑ Mg^{2+} (w/ renal insuff) [C, ?] **Disp:** Liq w/ AlOH 95 mg/Mg carbonate 358 mg/15 mL; Extra Strength liq AlOH 254 mg/Mg carbonate 237mg/15mL; chew tabs AlOH 160 mg/Mg carb 105 mg **SE:** constipation, D **Notes:** Doses qid are best given pc & hs; may affect absorption of some drugs, take 2-3 h apart to ↓ effect

Aluminum Hydroxide + Magnesium Hydroxide (Maalox) [OTC] **Uses:** *Hyperacidity* (peptic ulcer, hiatal hernia, etc) **Action:** Neutralizes gastric acid **Dose:** *Adults.* 10–20 mL or 2–4 tabs PO qid or PRN. *Peds.* 5–15 mL PO qid or PRN **Caution:** [C, ?] **Disp:** Tabs, susp **SE:** May cause ↑ Mg^{2+} in renal insuff, constipation, D **Notes:** Doses best given pc & hs

Aluminum Hydroxide + Magnesium Hydroxide & Simethicone (Mylanta, Mylanta II, Maalox Plus) [OTC] **Uses:** *Hyperacidity w/ bloating* **Action:** Neutralizes gastric acid & defoaming **Dose:** **Adults.** 10–20 mL or 2–4 tabs PO qid or PRN **Peds.** 5–15 mL PO qid or PRN; avoid in renal impair **Caution:** [C, ?] **Disp:** Tabs, susp, liquid **SE:** ↑ Mg²⁺ in renal insuff, D, constipation **Notes:** Mylanta II contains 2X Al & Mg hydroxide of Mylanta; may affect absorption of some drugs

Aluminum Hydroxide + Magnesium Trisilicate (Gaviscon, Regular Strength) [OTC]
Uses: *Relief of heartburn, upset or sour stomach, or acid indigestion* **Action:** Neutralizes gastric acid **Dose:** Chew 2–4 tabs qid; avoid in renal impair **Caution:** [C, ?] **Contra:** Mg²⁺, sensitivity **Disp:** AlOH 80 mg/Mg trisilicate 20 mg/tab **SE:** ↑ Mg²⁺ in renal insuff, constipation, D **Notes:** May affect absorption of some drugs

Amantadine (Symmetrel)
Uses: *Rx or prophylaxis influenza A, parkinsonism, & drug-induced EPS* (Note: Do not use for Influenza A in the US (increased resistance) **Action:** Prevents release of infectious viral nucleic acid into host cell; releases dopamine from intact dopaminergic terminals **Dose:** **Adults.** *Influenza A:* 200 mg/d PO or 100 mg PO bid. *Parkinsonism:* 100 mg PO qd–bid. **Peds.** *1–9 y:* 4.4–8.8 mg/kg/24 h to 150 mg/24 h max ÷ doses daily–bid. *10–12 y:* 100–200 mg/d in 1–2 ÷ doses; ↓ in renal impair **Caution:** [C, M] **Disp:** Caps 100 mg; tabs 100 mg; soln 50 mg/5 mL **SE:** Orthostatic ↓ BP, edema, insomnia, depression, irritability, hallucinations, dream abnormalities

Amifostine (Ethyol)
Uses: *Xerostomia prophylaxis during RT (head, neck, ovarian, non-small-cell lung CA); ↓ renal tox w/ repeated cisplatin* **Action:** Prodrug, dephosphorylated by alkaline phosphotase to active thiol metabolite **Dose:** 910 mg/m²/d 15-min IV inf 30 min prior to chemo **Caution:** [C, ?/–] **Disp:** 500 mg vials powder, reconstitute in NS **SE:** Transient ↓ BP (>60%), N/V, flushing w/ hot or cold chills, dizziness, ↓ Ca²⁺, somnolence, sneezing. **Notes:** Does not reduce the effectiveness of cyclophosphamide plus cisplatin chemo

Amikacin (Amikin)
Uses: *Serious gram(–) bacterial Infxns* & mycobacteria **Action:** Aminoglycoside; ↓ protein synthesis **Spectrum:** Good gram(–) bacterial coverage: Pseudomonas sp; Mycobacterium sp **Dose:** **Adults & Peds.** Conventional: 5–7.5 mg/kg/dose q 8 h, once daily: 15–20 mg/kg q 24 h ↑ interval w/ renal impair; *Neonates* <1200 g, 0–4 wk: 7.5 mg/kg/dose q12h–18h. *Postnatal age* <7 d, 1200–2000 g: 7.5 mg/kg/dose q12h; >2000 g: 10 mg/kg/dose q12h. *Postnatal age* >7 d, 1200–2000 g: 7 mg/kg/dose q8h; >2000 g: 7.5–10 mg/kg/dose q8h **Caution:** [C, +/–] avoid use w/ diuretics **Disp:** 50 mg/mL, 250 mg/mL **SE:** Nephro/oto/neurotox **Notes:** May be effective in gram(–) bacteria resistant to gentamicin & tobramycin; monitor renal Fxn and levels (Table 2) to adjust dose

Amiloride (Midamor)
Uses: *HTN, CHF, & thiazide-induced ↓ K⁺* **Action:** K⁺-sparing diuretic; interferes w/ K⁺/Na⁺ exchange in distal tubule **Dose:** **Adults.** 5–10 mg PO daily. **Peds.** 0.625 mg/kg/d; ↓ in renal impair **Caution:** [B, ?] **Contra:** ↑ K⁺, SCr > 1.5, BUN > 30 **Disp:** Tabs 5 mg **SE:** ↑ K⁺; HA, dizziness, dehydration, impotence **Notes:** monitor K+

Aminocaproic Acid (Amicar) **Uses:** *Excessive bleeding from systemic hyperfibrinolysis & urinary fibrinolysis* **Action:** ↓ fibrinolysis; via inhibition of TPA substances **Dose:** *Adults.* 5 g IV or PO (1st h) followed by 1–1.25 g/h IV or PO (max dose/d: 30 g) **Peds.** 100 mg/kg IV (1st h) then 1 g/m^2/h; max 18 g/m^2/d; ↓ in renal failure **Caution:** [C, ?] Upper urinary tract bleeding **Contra:** DIC **Disp:** Tabs 500, 1000 mg; syrup 250 mg/mL; inj 250 mg/mL **SE:** ↓ BP, bradycardia, dizziness, HA, fatigue, rash, GI disturbance, ↓ plt Fxn **Notes:** Administer for 8 h or until bleeding controlled; not for upper urinary tract bleeding

Amino-Cerv pH 5.5 Cream **Uses:** *Mild cervicitis,* postpartum cervicitis/cervical tears, postcauterization, postcryosurgery, & postconization **Action:** Hydrating agent; removes excess keratin in hyperkeratotic conditions **Dose:** 1 Applicatorful intravag hs for 2–4 wk **Caution:** [C, ?] Use in viral skin Infxn **Disp:** Vaginal cream **SE:** Transient stinging, local irritation **Notes:** AKA carbamide or urea; contains 8.34% urea, 0.5% sodium propionate, 0.83% methionine, 0.35% cystine, 0.83% inositol, & benzalkonium chloride

Aminoglutethimide (Cytadren) **Uses:** *Cushing syndrome* Adrenocortical carcinoma, breast CA & CAP **Action:** ↓ adrenal steroidogenesis & conversion of androgens to estrogens; aromatase inhibitor **Dose:** 750–1500 mg/d divided doses w/hydrocortisone 20–40 mg/d; ↓ in renal insuff **Caution:** [D, ?] **Disp:** Tabs 250 mg **SE:** Adrenal insuff ("medical adrenalectomy"), hypothyroidism, masculinization, ↓ BP, vomiting, rare hepatotox, rash, myalgia, fever

Aminophylline **Uses:** *Asthma, COPD* & bronchospasm **Action:** Relaxes smooth muscle (bronchi, pulmonary vessels); stimulates diaphragm **Dose:** *Adults. Acute asthma:* Load 6 mg/kg IV, then 0.4–0.9 mg/kg/h IV cont inf. *Chronic asthma:* 24 mg/kg/24 h PO or PR ÷ q6h. **Peds.** Load 6 mg/kg IV, then 1 mg/kg/h IV cont inf; ↓ in hepatic insuff & w/ certain drugs (macrolide & quinolone antibiotics, cimetidine, & propranolol) **Caution:** [C, +] Uncontrolled arrhythmias, Sz disorder, hyperthyroidism, peptic ulcers **Disp:** Tabs 100, 200 mg; soln 105 mg/5 mL, 90 mg/5 mL; supp 250, 500 mg; inj 25 mg/mL **SE:** N/V, irritability, tachycardia, ventricular arrhythmias, Szs **Notes:** Individualize dosage; follow levels (as theophylline, Table 2); aminophylline ≅85% theophylline; erratic rectal absorption

Amiodarone (Cordarone, Pacerone) **Uses:** *Recurrent VF or hemodynamically unstable VT,* supraventricular arrhythmias, AF **Action:** Class III antiarrhythmic (Table 12) **Dose:** *Adults.* Ventricular arrhythmias: IV: 15 mg/min for 10 min, then 1 mg/min for 6 h, then maint 0.5 mg/min cont. inf or *PO:* Load. 800–1600 mg/d PO for 1–3 wk. Maint: 600–800 mg/d PO for 1 mo, then 200–400 mg/d. *Supraventricular arrhythmias: IV:* 300 mg IV over 1 h, then 20 mg/kg for 24 h, then 600 mg PO qd for 1 wk, then maint 100–400 mg qd or PO: Load: 600–800 mg/d PO for 1–4 wk. Maint: Gradually ↓ to 100–400 mg PO QD. **Peds.** 10–15 mg/kg/24 h ÷ q12h PO for 7–10 d, then 5 mg/kg/24 h ÷ q12h or daily (infants/neonates require higher loading); ↓ w/liver insuff **Caution:** [D, –] **Contra:**

Sinus node dysfunction, 2nd-/3rd-degree AV block, sinus bradycardia (w/o pacemaker) **Disp:** Tabs 100, 200, 400 mg; inj 50 mg/mL **SE:** Pulmonary fibrosis, exacerbation of arrhythmias, prolongs QT interval; CHF, hypo/hyperthyroidism, ↑ LFTs, liver failure, corneal microdeposits, optic neuropathy/neuritis, peripheral neuropathy, photosensitivity **Notes:** Half-life 53 d; IV conc of >0.2 mg/mL via a central catheter; may require ↓ digoxin and warfarin dose

Amitriptyline (Elavil)
WARNING: Antidepressants may ↑ risk of suicidality; consider risks and benefits of use. Monitor patients closely **Uses:** *Depression,* peripheral neuropathy, chronic pain, tension HAs **Action:** TCA; ↓ reuptake of serotonin & norepinephrine by presynaptic neurons **Dose:** *Adults.* Initial, 30–50 mg PO hs, may ↑ to 300 mg hs. *Peds.* Not OK <12 y unless for chronic pain; initial 0.1 mg/kg PO hs, ↑ over 2–3 wk to 0.5–2 mg/kg PO hs; taper when D/C **Caution:** [D, +/–] NA glaucoma, hepatic impair **Contra:** W/ MAOIs, during acute MI recovery **Disp:** Tabs 10, 25, 50, 75, 100, 150 mg; inj 10 mg/mL **SE:** Strong anticholinergic SEs; OD may be fatal; urine retention, sedation, ECG changes, photosensitivity

Amlodipine (Norvasc)
Uses: *HTN, stable or unstable angina* **Action:** CCB; relaxes coronary vascular smooth muscle **Dose:** 2.5–10 mg/d PO; ↓ w/hepatic impair **Caution:** [C, ?] **Disp:** Tabs 2.5, 5, 10 mg **SE:** Peripheral edema, HA, palpitations, flushing **Notes:** Take w/o regard to meals

Amlodipine/Atorvastatin (Caduet)
Uses: * HTN, chronic stable/vasospastic angina, control cholesterol & triglycerides* **Action:** CCB & HMG-CoA reductase inhibitor **Dose:** Amlodipine 2.5–10 mg w/Atorvastatin 10–80 mg PO qd **Caution:** |X, –| **Contra:** Active liver Dz, ↑ LFT **Disp:** Tabs amlodipine/atorvastatin, 2.5/10, 2.5/20, 2.5/40, 5/10, 5/20, 5/40, 5/80, 10/10, 10/20, 10/40, 10/80 mg **SE:** Peripheral edema, HA, palpitations, flushing, myopathy, arthralgia, myalgia, GI upset **Notes:** Monitor LFTs

Ammonium Aluminum Sulfate [Alum] [OTC]
Uses: *Hemorrhagic cystitis when saline bladder irrigation fails* **Action:** Astringent **Dose:** 1–2% soln w/ constant NS bladder irrigation **Caution:** [+/–]**Disp:** Powder for reconstitution **SE:** Encephalopathy possible; obtain aluminum levels, especially in renal insuff; can precipitate & occlude catheters **Notes:** Safe to use w/o anesthesia & w/ vesicoureteral reflux

Amoxicillin (Amoxil, Polymox)
Uses: *Ear, nose, & throat, lower resp, skin, urinary tract Infxns resulting from susceptible gram(+) bacteria* endocarditis prophylaxis **Action:** β Lactam antibiotic; ↓ cell wall synthesis **Spectrum:** Gram(+) (Strep sp, Enterococcus sp); some gram(–) (*H. influenzae, E. coli, N. gonorrhoeae, H. pylori, & P. mirabilis*) **Dose:** *Adults.* 250–500 mg PO tid or 500–875 mg bid. *Peds.* 25–100 mg/kg/24 h PO ÷ q8h. 200–400 mg PO bid (equivalent to 125–250 mg tid); ↓ in renal impair **Caution:** [B, +] **Disp:** Caps 250, 500 mg; chew tabs 125, 200, 250, 400 mg; susp 50 mg/mL, 125, 200, 250 & 400 mg/5 mL; tabs 500, 875 mg **SE:** D; skin rash **Notes:** Cross hypersensitivity PCN; many strains of E. coli-resistant

Amoxicillin & Clavulanic Acid (Augmentin, Augmentin 600 ES, Augmentin XR) Uses: *Ear, lower resp, sinus, urinary tract, skin Infxns caused by β-lactamase-producing *H. influenzae*, *S. aureus*, & *E. coli** Action: Combo β-lactam antibiotic & β-lactamase inhibitor. *Spectrum:* Gram(+) same as amox alone, MSSA; gram(−) as w/ amox alone, β-lactamase-producing *H. influenzae*, *Klebsiella* sp, *M. catarrhalis* Dose: Adults. 250–500 mg PO q8h or 875 mg q12h; XR 2000 mg PO Q12H. Peds. 20–40 mg/kg/d as amoxicillin PO ÷ q8h or 45 mg/kg/d ÷ q12h; ↓ in renal impair; take w/ food Caution: [B, ?] Disp: Supplied (as amoxicillin/clavulanic acid): Tabs 250/125, 500/125, 875/125 mg; chew tabs 125/31.25, 200/28.5, 250/62.5, 400/57 mg; susp 125/31.25, 250/62.5, 200/28.5, 400/57 mg/5 mL; susp: ES 600/42.9mg/5mL; XR tab 1000/62.5 mg SE: Abdominal discomfort, N/V/D, allergic Rxn, vaginitis Notes: Do not substitute two 250-mg tabs for one 500-mg tab (OD of clavulanic acid)

Amphotericin B (Amphocin) Uses: *Severe, systemic fungal Infxns; oral & cutaneous candidiasis* Action: Binds ergosterol in the fungal membrane to alter permeability Dose: Adults & Peds. Test dose: 1 mg IV adults or 0.1 mg/kg to 1 mg IV in children; then 0.25–1.5 mg/kg/24 h IV over 2–6 h (range 25–50 mg/d or qod). Total dose varies w/ indication. PO: 1 mL qid. Topical: Apply bid–qid for 1–4 wk depending on Infxn; ↓ in renal impair Caution: [B, ?] Disp: Powder for inj 50 mg/vial; PO susp 100 mg/mL; cream, lotion, oint 3% SE: ↓ K+/Mg2+ from renal wasting; anaphylaxis reported, HA, fever, chills, nephrotoxicity, ↓ BP, anemia Notes: Monitor Cr/LFTs; pretreatment w/ APAP & antihistamines (Benadryl) minimizes adverse IV effects

Amphotericin B Cholesteryl (Amphotec) Uses: *Aspergillosis in pts intolerant/refractory to conventional amphotericin B,* systemic candidiasis Action: Binds sterols in the cell membrane, alters permeability Dose: Adults & Peds. Test dose 1.6–8.3 mg, over 15–20 min, then 3–4 mg/kg/d; 1 mg/kg/h inf; ↓ w/renal insuff Caution: [B, ?] Disp: Powder for inj 50 mg, 100 mg/vial SE: Anaphylaxis reported; fever, chills, HA, ↓ K+, ↓ Mg2+, nephrotox, ↓ BP, anemia Notes: Do not use in-line filter; monitor LFT & electrolytes

Amphotericin B Lipid Complex (Abelcet) Uses: *Refractory invasive fungal Infxn in pts intolerant to conventional amphotericin B* Action: Binds cell membrane sterols, alters permeability Dose: Adults & Peds. 5 mg/kg/d IV single daily dose; 2.5 mg/kg/h inf Caution: [B, ?] Disp: Inj 5 mg/mL SE: Anaphylaxis; fever, chills, HA, ↓ K+, ↓ Mg2+, nephrotox, ↓ BP, anemia Notes: Filter soln w/5-micron filter needle; do not mix in electrolyte-containing solns; if inf >2 h, manually mix bag

Amphotericin B Liposomal (AmBisome) Uses: *Refractory invasive fungal Infxn in pts intolerant to conventional amphotericin B, cryptococcal meningitis in HIV, empiric Rx for febrile neutropenia, visceral leishmaniasis* Action: Binds to sterols in cell membrane, changes membrane permeability Dose: Adults & Peds. 3–6 mg/kg/d, inf 60–120 min; ↓ in renal insuff Caution: [B, ?]

Disp: Powder for inj 50 mg **SE:** Anaphylaxis reported; fever, chills, HA, ↓ K⁺, ↓ Mg²⁺ nephrotox, ↓ BP, anemia **Notes:** Use no less than 1-micron filter

Ampicillin (Amcill, Omnipen) Uses:
Resp, GU, or GI tract Infxns, meningitis due to gram(−) & gram(+) bacteria; endocarditis prophylaxis **Action:** β-Lactam antibiotic; ↓ cell wall synthesis. *Spectrum:* Gram(+) (*Streptococcus* sp, *Staphylococcus* sp, *Listeria*); gram(−) (*Klebsiella* sp, *E. coli*, *H. influenzae*, *P. mirabilis*, *Shigella* sp, *Salmonella* sp) **Dose:** *Adults.* 500 mg–2 g IM or IV q6h or 250–500 mg PO q6h. *Peds.* Neonates <7 d: 50–100 mg/kg/24 h IV ÷ q8h. *Term infants:* 75–150 mg/kg/24 h ÷ q6–8h IV or PO. *Children >1 mo:* 100–200 mg/kg/24 h ÷ q4–6h IM or IV; 50–100 mg/kg/24 h ÷ q6h PO up to 250 mg/dose. *Meningitis:* 200–400 mg/kg/24 h ÷ q4–6h IV; ↓ in renal impair; take on empty stomach **Caution:** [B, M] Cross hypersensitivity w/ PCN **Disp:** Caps 250, 500 mg; susp 100 mg/mL (reconstituted as drops), 125 mg/5 mL, 250 mg/5 mL; powder for inj 125 mg, 250, 500 mg, 1 g, 2 g, 10 g/vial **SE:** D, skin rash, allergic Rxn **Notes:** Many strains of *E. coli*-resistant

Ampicillin–Sulbactam (Unasyn) Uses:
*Gynecologic, intraabdominal, skin Infxns caused by β-lactamase-producing strains of *S. aureus*, *Enterococcus*, *H. influenzae*, *P. mirabilis*, & *Bacteroides* sp* **Action:** Combo β-lactam antibiotic & a β-lactamase inhibitor. *Spectrum:* Gram(+) & gram(−) as for amp alone; also *Enterobacter*, *Acinetobacter*, *Bacteroides* **Dose:** *Adults.* 1.5–3 g IM or IV q6h. *Peds.* 100–200 mg ampicillin/kg/d (150–300 mg Unasyn) q6h; ↓ w/ renal insuff **Caution:** [B, M] **Disp:** Powder for inj 1.5, 3 g/vial, 15 g bulk package **SE:** Allergic Rxns, rash, D, inj site pain **Notes:** A 2:1 ratio ampicillin:sulbactam

Amprenavir (Agenerase) WARNING:
PO soln contra in children <4 y (potential tox from large volume of polypropylene glycol in formulation) **Uses:** *HIV Infxn* **Action:** Protease inhibitor; prevents virion maturation to mature virus **Dose:** *Adults.* 1200 mg bid. *Peds.* 20 mg/kg bid or 15 mg/kg tid to 2400 mg/d **Caution:** [C, ?] CDC recommends HIV-infected mothers not breast-feed (risk of HIV transmission); Hx sulfonamide allergy **Contra:** CYP450 3A4 substrates; soln <4 y, PRG, hepatic/renal insuff, disulfiram, or metronidazole **Disp:** Caps 50, 150 mg; soln 15 mg/mL **SE:** Life-threatening rash, hyperglycemia, hypertriglyceridemia, fat redistribution, N/V/D, depression **Notes:** Caps & soln contain vitamin E exceeding RDA; avoid high-fat meals; many drug interactions

Anakinra (Kineret) WARNING:
Associated w/ ↑ incidence of serious Infxn; D/C w/ serious Infxn **Uses:** *Reduce signs & Sxs of moderate/severe active RA, failed 1 or more DMARD* **Action:** Human IL-1 receptor antagonist **Dose:** 100 mg SQ qd **Caution:** [B, ?] **Contra:** Allergy to E. coli-derived proteins, active Infxn, <18 y **Disp:** 100-mg prefilled syringes **SE:** Neutropenia especially when used w/ TNF-blocking agents, inj site Rxn, Infxn

Anastrozole (Arimidex) Uses:
Breast CA: postmenopausal w/ metastatic breast CA, adjuvant Rx of postmenopausal w/ early hormone-receptor(+) breast CA **Action:** Selective nonsteroidal aromatase inhibitor, ↓ circ estradiol **Dose:**

1 mg/d **Caution:** [D, ?] **Contra:** PRG **Disp:** Tabs 1 mg **SE:** May ↑ cholesterol; D, HTN, flushing, ↑ bone & tumor pain, HA, somnolence **Notes:** No effect on adrenal corticosteroids or aldosterone

Anidulafungin (Eraxis) **Uses:** *Candidemia, esophageal candidiasis, and other Candida Infxn (peritonitis, intra-abdominal abscess)* **Action:** Echinocandin; ↓ cell wall synthesis *Spectrum: C. albicans, C. glabrata, C. parapsilosis,* and *C. tropicalis* **Dose:** Candidemia, others: 200 mg IV × 1, then 100 mg IV daily (Tx 14 days after last + culture); Esophageal candidiasis: 100 mg IV × 1, then 50 mg IV daily (Tx >14 d and 7 d after resolution of Sx); 1.1 mg/min max inf rate **Caution:** [C, ?/-] **Contra:** Echinocandin hypersensitivity **Disp:** Powder 50 mg/vial **SE:** Histamine-mediated infusion Rxns (urticaria, flushing, pruritus, rash, hypotension, dyspnea), fever, N/V/D, hypokalemia, HA, ↑LFTs, hepatitis, worsening hepatic failure **Notes:** ↓ inf rate to <1.1 mg/min w/inf Rxns

Anistreplase (Eminase) **Uses:** *AMI* **Action:** Thrombolytic; activates conversion of plasminogen to plasmin, ↑ thrombolysis **Dose:** 30 units IV over 2–5 min **Caution:** [C, ?] **Contra:** Active internal bleeding, Hx CVA, recent (<2 mo) intracranial or intraspinal surgery/trauma, intracranial neoplasm, AVM, aneurysm, bleeding diathesis, severe uncontrolled HTN **Disp:** Vials w/30 units **SE:** Bleeding, ↓ BP, hematoma **Notes:** Ineffective if readministered >5 d after the previous dose of anistreplase or streptokinase, or streptococcal Infxn (production of antistreptokinase Ab)

Anthralin (Anthra-Derm) **Uses:** *Psoriasis* **Action:** Keratolytic **Dose:** Apply qd **Caution:** [C, ?] **Contra:** Acutely inflamed psoriatic eruptions, erythroderma **Disp:** Cream, oint 0.1, 0.25, 0.4, 0.5, 1% **SE:** Irritation; hair/fingernails/skin discoloration

Antihemophilic Factor [AHF, Factor VIII] (Monoclate) **Uses:** *Classic hemophilia A, von Willebrand Dz* **Action:** Provides factor VIII needed to convert prothrombin to thrombin **Dose:** *Adults & Peds.* 1 AHF unit/kg ↑ factor VIII level ≈2%, Units required = (kg) (desired factor VIII ↑ as % nl) × (0.5); Prevent spontaneous hemorrhage = 5% nl; Hemostasis after trauma/surgery = 30% nl; Head injuries, major surgery, or bleeding = 80–100% nl **Caution:** [C, ?] **Disp:** Check each vial for units contained **SE:** Rash, fever, HA, chills, N/V **Notes:** Determine pt's % of nl factor VIII before dosing

Antithymocyte Globulin See Lymphocyte Immune Globulin, page 125

Apomorphine (Apokyn) WARNING: Do not administer IV **Uses:** *Acute, intermittent hypomobility ("off") episodes of Parkinson Dz* **Action:** Dopamine agonist **Dose:** *Adults.* 0.2-mL SQ test dose under medical supervision; if BP OK, initial 0.2 mL (2 mg) SQ during "off" periods; only 1 dose per "off" period; requires titration; 0.6 mL (6 mg)max single doses; use w/antiemetic; ↓ in renal impair **Caution:** [C, +/–] Avoid EtOH; antihypertensives, vasodilators, cardio or cerebrovascular Dz, hepatic impair **Contra:** 5HT3 antagonists, sulfite allergy

Disp: Inj 10 mg/mL, 3-mL pen cartridges; 2-mL amp **SE:** Emesis, syncope, QT prolongation, orthostatic ↓ BP, somnolence, ischemia, injection site Rxn, abuse potential, dyskinesia, fibrotic conditions, priapism **Notes:** Daytime somnolence may limit activities; trimethobenzamide 300 mg tid PO or other non-5HT3 antagonist antiemetic given 3 d prior to & up to 2 mo following initiation

Apraclonidine (Iopidine)
Uses: *Glaucoma, postop intraocular HTN* **Action:** α₂-Adrenergic agonist **Dose:** 1–2 gtt of 0.5% tid **Caution:** [C, ?] **Contra:** MAOI use **Disp:** 0.5, 1% soln **SE:** Ocular irritation, lethargy, xerostomia

Aprepitant (Emend)
Uses: *Prevents N/V assoc w/ emetogenic CA chemo (eg, cisplatin) (use in combo w/ other antiemetics)* **Action:** Substance P/neurokinin 1(NK₁) receptor antagonist **Dose:** 125 mg PO day 1, 1 h before chemo, then 80 mg PO q AM on days 2 & 3 **Caution:** [B, ?/–]; substrate & moderate inhibitor of CYP3A4; inducer of CYP2C9 (Table 13) **Contra:** Use w/ pimozide **Disp:** Caps 80, 125 mg **SE:** Fatigue, asthenia, hiccups **Notes:** ↓ Effectiveness of PO contraceptives; ↓ effect of warfarin

Aprotinin (Trasylol)
Uses: *↓/Prevent blood loss during CABG* **Action:** Protease inhibitor, antifibrinolytic **Dose:** 1-mL IV test dose. *High dose:* 2 million KIU load, 2 million KIU to prime pump, then 500,000 KIU/h until surgery ends. *Low dose:* 1 million KIU load, 1 million KIU to prime pump, then 250,000 KIU/h until surgery ends; 7 million KIU max total **Caution:** [B, ?] Thromboembolic Dz requiring anticoagulants or blood factor administration **Disp:** Inj 1.4 mg/mL (10,000 KIU/mL) **SE:** AF, MI, heart failure, dyspnea, postop renal dysfunction **Notes:** 1000/KIU = 0.14 mg of aprotinin

Ardeparin (Normiflo)
Uses: *Prevents DVT/PE following knee replacement* **Action:** LMW heparin **Dose:** 35–50 units/kg SQ q12h. Begin day of surgery, continue up to 14 d **Caution:** [C, ?] ↓ renal Fxn **Contra:** Active hemorrhage; allergy to pork products **Disp:** Inj 5000, 10,000 IU/0.5 mL **SE:** Bleeding, bruising, thrombocytopenia, pain at inj site, ↑ serum transaminases **Notes:** Lab monitoring usually not necessary

Argatroban (Acova)
Uses: *Prevent/Tx thrombosis in HIT, PCI in pts w/ risk of HIT* **Action:** Anticoagulant, direct thrombin inhibitor **Dose:** 2 mcg/kg/min IV; adjust until aPTT 1.5–3 × baseline not to exceed 100 s; 10 mcg/kg/min max; ↓ w/hepatic impair **Caution:** [B, ?] Avoid PO anticoagulants, ↑ bleeding risk; avoid use w/thrombolytics **Contra:** Overt major bleed **Disp:** Inj 100 mg/mL **SE:** AF, cardiac arrest, cerebrovascular disorder, ↓BP, VT, N/V/D, sepsis, cough, renal tox, ↓ Hgb **Notes:** Steady state in 1–3 h

Aripiprazole (Abilify)
WARNING: Increased mortality in elderly with dementia-related psychosis **Uses:** *Schizophrenia* **Action:** Dopamine & serotonin antagonist **Dose:** Adults. 10–15 mg PO qd; ↓ dose w/CYP3A4 or CYP2D6 inhibitors (Table 13); ↑ dose w/inducer of CYP3A4 **Caution:** [C, –] **Disp:** Tabs 2, 5, 10, 15, 20, 30 mg; soln 1 mg/ml **SE:** Neuroleptic malignant syndrome, tardive dyskinesia, orthostatic ↓ BP, cognitive & motor impair, hyperglycemia

Artificial Tears (Tears Naturale) [OTC] Uses: *Dry eyes* Action: Ocular lubricant Dose: 1–2 gtt tid–qid Disp: OTC soln

L-Asparaginase (Elspar, Oncaspar) Uses: *ALL* (in combo w/ other agents) Action: Protein synthesis inhibitor Dose: 500–20,000 IU/m²/d for 1–14 d (Per protocols) Caution: [C, ?] Contra: Active/Hx pancreatitis In powder for reconstitution 10,000 units SE: Allergy 20–35% (from urticaria to anaphylaxis test dose recommended); rare GI tox (mild nausea/anorexia, pancreatitis)

Aspirin (Bayer, Ecotrin, St. Joseph's) [OTC] Uses: *Angina, CABG, PTCA, carotid endarterectomy, ischemic stroke, TIA, MI, arthritis, pain,* HA, *fever, * inflammation, Kawasaki Dz Action: Prostaglandin inhibitor Dose: *Adults.* Pain, fever: 325–650 mg q4–6h PO or PR. RA: 3–6 g/d PO in ÷ doses. *Plt inhibitor:* 81–325 mg PO qd. *Prevent MI:* 81–325 mg PO qd. *Peds. Antipyretic:* 10–15 mg/kg/dose PO or PR q4h up to 80 mg/kg/24 h. RA: 60–100 mg/kg/24 h PO ÷ q4–6h (keep levels between 15 & 30 mg/dL); avoid w/ CrCl <10 mL/min, severe liver Dz Caution: [C, M] Linked to Reye's syndrome; avoid w/viral illness in children Contra: Allergy to ASA, chickenpox/flu Sxs, syndrome of nasal polyps, asthma, rhinitis Disp: Tabs 325, 500 mg; chew tabs 81 mg; EC tabs 81,162, 325, 500, 650, 975 mg; SR tabs 650, 800 mg; effervescent tabs 325, 500 mg; supp 125, 200, 300, 600 mg SE: GI upset & erosion Notes: D/C 1 wk prior to surgery to ↓ bleeding; avoid/limit EtOH

Aspirin & Butalbital Compound (Fiorinal) [C-III] Uses: *Tension HA,* pain Action: Combo barbiturate & analgesic Dose: 1–2 PO q4h PRN, max 6 tabs/d; avoid w/ CrCl <10 mL/min & severe liver Dz Caution: [C (D w/ prolonged use or high doses at term), ?] Contra: ASA allergy, GI ulceration, bleeding disorder, porphyria, syndrome of nasal polyps, angioedema, & bronchospasm to NSAIDs Disp: Caps (Fiorgen PF, Lanorinal), Tabs (Lanorinal) ASA 325 mg/butalbital 50 mg/caffeine 40 mg SE: Drowsiness, dizziness, GI upset, ulceration, bleeding Notes: Butalbital habit-forming; avoid or limit EtOH intake

Aspirin + Butalbital, Caffeine, & Codeine (Fiorinal + Codeine) [C-III] Uses: Mild *pain*, HA, especially when associated w/ stress Action: Sedative analgesic, narcotic analgesic Dose: 1–2 tabs (caps) PO q4–6h PRN max 6/day Caution: [D, ?] Contra: Allergy to ASA and codeine Disp: Cap/tab contains 325 mg ASA, 40 mg caffeine, 50 mg of butalbital, 30 mg of codeine SE: Drowsiness, dizziness, GI upset, ulceration, bleeding; avoid or limit ETOH

Aspirin + Codeine (Empirin No. 3,4) [C-III] Uses: Mild to *moderate pain* Action: Combined effects of ASA & codeine Dose: *Adults.* 1–2 tabs PO q4–6h PRN. *Peds.* ASA 10 mg/kg/dose; codeine 0.5–1 mg/kg/dose q4h Caution: [D, M] Contra: Allergy to ASA/codeine, PUD, bleeding, anticoagulant Rx, children w/ chickenpox or flu Sxs Disp: Tabs 325 mg of ASA & codeine (Codeine in No. 3 = 30 mg, No. 4 = 60 mg) SE: Drowsiness, dizziness, GI upset, ulceration, bleeding

Atazanavir (Reyataz) WARNING: Hyperbilirubinemia may require drug D/C Uses: *HIV-1 Infxn* Action: Protease inhibitor Dose: 400 mg PO qd w/ food; when given w/ efavirenz 600 mg, administer atazanavir 300 mg + ritonavir 100 mg once/d; separate doses from buffered didanosine administration; ↓ in hepatic impair Caution: [B, –]; ↑ levels of statins, sildenafil, antiarrhythmics, warfarin, cyclosporine, TCAs; atazanavir ↓ by St. John's wort Contra: Use w/midazolam, triazolam, ergots, cisapride, pimozide Disp: Caps 100, 150, 200 mg SE: HA, N/V/D, rash, abdominal pain, DM, photosensitivity, ↑ PR interval Notes: May have less adverse effect on cholesterol

Atenolol (Tenormin) Uses: *HTN, angina, MI* Action: Competitively blocks β adrenergic receptors, β₁ Dose: *HTN & angina:* 50–100 mg/d PO. *AMI:* 5 mg IV ×2 over 10 min, then 50 mg PO bid if tolerated; ↓ in renal impair Caution: [D, M] DM, bronchospasm; abrupt D/C can exacerbate angina & ↑ MI risk Contra: Bradycardia, cardiogenic shock, cardiac failure, 2nd-/3rd-degree AV block Disp: Tabs 25, 50, 100 mg; inj 5 mg/10 mL SE: Bradycardia, ↓ BP, 2nd-/3rd-degree AV block, dizziness, fatigue

Atenolol & Chlorthalidone (Tenoretic) Uses: *HTN* Action: β Adrenergic blockade w/ diuretic Dose: 50–100 mg/d PO; ↓ in renal impair Caution: [D, M] DM, bronchospasm Contra: See atenolol; anuria, sulfonamide cross-sensitivity Disp: Tenoretic 50: Atenolol 50 mg/chlorthalidone 25 mg; Tenoretic 100: Atenolol 100 mg/chlorthalidone 25 mg SE: Bradycardia, ↓ BP, 2nd- or 3rd-degree AV block, dizziness, fatigue, ↓ K⁺, photosensitivity

Atomoxetine (Strattera) WARNING: Severe liver injury may occur in rare cases. DC w/jaundice or ↑LFT Increased frequency of suicidal thinking Uses: * ADHD* Action: Selective norepinephrine reuptake inhibitor Dose: *Adults & children >70 kg:* 40 mg × 3 days, ↑ to 80–100 mg ÷ daily–bid. *Peds <70 kg:* 0.5 mg/kg × 3 d, then ↑ 1.2 mg/kg max daily or bid Caution: [C, ? /] Contra: NA glaucoma, use w/ or w/in 2 wk of D/C an MAOI Disp: Caps 10, 18, 25, 40, 60 mg SE: ↑ BP, tachycardia, weight loss, sexual dysfunction Notes: ↓ dose w/ hepatic insuff or in combo w/ inhibitors of CYP2D6 (Table 13)

Atorvastatin (Lipitor) Uses: *↑ cholesterol & triglycerides* Action: HMG-CoA reductase inhibitor Dose: Initial 10 mg/d, may ↑ to 80 mg/d Caution: [X, –] Contra: Active liver Dz, unexplained ↑ LFT Disp: Tabs 10, 20, 40, 80 mg SE: Myopathy, HA, arthralgia, myalgia, GI upset Notes: Monitor LFTs, instruct patient to report unusual muscle pain or weakness

Atovaquone (Mepron) Uses: *Rx & prevention PCP* Action: ↓ nucleic acid & ATP synthesis Dose: Rx: 750 mg PO bid for 21 d. *Prevention:* 1500 mg PO once/d (w/ meals) Caution: [C, ?] Disp: Suspension 750 mg/5 mL SE: Fever, HA, anxiety, insomnia, rash, N/V

Atovaquone/Proguanil (Malarone) Uses: *Prevention or Rx P. falciparum malaria* Action: Antimalarial Dose: *Adults: Prevention:* 1 tab PO 2 d before, during, & 7 d after leaving endemic region; *Rx:* 4 tabs PO single dose qd ×

3 d. *Peds.* See insert **Caution:** [C, ?] **Contra:** CrCl <30 mL/min **Disp:** Tab atovaquone 250 mg/proguanil 100 mg; peds 62.5/25 mg **SE:** HA, fever, myalgia

Atracurium (Tracrium) Uses: * Anesthesia adjunct to facilitate ET intubation* **Action:** Nondepolarizing neuromuscular blocker **Dose:** *Adults & Peds.* 0.4–0.5 mg/kg IV bolus, then 0.08–0.1 mg/kg q20–45 min PRN **Caution:** [C, ?] **Disp:** Inj 10 mg/mL **SE:** Flushing **Notes:** Pt must be intubated & on controlled ventilation; use adequate amounts of sedation & analgesia

Atropine Uses: *Preanesthetic; symptomatic bradycardia & asystole* **Action:** Antimuscarinic agent; blocks acetylcholine at parasympathetic sites **Dose:** *Adults.* ECC: 0.5–1 mg IV q3–5min. *Preanesthetic:* 0.3–0.6 mg IM. *Peds.* ECC: 0.01–0.03 mg/kg IV q2–5min, max 1 mg, min dose 0.1 mg. *Preanesthetic:* 0.01 mg/kg/dose SC/IV (max 0.4 mg) **Caution:** [C, +] **Contra:** Glaucoma **Disp:** Tabs 0.3, 0.4, 0.6 mg; inj 0.05, 0.1, 0.3, 0.4, 0.5, 0.8, 1 mg/mL; ophth sol 0.5, 1, 2%; ophth oint 1% **SE:** Blurred vision, urinary retention, constipation, dried mucous membranes

Azathioprine (Imuran) Uses: *Adjunct to prevent renal transplant rejection, RA,* SLE **Action:** Immunosuppressive; antagonizes purine metabolism **Dose:** *Adults & Peds.* 1–3 mg/kg/d IV or PO; ↓ w/renal insuff) **Caution:** [D, ?] **Contra:** PRG **Disp:** Tabs 50 mg; inj 100 mg powder for reconstitution. **SE:** GI intolerance, fever, chills, leukopenia, thrombocytopenia; chronic use may ↑ neoplasia **Notes:** Handle inj w/ cytotoxic precautions; interaction w/ allopurinol; do not administer live vaccines on drug

Azelastine (Astelin, Optivar) Uses: *Allergic rhinitis (rhinorrhea, sneezing, nasal pruritus); allergic conjunctivitis* **Action:** Histamine H₁-receptor antagonist **Dose:** *Nasal:* 2 sprays/nostril bid. *Ophth:* 1 gt into each affected eye bid **Caution:** [C, ?/–] **Contra:** Component sensitivity **Disp:** Nasal 137 mcg/spray; ophth soln 0.05% **SE:** Somnolence, bitter taste

Azithromycin (Zithromax) Uses: *Community-acquired pneumonia, pharyngitis, otitis media, skin Infxns, nongonococcal urethritis, & PID; Rx & prevention of MAC in HIV* **Action:** Macrolide antibiotic; ↓ protein synthesis. *Spectrum: Chlamydia, H. ducreyi, H. influenzae, Legionella, M. catarrhalis, M. pneumoniae, M. hominis, N. gonorrhoeae, S. aureus, S. agalactiae, S. pneumoniae, S. pyogenes* **Dose:** *Adults.* PO: Resp tract Infxns: 500 mg day 1, then 250 mg/d PO × 4 d; 500 mg/d PO × 3 days; or 2 g PO × 1. *Nongonococcal urethritis:* 1 g PO single dose. *Prevention of MAC:* 1200 mg PO once/wk. IV: 500 mg × 2 d, then 500 mg PO ×7–10 d. *Peds. Otitis media:* 10 mg/kg PO day 1, then 5 mg/kg/d days 2–5. *Pharyngitis:* 12 mg/kg/d PO × 5 d (take susp on an empty stomach; tabs may be taken w/wo food) **Caution:** [B, +] **Disp:** Tabs 250, 500, 600 mg; Z-Pack (5-day); Tri-Pak (500-mg tabs × 3); susp 1-g; single-dose packet Zmax XR suspension (2 gm); susp 100, 200 mg/5 mL; powder for reconstitution 500 mg **SE:** GI upset

Aztreonam (Azactam) Uses: *Aerobic gram(–) UTIs, lower resp, intraabdominal, skin, gynecologic Infxns & septicemia* **Action:** Monobactam. ↓ Cell wall synthesis. Spectrum: Gram(–) (*Pseudomonas, E. coli, Klebsiella, H. influen-*

zae, Serratia, Proteus, Enterobacter, Citrobacter) **Dose:** *Adults.* 1–2 g IV/IM q6–12h. **Peds.** Premature: 30 mg/kg/dose IV q12h. *Term & children:* 30 mg/kg/dose q6–8h; ↓ in renal impair **Caution:** [B, +] **Disp:** Inj (soln), 1 g, 2 g Inj powder for reconstitution 500 mg 1 g, 2 g **SE:** N/V/D, rash, pain at injection site **Notes:** No gram(+) or anaerobic activity; OK in PCN-allergic pts

Bacitracin, Ophthalmic (AK-Tracin Ophthalmic); Bacitracin & Polymyxin B, Ophthalmic (AK Poly Bac Ophthalmic, Polysporin Ophthalmic); Bacitracin, Neomycin, & Polymyxin B, Ophthalmic (AK Spore Ophthalmic, Neosporin Ophthalmic); Bacitracin, Neomycin, Polymyxin B, & Hydrocortisone, Ophthalmic (AK Spore HC Ophthalmic, Cortisporin Ophthalmic) Uses: *Steroid-responsive inflammatory ocular conditions* **Action:** Topical antibiotic w/antiinflammatory **Dose:** Apply q3–4h into conjunctival sac **Caution:** [C, ?] **Contra:** Viral, mycobacterial, fungal eye Infxn **Disp:** See Bacitracin, Topical equivalents, below

Bacitracin, Topical (Baciguent); Bacitracin & Polymyxin B, Topical (Polysporin); Bacitracin, Neomycin, & Polymyxin B, Topical (Neosporin Ointment); Bacitracin, Neomycin, Polymyxin B, & Hydrocortisone, Topical (Cortisporin); Bacitracin, Neomycin, Polymyxin B, & Lidocaine, Topical (Clomycin) Uses: Prevent/Rx of *minor skin Infxns* **Action:** Topical antibiotic w/ added components (anti-inflammatory & analgesic) **Dose:** Apply sparingly bid-qid **Caution:** [C, ?] **Disp:** Bacitracin 500 U/g oint; Bacitracin 500 U/polymyxin B sulfate 10,000 U/g oint & powder; Bacitracin 400 U/neomycin 3.5 mg/polymyxin B 5000 U/g oint Bacitracin 400 U/neomycin 3.5 mg/polymyxin B/10,000 U/hydrocortisone 10 mg/g oint; Bacitracin 500 U/neomycin 3.5 mg/polymyxin B 5000 U/lidocaine 40 mg/g oint **Notes:** Systemic & irrigation forms available, but not generally used due to potential tox

Baclofen (Lioresal) Uses: *Spasticity due to severe chronic disorders (eg, MS, ALS, or spinal cord lesions).* trigeminal neuralgia, hiccups **Action:** Centrally acting skeletal muscle relaxant; ↓ transmission of monosynaptic & polysynaptic cord reflexes **Dose:** *Adults.* Initial, 5 mg PO tid; ↑ q3d to effect; max 80 mg/d. *Intrathecal:* via implantable pump **Peds.** 2–7 y: 10–15 mg/d ÷ q8h; titrate, max 40 mg/d. *>8 y:* Max 60 mg/d. *II:* via implantable pump; ↓ in renal impair; w/ food or milk **Caution:** [C, +] Epilepsy, neuropsychiatric disturbances; withdrawal w/ abrupt D/C **Disp:** Tabs 10, 20 mg; IT inj 50 mcg/mL 10 mg/20 mL, 10 mg/5 mL **SE:** Dizziness, drowsiness, insomnia, ataxia, weakness, ↓ BP

Balsalazide (Colazal) Uses: *Ulcerative colitis* **Action:** 5-ASA derivative, anti-inflammatory, ↓ leukotriene synthesis **Dose:** 2.25 g (3 caps) tid × 8–12 wk **Caution:** [B, ?] Severe renal/hepatic failure **Contra:** Mesalamine or salicylates hypersensitivity **Disp:** Caps 750 mg **SE:** Dizziness, HA, nausea, agranulocytosis, pancytopenia, renal impair, allergic Rxns **Notes:** Daily dose of 6.75 g = to 2.4 g mesalamine

Basiliximab (Simulect) Uses: *Prevent acute transplant rejection* Action: IL-2 receptor antagonists Dose: *Adults.* 20 mg IV 2 h before transplant, then 20 mg IV 4 d post. *Peds.* 12 mg/m^2 ↑ to max of 20 mg 2 h prior to transplant; the same dose IV 4 d post Caution: [B, ?/–] Contra: Hypersensitivity to Murine proteins Disp: Inj: powder for reconstitution 10, 20 mg SE: Edema, HTN, HA, dizziness, fever, pain, Infxn, GI effects, electrolyte disturbances Notes: Murine/human MoAb

BCG [Bacillus Calmette-Guérin] (TheraCys, Tice BCG) Uses: *Bladder carcinoma (superficial),* TB prophylaxis Action: Immunomodulator Dose: Bladder CA, 1 vial prepared & instilled in bladder for 2 h. Repeat once/wk for 6 wk; then 1 treatment at 3, 6, 12, 18, & 24 mo after initial therapy Caution: [C, ?] Asthma, do not administer w/traumatic catheterization or UTI Contra: Immunosuppression, UTI, steroid use, acute illness, fever of unknown origin Disp: Inj 81 mg (10.5 ± 8.7 × 10^8 CFU vial) (TheraCys), 50 mg (1–8 × 10^8 CFU/vial) (Tice BCG) SE: *Intravesical:* Hematuria, urinary frequency, dysuria, bacterial UTI, rare BCG sepsis Notes: Routine US adult BCG immunization not rec; occasionally used in high-risk children who are PPD(–) & cannot take INH

Becaplermin (Regranex Gel) Uses: Adjunct to local wound care w/*diabetic foot ulcers* Action: Recombinant PDGF, enhances granulation tissue Dose: Based on lesion; 11/3-in. ribbon from 2-g tube, 2/3-in. ribbon from 7.5- or 15-g tube/in.^{2} of ulcer; apply & cover w/moist gauze; rinse after 12 h; do not reapply; repeat in 12 h Caution: [C, ?] Contra: Neoplasm/or active site Infxn Disp: 0.01% gel in 2-, 7.5-, 15-g tubes SE: Erythema, local pain Notes: Use w/ good wound care; wound must be vascularized

Beclomethasone (Beconase, Vancenase Nasal Inhaler) Uses: *Allergic rhinitis* refractory to antihistamines & decongestants; *nasal polyps* Action: Inhaled steroid Dose: *Adults.* 1 spray intranasal bid–qid. *Aqueous inhal:* 1–2 sprays/nostril twice daily. *Peds 6–12 y.* 1 spray intranasal tid Caution: [C, ?] Disp: Nasal met-dose inhaler SE: Local irritation, burning, epistaxis Notes: Nasal spray delivers 42 mcg/dose & 84 mcg/dose

Beclomethasone (QVAR) Uses: Chronic *asthma* Action: Inhaled corticosteroid Dose: *Adults & Peds.* 1–4 inhal bid (Rinse mouth/throat after) Caution: [C, ?] Contra: Acute asthma Disp: PO met-dose inhaler; 40, 80 mcg/inhal SE: HA, cough, hoarseness, oral candidiasis Notes: Not effective for acute asthma

Belladonna & Opium Suppositories (B & O Supprettes) [C-II] Uses: *Bladder spasms; moderate/severe pain* Action: Antispasmodic, analgesic Dose: 1 supp PR q6h PRN; 15A = 30 mg powdered opium/16.2 mg belladonna extract; 16A = 60 mg powdered opium/16.2 mg belladonna extract Caution: [C, ?] Disp: Supp 15A, 16A SE: Anticholinergic (sedation, urinary retention, constipation)

Benazepril (Lotensin) Uses: *HTN,* DN, CHF Action: ACE inhibitor Dose: 10–40 mg/d PO Caution: [C (1st tri), D (2nd & 3rd tri), +] Contra: Angioedema, Hx edema Disp: Tabs 5, 10, 20, 40 mg SE: Symptomatic ↓ BP w/ diuretics; dizziness, HA, ↑ K$^+$, nonproductive cough

Benzocaine & Antipyrine (Auralgan) Uses: *Analgesia in severe otitis media* Action: Anesthetic w/ local decongestant Dose: Fill ear & insert a moist cotton plug; repeat 1–2 h PRN Caution: [C, ?] Contra: w/ perforated eardrum Disp: Soln SE: Local irritation

Benzonatate (Tessalon Perles) Uses: Symptomatic relief of *cough* Action: Anesthetizes the stretch receptors in the resp passages Dose: *Adults & Peds >10 y.* 100 mg PO tid Caution: [C, ?] Disp: Caps 100, 200 mg SE: Sedation, dizziness, GI upset Notes: Do not chew or puncture the caps

Benztropine (Cogentin) Uses: *Parkinsonism & drug-induced extrapyramidal disorders* Action: Partially blocks striatal cholinergic receptors Dose: *Adults.* 0.5–6 mg PO, IM, or IV in ÷ doses/d. *Peds >3 y.* 0.02–0.05 mg/kg/dose 1–2/d Caution: [C, ?] Contra: < 3 y Disp: Tabs 0.5, 1, 2 mg; inj 1 mg/mL SE: Anticholinergic side effects Notes: Physostigmine 1–2 mg SC/IV to reverse severe Sxs

Beractant (Survanta) Uses: *Prevention & Rx of RDS in premature infants* Action: Replaces pulmonary surfactant Dose: 100 mg/kg via ET tube; may repeat 3× q6h; max 4 doses/48 h Disp: Susp 25 mg of phospholipid/mL SE: Transient bradycardia, desaturation, apnea Notes: Administer via 4-quadrant method

Betaxolol (Kerlone) Uses: *HTN* Action: Competitively blocks β-adrenergic receptors, β1 Caution: [C (1st tri), D (2nd or 3rd tri), +/–] Contra: Sinus bradycardia, AV conduction abnormalities, cardiac failure Dose: 10–20 mg/d Disp: Tabs 10, 20 mg SE: Dizziness, HA, bradycardia, edema, CHF

Betaxolol, Ophthalmic (Betoptic) Uses: Glaucoma Action: Competitively blocks β-adrenergic receptors, β1 Dose: 1–2 gtt bid Caution: [C (1st tri), D (2nd or 3rd tri), ?/–] Disp: Soln 0.5%; susp 0.25% SE: Local irritation, photophobia

Bethanechol (Urecholine, Duvoid, others) Uses: *Neurogenic bladder atony w/ retention,* acute *postop* & postpartum functional *(nonobstructive)* urinary retention* Action: Stimulates cholinergic smooth muscle receptors in bladder & GI tract Dose: *Adults.* 10–50 mg PO tid–qid or 2.5–5 mg SQ tid–qid & PRN. *Peds.* 0.6 mg/kg/24 h PO ÷ tid–qid or 0.15–2 mg/kg/d SQ ÷ 3–4× (take on empty stomach) Caution: [C, ?/–] Contra: BOO, PUD, epilepsy, hyperthyroidism, bradycardia, COPD, AV conduction defects, parkinsonism, ↓ BP, vasomotor instability Disp: Tabs 5, 10, 25, 50 mg; inj 5 mg/mL SE: Abdominal cramps, D, salivation, ↓BP Notes: Do not use IM/IV

Bevacizumab (Avastin) WARNING: Associated w/ GI perforation, wound dehiscence, & fatal hemoptysis Uses: * Metastatic Colorectal Ca, w/ 5-FU* Nonsquamous NSCLC w/ paclitaxel and carboplatin Action: Vascular endothelial GF inhibitor Dose: *Adults.* 5 mg/kg IV q14d; 1st dose over 90 min; 2nd over 60 min, 3rd over 30 min if tolerated Caution: [C, –] Do not use w/in 28 d of surgery if time for separation of drug & anticipated surgical procedures is unknown; D/C w/ serious adverse events Disp: 100 mg/4 mL, 400 mg/16 mL vials SE: Wound dehiscence, GI perforation, hemoptysis, hemorrhage, HTN, proteinuria, CHF, inf Rxns, D, leucopenia, thromboembolism **Notes:** Monitor for ↑ BP & proteinuria

Bicalutamide (Casodex) **Uses:** *Advanced CAP (metastatic)* (w/ GnRH agonists [eg, leuprolide, goserelin]) **Action:** Nonsteroidal antiandrogen **Dose:** 50 mg/d **Caution:** [X, ?] **Contra:** Women **Disp:** Caps 50 mg **SE:** Hot flashes, loss of libido, impotence, D/N/V, gynecomastia, & LFT elevation

Bicarbonate See Sodium Bicarbonate, page 172

Bisacodyl (Dulcolax) [OTC] **Uses:** *Constipation; preop bowel prep* **Action:** Stimulates peristalsis **Dose:** *Adults.* 5–15 mg PO or 10 mg PR PRN. *Peds.* <2 y: 5 mg PR PRN. >2 y: 5 mg PO or 10 mg PR PRN (do not chew tabs or give w/in 1 h of antacids or milk) **Caution:** [B, ?] **Contra:** Acute abdomen or bowel obstruction, appendicitis, gastroenteritis **Disp:** EC tabs 5 mg; DR Tab 5 mg; supp 10 mg **SE:** Abdominal cramps, proctitis, & inflammation w/ suppositories

Bismuth Subsalicylate (Pepto-Bismol) [OTC] **Uses:** Indigestion, nausea, & *D;* combo for Rx of *H. pylori Infxn* **Action:** Antisecretory & anti-inflammatory **Dose:** *Adults.* 2 tabs or 30 mL PO PRN (max 8 doses/24 h). *Peds.* 3–6 y: 1/3 tab or 5 mL PO PRN (max 8 doses/24 h). 6–9 y: 2/3 tab or 10 mL PO PRN (max 8 doses/24 h). 9–12 y: 1 tab or 15 mL PO PRN (max 8 doses/24 h) **Caution:** [C, D (3rd tri), –] Avoid in renal failure **Contra:** Influenza or chickenpox (↑ risk of Reye's syndrome), ASA allergy **Disp:** Chew tabs 262 mg; Caplets 262 mg, liq 262, 525 mg/15 mL **SE:** May turn tongue & stools black

Bisoprolol (Zebeta) **Uses:** *HTN* **Action:** Competitively blocks β_1-adrenergic receptors **Dose:** 5–10 mg/d (max dose 20 mg/d); ↓ w/renal impair **Caution:** [C (D 2nd & 3rd tri), +/–] **Contra:** Sinus bradycardia, AV conduction abnormalities, cardiac failure **Disp:** Tabs 5, 10 mg **SE:** Fatigue, lethargy, HA, bradycardia, edema, CHF **Notes:** Not dialyzed

Bitolterol (Tornalate) **Uses:** Prophylaxis & Rx of *asthma* & reversible bronchospasm **Action:** Sympathomimetic bronchodilator; stimulates pulmonary β_2-adrenergic receptors **Dose:** *Adults & Peds >12 y.* 2 inhal q8h **Caution:** [C, ?] **Disp:** Aerosol 0.8% **SE:** Dizziness, nervousness, trembling, HTN, palpitations

Bivalirudin (Angiomax) **Uses:** *Anticoagulant w/ ASA in unstable angina undergoing PTCA, PCI or in patients undergoing PCI w/ or at risk of HIT/HITTS* **Action:** Anticoagulant, thrombin inhibitor **Dose:** 0.75 mg/kg IV bolus, then 1.75 mg/kg/h for duration of procedure and up to 4 h post; check ACT 5 min after bolus, may repeat 0.3 mg/kg bolus if necessary (give w/ aspirin 300–325 mg/d; start pre-PTCA) **Caution:** [B, ?] **Contra:** Major bleeding **Disp:** Powder 250 mg for inj **SE:** Bleeding, back pain, nausea, HA

Bleomycin Sulfate (Blenoxane) **Uses:** *Testis CA; Hodgkin Dz & NHLs; cutaneous lymphomas; & squamous cell CA (head & neck, larynx, cervix, skin, penis); sclerosing agent for malignant pleural effusion* **Action:** Induces breakage (scission) of DNA **Dose:** (Per protocols); ↓ in renal impair **Caution:** [D, ?] Severe pulmonary Dz **Disp:** Inj: Powder for reconstitution 15, 30 units **SE:**

Hyperpigmentation (skin staining) & allergy (rash to anaphylaxis); fever in 50%; lung tox (idiosyncratic & dose related); pneumonitis may progress to fibrosis; Raynaud phenomenon, N/V **Notes:** Test dose 1 mg (U) OK, especially in lymphoma pts; lung tox w/ total dose >400 mg (U)

Bortezomib (Velcade) **WARNING:** May worsen preexisting neuropathy **Uses:** *Progression of multiple myeloma despite one previous Rx* **Action:** Proteasome inhibitor **Dose:** 1.3 mg/m^2 bolus IV 2×/wk × 2 wk, w/ 10-day rest period (= 1 cycle); ↓ w/hematologic tox, neuropathy **Caution:** [D, ?/–] w/ drugs metabolized via CYP450 (Table 13) **Disp:** 3.5-mg vial **SE:** Asthenia, GI upset, anorexia, dyspnea, HA, orthostatic ↓ BP, edema, insomnia, dizziness, rash, pyrexia, arthralgia, neuropathy

Brimonidine (Alphagan) **Uses:** *Open-angle glaucoma, ocular HTN* **Action:** α$_2$-Adrenergic agonist **Dose:** 1 gtt in eye(s) tid (wait 15 min to insert contacts) **Caution:** [B, ?] **Contra:** MAOI therapy **Disp:** 0.2% soln **SE:** Local irritation, HA, fatigue

Brinzolamide (Azopt) **Uses:** *Open-angle glaucoma, ocular HTN* **Action:** Carbonic anhydrase inhibitor **Dose:** 1 gh in eye(s) tid **Caution:** [C, ?] **Disp:** 1% susp **SE:** Blurred vision, dry eye, blepharitis, taste disturbance

Bromocriptine (Parlodel) **Uses:** *Parkinson Dz, hyperprolactinemia, acromegaly, pituitary tumors* **Action:** Direct-acting on the striatal dopamine receptors; ↓ prolactin secretion **Dose:** Initial, 1.25 mg PO bid; titrate to effect, w/food **Caution:** [C, ?] **Contra:** Severe ischemic heart Dz or PVD **Disp:** Tabs 2.5 mg; caps 5 mg **SE:** ↓ BP, Raynaud phenomenon, dizziness, N, hallucinations

Budesonide (Rhinocort Aqua, Pulmicort) **Uses:** *Allergic & nonallergic rhinitis, asthma* **Action:** Steroid **Dose:** Adults: Intranasal: 1–4 sprays/nostril/d; Turbuhaler 1–4 inhal bid; Peds: intranasal 1–2 sprays/nostril/d; Turbuhaler 1–2 inhal bid, Respules: 0.25–0.5 mg QD or bid (Rinse mouth after PO use) **Caution:** [C, ?/–] **Disp:** Met-dose Turbuhaler, 200 mcg/inhalation; Respules 0.25 mg/mL, 0.5 mL; Rhinocort Aqua 32 mcg/spray **SE:** HA, cough, hoarseness, *Candida* Infxn, epistaxis

Bumetanide (Bumex) **Uses:** *Edema from CHF, hepatic cirrhosis, & renal Dz* **Action:** Loop diuretic; ↓ reabsorption of Na$^+$ & Cl$^-$, in ascending loop of Henle & the distal tubule **Dose:** *Adults.* 0.5–2 mg/d PO; 0.5–1 mg IV/IM q8–24h (max 10 mg/d) for PO and IV. *Peds.* 0.015–0.1 mg/kg/d PO, q24h–24h **Caution:** [D, ?] **Contra:** Anuria, hepatic coma, severe electrolyte depletion **Disp:** Tabs 0.5, 1, 2 mg; inj 0.25 mg/mL **SE:** ↓ K$^+$, ↓ Na$^+$, ↑ creatinine, ↑ uric acid, dizziness, ototox **Notes:** Monitor fluid & electrolytes

Bupivacaine (Marcaine) **Uses:** *Local, regional, & spinal anesthesia, local & regional analgesia* **Action:** Local anesthetic **Dose:** *Adults & Peds.* Dose dependent on procedure (ie, tissue vascularity, depth of anesthesia, etc) (Table 3) **Caution:** [C, ?] **Contra:** Severe bleeding, ↓ BP, shock & arrhythmias, local Infxns at anesthesia site, septicemia **Disp:** Inj 0.25, 0.5, 0.75% **SE:** ↓ BP, bradycardia, dizziness, anxiety

Buprenorphine (Buprenex) [C-V]   Uses: *Moderate/severe pain* Action: Opiate agonist–antagonist Dose: 0.3–0.6 mg IM or slow IV push q6h PRN Caution: [C, ?/–] Disp: 0.3 mg/mL SE: Sedation, ↓ BP, resp depression Notes: Withdrawal if opioid-dependent

Bupropion (Wellbutrin, Wellbutrin SR, Wellbutrin XL, Zyban)   WARNING: Closely monitor for worsening depression or emergence of suicidality Uses: *Depression, adjunct to smoking cessation* Action: Weak inhibitor of neuronal uptake of serotonin & norepinephrine; ↓ neuronal dopamine reuptake Dose: Depression: 100–450 mg ÷ bid–tid; SR 100–200 mg bid; XL 150–300 mg qd. Smoking cessation: 150 mg/d × 3 d, then 150 mg bid ×8–12 wk; ↓renal/hepatic impair Caution: [B, ?/–] Contra: Sz disorder, Hx anorexia nervosa or bulimia, MAOI, abrupt D/C of EtOH or sedatives Disp: Tabs 75, 100 mg; SR tabs 100, 150, 200 mg; XL tabs 150, 300 mg; Zyban 150 mg tabs SE: Szs, agitation, insomnia, HA, tachycardia Notes: Avoid EtOH & other CNS depressants

Buspirone (BuSpar)   WARNING: Closely monitor for worsening depression or emergence of suicidality Uses: *Short-term relief of *anxiety* Action: Antianxiety; antagonizes CNS serotonin receptors Dose: Initial: 7.5 mg PO bid; ↑ by 5 mg q 2–3 days to effect; usual 20–30 mg/d; max 60 mg/d; ↓ w/severe hepatic/renal insuff Caution: [B, ?/–] Disp: Tabs dividose 5, 7.5, 10, 15, 30 mg SE: Drowsiness, dizziness; HA, N Notes: No abuse potential or physical/psychologic dependence

Busulfan (Myleran, Busulfex)   Uses: *CML,* preparative regimens for allogeneic & ABMT in high doses Action: Alkylating agent Dose: (per protocol) Caution: [D, ?] Disp: Tabs 2 mg, inj 60 mg/10 mL SE: Myelosuppression, pulmonary fibrosis, nausea (w/high-dose), gynecomastia, adrenal insuff, & skin hyperpigmentation

Butorphanol (Stadol) [C-IV]   Uses: *Anesthesia adjunct, pain* & migraine HA Action: Opiate agonist–antagonist w/ central analgesic actions Dose: 1–4 mg IM or IV q3–4h PRN. ↓ in renal impair Caution: [C (D if high doses or prolonged periods at term), +] Disp: Inj 2 mg/mL SE: Drowsiness, dizziness, nasal congestion Notes: May induce withdrawal in opioid dependency

Calcipotriene (Dovonex)   Uses: *Plaque psoriasis* Action: Keratolytic Dose: Apply bid Caution: [C, ?] Contra: ↑ Ca²⁺; vitamin D tox; do not apply to face Disp: Cream; oint; soln 0.005% SE: Skin irritation, dermatitis

Calcitonin (Fortical, Miacalcin)   Uses: *Paget Dz of bone, ↑ Ca²⁺,* osteogenesis imperfecta, *postmenopausal osteoporosis* Action: Polypeptide hormone Dose: Paget Dz: 100 units/d IM/SC initial, 50 units/d or 50–100 units q1–3d maint. ↑ Ca²⁺ 4 units/kg IM/SC q12h; ↑ to 8 units/kg q12h, max q6h. Osteoporosis: 100 units/d IM/SQ; intranasal 200 units = 1 nasal spray/d Caution: [C, ?] Disp: Spray, nasal 200 units/activation; inj, salmon 200 units/mL (2 mL) SE: Facial flushing, nausea, injection site edema, nasal irritation, polyuria Notes: For nasal spray alternate nostrils daily

Calcitriol (Rocaltrol, Calcijex) Uses: *Reduction of ↑ PTH levels, ↓ Ca^{2+} on dialysis* Action: 1,25-Dihydroxycholecalciferol (vitamin D analog) Dose: *Adults.* Renal failure: 0.25 mcg/d PO, ↑ 0.25 mcg/d q4–6wk PRN; 0.5 mcg 3×/wk IV, ↑ PRN. *Hypoparathyroidism:* 0.5–2 mcg/d. *Peds.* Renal failure: 15 ng/kg/d, ↑ PRN; maint 30–60 ng/kg/d. *Hypoparathyroidism: <5 y,* 0.25–0.75 mcg/d. *>6 y,* 0.5–2 mcg/d Caution: [C, ?] Contra: ↑ Ca^{2+}; vitamin D tox Disp: Inj 1, 2 mcg/mL (in 1-mL); caps 0.25, 0.5 mcg; sol 1 mcg/mL SE: ↑ Ca^{2+} possible Notes: Monitor to keep Ca^{2+} WNL

Calcium Acetate (PhosLo) Uses: *ESRD-associated hyperphosphatemia* Action: Ca^{2+} supl w/o aluminum to ↓ PO_4^{-2} Dose: 2–4 tabs PO w/ meals Caution: [C, ?] Contra: ↑ Ca^{2+} Disp: Gelcap 667 mg; Inj 0.5 mEq/mL SE: Can ↑ Ca^{2+}, hypophosphatemia, constipation Notes: Monitor Ca^{2+}

Calcium Carbonate (Tums, Alka-Mints) [OTC] Uses: *Hyperacidity associated w/ peptic ulcer Dz, hiatal hernia,* etc Action: Neutralizes gastric acid Dose: 500 mg–2 g PO PRN; ↓ in renal impair Caution: [C, ?] Disp: Chew tabs 350, 420, 500, 550, 750, 850 mg; susp SE: ↑ Ca^{2+}, hypophosphatemia, constipation

Calcium Glubionate (Neo-Calglucon) [OTC] Uses: *Rx & prevent calcium deficiency* Action: Ca^{2+} supl Dose: *Adults.* 6–18 g/d ÷ doses. *Peds.* 600–2000 mg/kg/d ÷ qid (9 g/d max); ↓ in renal impair Caution: [C, ?] Contra: ↑ Ca^{2+} Disp: OTC syrup 1.8 g/5 mL = Ca 115 mg/5 mL SE: ↑ Ca^{2+}, hypophosphatemia, constipation

Calcium Salts (Chloride, Gluconate, Gluceptate) Uses: *Ca^{2+} replacement,* VF, Ca^{2+} blocker tox, Mg^{2+} intox, tetany, *hyperphosphatemia in ESRD* Action: Ca^{2+} supl/replacement Dose: *Adults.* Replacement: 1–2 g/d PO. *Cardiac emergencies:* CaCl 0.5–1 g IV q 10 min or Ca gluconate 1–2 g IV q 10 min. *Tetany.* 1 g CaCl over 10–30 min; repeat in 6 h PRN. *Peds.* Replacement: 200–500 mg/kg/24 h PO or IV ÷ qid. *Cardiac emergency:* 100 mg/kg/dose IV gluconate salt q 10 min. *Tetany:* 10 mg/kg CaCl over 5–10 min; repeat in 6 h or use inf (200 mg/kg max). *Adult & Peds.* ↓ Ca^{2+} due to citrated blood inf: 0.45 mEq Ca/100 mL citrated blood inf (↓ in renal impair) Caution: [C, ?] Contra: ↑ Ca^{2+} Disp: CaCl inj 10% = 100 mg/mL = Ca 27.2 mg/mL = 10-mL amp; Ca gluconate inj 10% = 100 mg/mL = Ca 9 mg/mL; tabs 500 mg = 45 mg Ca, 650 mg = 58.5 mg Ca, 975 mg = 87.75 mg Ca, 1 g = 90 mg Ca; Ca gluceptate inj 220 mg/mL = 18 mg/mL Ca SE: Bradycardia, cardiac arrhythmias, ↑ Ca^{2+} Notes: CaCl 270 mg (13.6 mEq) elemental Ca/g, & calcium gluconate 90 mg (4.5 mEq) Ca/g. RDA for Ca: Adults = 800 mg/d; Peds = <6 mo 360 mg/d, 6 mo–1 y 540 mg/d, 1–10 y 800 mg/d, 10–18 y 1200 mg/d

Calfactant (Infasurf) Uses: *Prevention & Rx of RSD in infants* Action: Exogenous pulmonary surfactant Dose: 3 mL/kg instilled into lungs. Can retreat for a total of 3 doses given 12 h apart Caution: [?, ?] Disp: Intratracheal susp 35

mg/mL **SE:** Monitor for cyanosis, airway obstruction, bradycardia during administration

Candesartan (Atacand) Uses: *HTN,* DN, CHF **Action:** Angiotensin II receptor antagonist **Dose:** 4–32 mg/d (usual 16 mg/d) **Caution:** [X, –] **Contra:** Primary hyperaldosteronism; bilateral renal artery stenosis **Disp:** Tabs 4, 8, 16, 32 mg **SE:** Dizziness, HA, flushing, angioedema

Capsaicin (Capsin, Zostrix, others) [OTC] Uses: Pain due to *postherpetic neuralgia,* chronic neuralgia, *arthritis, diabetic neuropathy,* postop pain, psoriasis, intractable pruritus **Action:** Topical analgesic **Dose:** Apply tid–qid **Caution:** [?, ?] **Disp:** OTC creams; gel; lotions; roll-ons **SE:** Local irritation, neurotox, cough

Captopril (Capoten, others) Uses: *HTN, CHF, MI,* LVD, DN **Action:** ACE inhibitor **Dose:** *Adults.* HTN: Initial, 25 mg PO bid–tid; ↑ to maint q1–2wk by 25-mg increments/dose (max 450 mg/d) to effect. *CHF:* Initial, 6.25–12.5 mg PO tid; titrate PRN LVD: 50 mg PO tid. *DN:* 25 mg PO tid. **Peds.** Infants <2 mo: 0.05–0.5 mg/kg/dose PO q8–24h. *Children:* Initial, 0.3–0.5 mg/kg/dose PO; ↑ to 6 mg/kg/d max (1 h before meals) **Caution:** [C (1st tri); D (2nd & 3rd tri); unknown effects in renal impair +] **Contra:** Hx angioedema **Disp:** Tabs 12.5, 25, 50, 100 mg **SE:** Rash, proteinuria, cough, ↑ K⁺

Carbamazepine (Tegretol XR, Carbatrol, Epitol) WARNING: Aplastic anemia & agranulocytosis have been reported w/ carbamazepine Uses: *Epilepsy, trigeminal neuralgia,* EtOH withdrawal **Action:** Anticonvulsant **Dose:** *Adults.* Initial, 200 mg PO bid; or 100 mg 4 times/day q susp; ↑ by 200 mg/d; usual 800–1200 mg/d ÷ doses. **Peds.** <6 y: 5 mg/kg/d, ↑ to 10–20 mg/kg/d ÷ in 2–4 doses. *6–12 y:* Initial, 100 mg PO bid or 10 mg/kg/24 h PO ÷ qd–bid; ↑ to maint 20–30 mg/kg/24 h ÷ tid–qid; ↓ in renal impair (take w/ food) **Caution:** [D, +] **Contra:** MAOI use, Hx BM suppression **Disp:** Tabs 200 mg; chew tabs 100 mg; xr tabs 100, 200, 400 mg; Caps ER 100, 200, 300 mg; susp 100 mg/5 mL **SE:** Drowsiness, dizziness, blurred vision, N/V, rash, ↓ Na⁺, leukopenia, agranulocytosis **Notes:** Monitor CBC & serum levels (Table 2, page 210), generic products not interchangeable

Carbidopa/Levodopa (Sinemet, Parcopa) Uses: *Parkinson Dz* **Action:** ↑ CNS dopamine levels **Dose:** 25/100 mg bid–qid; ↑ as needed (max 200/2000 mg/d) **Caution:** [C, ?] **Contra:** NA glaucoma, suspicious skin lesion (may activate melanoma), melanoma, MAOI use **Disp:** Tabs (mg carbidopa/mg levodopa) 10/100, 25/100, 25/250; tabs SR (mg carbidopa/mg levodopa) 25/100, 50/200; ODT (oral disintegrating tab) 10/100, 25/100, 25/250. **SE:** Psychiatric disturbances, orthostatic ↓ BP, dyskinesias, cardiac arrhythmias

Carboplatin (Paraplatin) Uses: *Ovarian, lung, head & neck, testicular, urothelial,* & brain *CA, NHL** & allogeneic & ABMT in high doses **Action:** DNA cross-linker; forms DNA-platinum adducts **Dose:** 360 mg/m² (ovarian carcinoma); AUC dosing 4–7 mg/mL (Culvert formula: mg = AUC × [25 + calculated

GFR]); adjust based on pretreatment plt count, CrCl, & BSA (Egorin formula); up to 1500 mg/m² used in ABMT setting (per protocols) **Caution:** [D, ?] **Contra:** Severe BM suppression, excessive bleeding **Disp:** Inj 50, 150, 450 mg **SE:** Myelosuppression, N/V/D, nephrotox, hematuria, neurotox, ↑ LFTs **Notes:** Physiologic dosing based on either Culvert or Egorin formula allows ↑ doses w/ ↓ tox

Carisoprodol (Soma) **Uses:** *Adjunct to sleep & physical therapy to relieve painful musculoskeletal conditions* **Action:** Centrally acting muscle relaxant **Dose:** 350 mg PO tid–qid **Caution:** [C, M] Tolerance may result; w/ renal/hepatic impair **Contra:** Allergy to meprobamate; acute intermittent porphyria **Disp:** Tabs 350 mg **SE:** CNS depression, drowsiness, dizziness, tachycardia **Notes:** Avoid EtOH & other CNS depressants; available in combo w/ ASA or codeine.

Carmustine [BCNU] (BiCNU, Gliadel) **Uses:** *Primary brain tumors, melanoma, Hodgkin's lymphoma & NHLs, multiple myeloma, & induction for allogeneic & ABMT in high doses; adjunct to surgery in pts w/ recurrent glioblastoma* **Action:** Alkylating agent; nitrosourea forms DNA cross-links to inhibit DNA synthesis **Dose:** 150–200 mg/m² q6–8wk single or ÷ dose qd inj over 2 d; 20–65 mg/m² q4–6wk; 300–900 mg/m² in BMT (per protocols) **Caution:** [D, ?] ↓ WBC, RBC, plt counts, renal/hepatic impair **Contra:** Myelosuppression, PRG **Disp:** Inj 100 mg/vial; wafer: 7.7 mg **SE:** ↓BP, N/V, myelosuppression (WBC & plt), phlebitis, facial flushing, hepatic/renal dysfunction, pulmonary fibrosis, optic neuroretinitis; hematologic tox may persist 4–6 wk after dose **Notes:** Do not give course more frequently than q6wk (cumulative tox); check baseline PFTs

Carteolol (Cartrol, Ophthalmic) **Uses:** *HTN, ↑ intraocular pressure, chronic open-angle glaucoma* **Action:** Blocks β-adrenergic receptors (β₁, β₂), mild ISA **Dose:** PO 2.5–5 mg/d; ophth 1 gt in eye(s) bid; ↓ in renal impair **Caution:** [C (1st tri); D (2nd & 3rd tri), ?/–] Cardiac failure, asthma **Contra:** Sinus bradycardia; heart block >1st degree; bronchospasm **Disp:** Tabs 2.5, 5 mg; ophth soln 1% **SE:** Drowsiness, sexual dysfunction, bradycardia, edema, CHF; ocular: conjunctival hyperemia, anisocoria, keratitis, eye pain **Notes:** No value in CHF

Carvedilol (Coreg) **Uses:** *HTN, CHF, MI* **Action:** Blocks adrenergic receptors, β₁, β₂, α **Dose:** *HTN:* 6.25–12.5 mg bid. *CHF:* 3.125–25 mg bid; w/ food to minimize ↓ BP **Caution:** [C (1st tri); D (2nd & 3rd tri), ?/–] Bradycardia, asthma, diabetes **Contra:** Decompensated cardiac failure, 2nd-/3rd-degree heart block, SSS, severe hepatic impair **Disp:** Tabs 3.125, 6.25, 12.5, 25 mg **SE:** Dizziness, fatigue, hyperglycemia, bradycardia, edema, hypercholesterolemia **Notes:** Do not D/C abruptly; ↑ digoxin levels

Caspofungin (Cancidas) **Uses:** *Invasive aspergillosis refractory/intolerant to standard therapy, esophageal candidiasis* **Action:** Echinocandin; ↓ fungal cell wall synthesis; highest activity in regions of active cell growth **Dose:** 70 mg IV load day 1, 50 mg/d IV; slow inf; ↓ in hepatic impair **Caution:** [C, ?/–] Do not use w/ cyclosporine; not studied as initial therapy **Contra:** Allergy to any component **Disp:** Inj 50, 70 mg **SE:** Fever, HA, N/V, thrombophlebitis at site, ↑ LFTs **Notes:** Monitor during inf; limited experience beyond 2 wk of therapy

Cefaclor (Raniclor) **Uses:** * Bacterial Infxns of the upper & lower resp tract, skin, bone, urinary tract, abdomen, gynecologic system* **Action:** 2nd-gen cephalosporin; ↓ cell wall synthesis. Spectrum: More gram(−) activity than 1st-gen cephalosporins; effective against gram(+) (S. aureus); good gram(−) coverage against Haemophilus influenzae **Dose:** *Adults.* 250–500 mg PO bid; XR 375–500 mg bid. *Peds.* 20–40 mg/kg/d PO ÷ 8–12 h; ↓ renal impair **Caution:** [B, +] **Contra:** Cephalosporin allergy **Disp:** Caps 250, 500 mg; Chew tabs 125, 187, 250, 375 mg; susp 125, 187, 250, 375 mg/5 mL **SE:** D, rash, eosinophilia, ↑ transaminases

Cefadroxil (Duricef) **Uses:** *Infxns of skin, bone, upper & lower resp tract, urinary tract* **Action:** 1st-gen cephalosporin; ↓cell wall synthesis. *Spectrum:* Good gram(+) coverage (group A β-hemolytic *Strep, Staph*); gram(−) (*E. coli, Proteus, Klebsiella*) **Dose:** *Adults.* 1–2 g/d PO, 2 ÷ doses *Peds.* 30 mg/kg/d ÷ bid; ↓in renal impair **Caution:** [B, +] Contra: Cephalosporin allergy **Disp:** Caps 500 mg; tabs 1 g; susp 250, 500 mg/5 mL **SE:** N/V/D, rash, eosinophilia, ↑ transaminases

Cefazolin (Ancef) **Uses:** * Infxns of skin, bone, upper & lower resp tract, urinary tract* **Action:** 1st-gen cephalosporin; ↓cell wall synthesis. *Spectrum:* Good coverage gram(+) bacilli & cocci, (*Strep, Staph* [except *Enterococcus*]); some gram(−) (*E. coli, Proteus, Klebsiella*) **Dose:** *Adults.* 1–2 g IV q8h *Peds.* 25–100 mg/kg/d IV ÷ q6–8h; ↓ in renal impair **Caution:** [B, +] **Contra:** Cephalosporin allergy **Disp:** Premixed infusion 500 mg, 1 g, Inj: 500 mg, 1, 10, 20 g **SE:** D, rash, eosinophilia, elevated transaminases, pain at inj site **Notes:** Widely used for surgical prophylaxis

Cefdinir (Omnicef) **Uses:** *Infxns of the resp tract, skin, bone, & urinary tract* **Action:** 3rd-gen cephalosporin; ↓ cell wall synthesis Spectrum: Wide range of gram(+) & gram(−) organisms; more active than cefaclor & cephalexin against Streptococcus, Staphylococcus; some anaerobes **Dose:** *Adults.* 300 mg PO bid or 600 mg/d PO. *Peds.* 7 mg/kg PO bid or 14 mg/kg/d PO; ↓ in renal impair **Caution:** [B, +] In PCN-sensitive pts, serum sicknesslike Rxns reported **Contra:** Hypersensitivity to cephalosporins **Disp:** Caps 300 mg; susp 125, 250 mg/5 mL **SE:** Anaphylaxis, D, rare pseudomembranous colitis

Cefditoren (Spectracef) **Uses:** *Acute exacerbations of chronic bronchitis, pharyngitis, tonsillitis; skin Infxns* **Action:** 3rd-gen cephalosporin; ↓ cell wall synthesis. Spectrum: Good gram(+) (*Strep & Staph*); gram(−) (*Haemophilus influenzae & Moraxella catarrhalis*) **Dose:** *Adults & Peds >12 y.* Skin: 200 mg PO bid × 10 days. *Chronic bronchitis, pharyngitis, tonsillitis:* 400 mg PO bid × 10 days; avoid antacids w/in 2 h; take w/ meals; ↓ in renal impair **Caution:** [B, ?] Renal/hepatic impair **Contra:** Cephalosporin/PCN allergy, milk protein, or carnitine deficiency **Disp:** 200-mg tabs **SE:** HA, N/V/D, colitis, nephrotox, hepatic dysfunction, Stevens–Johnson syndrome, toxic epidermal necrolysis, allergy Rxns **Notes:** Causes renal excretion of carnitine; tablets contain milk protein

Cefepime (Maxipime) Uses: *UTI, pneumonia, febrile neutropenia, skin/soft tissue Infxns* **Action:** 4th-gen cephalosporin; ↓ cell wall synthesis. *Spectrum.* gram(+) S. pneumoniae, S. aureus, gram(−)K. pneumoniae, E. coli, P. aeruginosa, & Enterobacter sp **Dose:** *Adults.* 1–2 g IV q12h. *Peds.* 50 mg/kg q8h for febrile neutropenia; 50 mg/kg bid for skin/soft tissue Infxns; ↓ in renal impair **Caution:** [B, +] **Contra:** Cephalosporin allergy **Disp:** Inj 500 mg, 1, 2 g **SE:** Rash, pruritus, N/V/D, fever, HA, (+) Coombs' test w/o hemolysis **Notes:** Administered as IM or IV

Cefixime (Suprax) Uses: *Infxns of the resp tract, skin, bone, & urinary tract* **Action:** 3rd-gen cephalosporin; ↓ cell wall synthesis. Spectrum: S. pneumoniae, S. pyogenes, H. influenzae, & enterobacteria. **Dose:** *Adults.* 400 mg PO qd–bid. *Peds.* 8 mg/kg/d PO ÷ qd–bid; ↓ in renal impair **Caution:** [B, +] **Contra:** Cephalosporin allergy **Disp:** Susp 100 mg/5 mL **SE:** N/V/D, flatulence, & abdominal pain **Notes:** Monitor renal & hepatic Fxn; use susp for otitis media

Cefmetazole (Zefazone) Uses: *Rx Infxns of the upper & lower resp tract, skin, bone, urinary tract, abdomen, & gynecologic system* **Action:** 2nd-gen cephalosporin; ↓ cell wall synthesis. Spectrum: Gram(+) against S. aureus; gram(−) activity & some anaerobic activity; use in mixed aerobic–anaerobic Infxns where *Bacteroides fragilis* likely **Dose:** *Adults.* 2 g IV q6–12h; ↓ in renal impair **Caution:** [B, +] **Contra:** Cephalosporin allergy **Disp:** Inj 1, 2 g **SE:** Eosinophilia, leukopenia, N/V/D, ↑ LFTs, bleeding risk, rash, pseudomembranous colitis, disulfiram Rxn **Notes:** Avoid EtOH; safety not established in children

Cefonicid (Monocid) Uses: *Rx bacterial Infxns (resp tract, skin, bone & joint, urinary tract, gynecologic, sepsis)* **Action:** 2nd-gen cephalosporin; ↓ cell wall synthesis. Spectrum: Gram(+) including MSSA & many streptococci, gram(−) bacilli including E. coli, Klebsiella, P. mirabilis, H. influenzae, & Moraxella **Dose:** 0.5–2 g/24 h IM/IV; ↓ in renal impair **Caution:** [B, +] **Contra:** Cephalosporin allergy **Disp:** Powder for inj 500 mg, 1 g, 10 g **SE:** D, rash, ↑ plts, eosinophilia, ↑ transaminases

Cefoperazone (Cefobid) Uses: *Rx Infxns of the resp, skin, urinary tract, sepsis* **Action:** 3rd-gen cephalosporin; ↓ bacterial cell wall synthesis. *Spectrum:* Gram(−) (e.g. E. coli, Klebsiella); variable against *Streptococcus* & *Staphylococcus* sp; active P. aeruginosa but < ceftazidime **Dose:** *Adults.* 2–4 g/d IM/IV ÷ q 8–12h (12 g/d max). *Peds.* (not approved) 100–150 mg/kg/d IM/IV ÷ bid–tid (12 g/d max); ↓ in renal/hepatic impair **Caution:** [B, +] May ↑ risk of bleeding **Contra:** Cephalosporin allergy **Disp:** Powder for inj 1, 2, 10 g **SE:** D, rash, eosinophilia, ↑ LFTs, hypoprothrombinemia, & bleeding (due to MTT side chain) **Notes:** May interfere w/ warfarin

Cefotaxime (Claforan) Uses: *Rx Infxns of resp tract, skin, bone, urinary tract, meningitis, sepsis* **Action:** 3rd-gen cephalosporin; ↓ cell wall synthesis. *Spectrum:* Most gram(−) (not *Pseudomonas*), some gram(+) cocci (not

Enterococcus); many PCN-resistant pneumococci **Dose:** *Adults.* 1–2 g IV q4–12h. *Peds.* 50–200 mg/kg/d IV ÷ q 4–12h; ↓ dose renal/hepatic impair **Caution:** [B, +] Arrhythmia associated w/ rapid inj; caution in colitis **Contra:** Cephalosporin allergy **Disp:** Powder for inj 500 mg, 1, 2, 10, 20 g **SE:** D, rash, pruritus, colitis, eosinophilia, ↑ transaminases

Cefotetan (Cefotan) **Uses:** *Rx Infxns of the upper & lower resp tract, skin, bone, urinary tract, abdomen, & gynecologic system* **Action:** 2nd-gen cephalosporin; ↓cell wall synthesis. *Spectrum:* Less active against gram(+); anaerobes including *B. fragilis;* gram(–), including *E. coli, Klebsiella, & Proteus* **Dose:** *Adults.* 1–2 g IV q12h. *Peds.* 20–40 mg/kg/d IV ÷ q12h; ↓ w/renal impair **Caution:** [B, +] May ↑ bleeding risk; w/Hx of PCN allergies, w/ other nephrotoxic drugs **Contra:** Cephalosporin allergy **Disp:** Powder for inj 1, 2, 10 g **SE:** D, rash, eosinophilia, ↑ transaminases, hypoprothrombinemia, & bleeding (due to MTT side chain) **Notes:** May interfere w/ warfarin

Cefoxitin (Mefoxin) **Uses:** *Rx Infxns of the upper & lower resp tract, skin, bone, urinary tract, abdomen, & gynecologic system* **Action:** 2nd-gen cephalosporin; ↓ cell wall synthesis. *Spectrum:* Good gram(–) against enteric bacilli (ie, *E. coli, Klebsiella, & Proteus*); anaerobic activity against *B. fragilis* **Dose:** *Adults.* 1–2 g IV q6–8h. *Peds.* 80–160 mg/kg/d ÷ q4–6h; ↓in renal impair **Caution:** [B, +] **Contra:** Cephalosporin allergy **Disp:** Powder for inj 1, 2, 10 g **SE:** D, rash, eosinophilia, ↑ transaminases

Cefpodoxime (Vantin) **Uses:** *Rx resp, skin, & urinary tract Infxns* **Action:** 3rd-gen cephalosporin; ↓ cell wall synthesis. *Spectrum:* *S. pneumoniae* or non-β-lactamase-producing *H. influenzae;* acute uncomplicated *N. gonorrhoeae;* some uncomplicated gram(–) (*E. coli, Klebsiella, Proteus*) **Dose:** *Adults.* 200–400 mg PO q12h. *Peds.* 10 mg/kg/d PO ÷ bid; ↓ in renal impair, take w/ food **Caution:** [B, +] **Contra:** Cephalosporin allergy **Disp:** Tabs 100, 200 mg; susp 50, 100 mg/5 mL **SE:** D, rash, HA, eosinophilia, elevated transaminases **Notes:** Drug interactions w/ agents that ↑ gastric pH

Cefprozil (Cefzil) **Uses:** *Rx resp tract, skin, & urinary tract Infxns* **Action:** 2nd-gen cephalosporin; ↓ cell wall synthesis. *Spectrum:* Active against MSSA, strep, & gram(–) bacilli (*E. coli, Klebsiella, P. mirabilis, H. influenzae, Moraxella*) **Dose:** *Adults.* 250–500 mg PO daily–bid. *Peds.* 7.5–15 mg/kg/d PO ÷ bid; ↓ in renal impair **Caution:** [B, +] **Contra:** Cephalosporin allergy **Disp:** Tabs 250, 500 mg; susp 125, 250 mg/5 mL **SE:** D, dizziness, rash, eosinophilia, ↑ transaminases **Notes:** Use higher doses for otitis & pneumonia

Ceftazidime (Fortaz, Tazicef) **Uses:** *Rx resp tract, skin, bone, urinary tract Infxns, meningitis, & septicemia* **Action:** 3rd-gen cephalosporin; ↓ cell wall synthesis. *Spectrum:* *P. aeruginosa* sp, good gram(–) activity **Dose:** *Adults.* 500–2 g IV q8–12h. *Peds.* 30–50 mg/kg/dose IV q8h; ↓ in renal impair **Caution:** [B, +] **Contra:** Cephalosporin allergy **Disp:** Powder for inj 500 mg, 1, 2, 6g **SE:** D, rash, eosinophilia, ↑ transaminases

Ceftibuten (Cedax) Uses: *Rx resp tract, skin, urinary tract Infns & otitis media* Action: 3rd-gen cephalosporin; ↓ cell wall synthesis. *Spectrum: H. influenzae & M. catarrhalis;* weak against *S. pneumoniae* Dose: Adults. 400 mg/d PO. Peds. 9 mg/kg/d PO; ↓ in renal impair; take on empty stomach Caution: [B, +] Contra: Cephalosporin allergy Disp: Caps 400 mg; susp 90mg/5 mL SE: D, rash, eosinophilia, ↑ transaminases

Ceftizoxime (Cefizox) Uses: *Rx resp tract, skin, bone, & urinary tract Infns, meningitis, septicemia* Action: 3rd-gen cephalosporin; ↓ cell wall synthesis. *Spectrum:* Good gram(−) bacilli (not *Pseudomonas*), some gram(+) cocci (not *Enterococcus*), & some anaerobes Dose: Adults. 1–2 g IV q8–12h. Peds. 150–200 mg/kg/d IV ÷ q6–8h; ↓ in renal impair Caution: [B, +] Contra: Cephalosporin allergy Disp: Inj 1, 2, 10 g SE: D, fever, rash, eosinophilia, thrombocytosis, ↑ transaminases

Ceftriaxone (Rocephin) Uses: *Resp tract (pneumonia), skin, bone, urinary tract Infns, meningitis, & septicemia;* * Action: 3rd-gen cephalosporin; ↓ cell wall synthesis. Spectrum: Moderate gram(+); excellent against β-lactamase producers Dose: Adults. 1–2 g IV/IM q12–24h. Peds. 50–100 mg/kg/d IV/IM ÷ q12–24h; ↓ in renal impair Caution: [B, +] Contra: Cephalosporin allergy; hyperbilirubinemic neonates (displaces bilirubin from binding sites) Disp: Powder for inj 250 mg, 500 mg, 1, 2, 10 g SE: D, rash, leukopenia, thrombocytosis, eosinophilia, ↑ transaminases

Cefuroxime (Ceftin [PO], Zinacef [parenteral]) Uses: *Upper & lower resp tract, skin, bone, urinary tract Infns, abdomen, gynecologic Infns* Action: 2nd-gen cephalosporin; ↓ cell wall synthesis Spectrum: Staphylococci, group B streptococci, H. influenzae, E. coli, Enterobacter, Salmonella, & Klebsiella Dose: Adults. 750 mg–1.5 g IV q8h or 250 500 mg PO bid. Peds. 100–150 mg/kg/d IV ÷ q8h or 20–30 mg/kg/d PO ÷ bid; ↓ in renal impair; take w/ food Caution: [B, +] Contra: Cephalosporin allergy Disp: Tabs 125, 250, 500 mg; susp 125, 250 mg/5 mL; powder for inj 750 mg, 1.5, 7.5 g SE: D, rash, eosinophilia, ↑ LFTs Notes: Cefuroxime film-coated tabs & susp not bioequivalent; do not substitute on a mg/mg basis; IV crosses blood–brain barrier

Celecoxib (Celebrex) WARNING: ↑ Risk of serious CV thrombotic events, MI & stroke, which can be fatal; ↑ risk of serious GI adverse events including bleeding, ulceration, & perforation of the stomach or intestines, which can be fatal Uses: *Osteoarthritis & RA, ankylosing spondylitis*; acute pain, primary dysmenorrhea; preventive in familial adenomatous polyposis Action: NSAID; ↓ the COX-2 pathway Dose: 100–200 mg/d or bid PO; FAP: 400 mg po bid; ↓ in hepatic impair; take w/ food/milk Caution: [C/D (3rd tri), ?] Caution in renal impair Contra: Allergy to sulfonamides, periop CABG Disp: Caps 100, 200 400 mg SE: see Warning; GI upset, HTN, edema, renal failure, HA Notes: Watch for Sxs of GI bleeding; no effect on plt/bleeding time; can affect drugs metabolized by P-450 pathway

Cephalexin (Keflex, Pranixine disperdose) Uses: *Skin, bone, upper/lower resp tract, urinary tract Infxns* Action: 1st-gen cephalosporin; ↓ cell wall synthesis. *Spectrum: Strep, Staph, E. coli, Proteus, & Klebsiella* Dose: *Adults.* 250–500 mg PO qid. *Peds.* 25–100 mg/kg/d PO ÷ qid; ↓ in renal impair; (on empty stomach) Caution: [B, +] Contra: Cephalosporin allergy Disp: Caps 250, 500 mg; tabs for oral susp 125, 250 mg; susp 125, 250 mg/5 mL SE: D, rash, eosinophilia, ↑ LFTs

Cephradine (Velosef) Uses: *Respiratory, GU, GI, skin, soft tissue, bone, & joint Infxns* Action: 1st-gen cephalosporin; ↓ cell wall synthesis. *Spectrum:* Gram(+) bacilli & cocci (not *Enterococcus*); some gram(–) (*E. coli, Proteus, & Klebsiella*) Dose: *Adults.* 250–500 mg q6–12h (8 g/d max) *Peds >9 mo.* 25–100 mg/kg/d ÷ bid–qid (4 g/d max); ↓ in renal impair Caution: [B, +] Contra: Cephalosporin allergy Disp: Caps 250, 500 mg; powder for susp 250 mg/5 mL, inj SE: Rash, eosinophilia, ↑ LFTs, N/V/D

Cetirizine (Zyrtec, Zyrtec D) Uses: *Allergic rhinitis & other allergic Sxs including urticaria* Action: Nonsedating antihistamine Dose: *Adults & Children >6 y.* 5–10 mg/d. Zyrtec D 5/120 mg PO bid whole *Peds.* 6–11 mo: 2.5 mg qd. *12–23 mo:* 2.5 mg qd–bid; ↓ in renal/hepatic impair Caution: [B, ?/–] Elderly & nursing mothers; >10 mg/d may cause drowsiness Contra: Allergy to cetirizine, hydroxyzine Disp: Tabs 5, 10 mg; Chew Tabs 5, 10 mg; syrup 5 mg/5 mL; Zyrtec D: Tabs 5/120 mg (cetirizine/pseudoephedrine) SE: HA, drowsiness, xerostomia Notes: Can cause sedation

Cetuximab (Erbitux)   WARNING: Severe inf Rxns including rapid onset of airway obstruction (bronchospasm, stridor, hoarseness), urticaria, & hypotension. Permanent D/C is required Uses: *EGFR-expressing metastatic colorectal CA w/wo irinotecan, unresectable head/neck SCC w/RT; monotherapy in met head/neck cancer* Action: Human/mouse recombinant MoAb; binds EGFR, ↓ tumor cell growth Dose: Per protocol; load 400 mg/m² IV over 2 h; 250 mg/m² given over 1 h 1 × wk Caution: [C, –] Disp: Inj 100 mg/ 50 mL SE: Acneform rash, asthenia/malaise, N/V/D, abdominal pain, alopecia, inf Rxn, dermatologic tox, interstitial lung disease, fever, sepsis, dehydration, kidney failure, PE Notes: Assess tumor for EGFR before Rx; pretreat w/ diphenhydramine; w/ mild SE ↓ inf rate by 50%; limit sun exposure

Charcoal, Activated (Superchar, Actidose, Liqui-Char) Uses: *Emergency poisoning by most drugs & chemicals (see Contra)* Action: Adsorbent detoxicant Dose: Give w/ 70% sorbitol (2 mL/kg); repeated use of sorbitol not OK *Adults.* Acute intox: 30–100 g/dose. GI dialysis: 20–50 g q6h for 1–2 d. *Peds 1–12 y.* Acute intox: 1–2 g/kg/dose. GI dialysis: 5–10 g/dose q4–8h Caution: [C, ?] May cause vomiting (hazardous w/ petroleum & caustic ingestions); do not mix w/ dairy Contra: Not effective for cyanide, mineral acids, caustic alkalis, organic solvents, iron, EtOH, methanol poisoning, Li; do not use sorbitol in pts w/ fructose intolerance Disp: Powder, liq, caps SE: Some liq dosage forms in sorbitol base (a cathartic); V/D, black stools, constipation Notes: Charcoal w/ sorbitol not OK in children <1 y; monitor for ↓ K⁺ & Mg²⁺; protect airway in lethargic/comatose pts

Chloral Hydrate (Aquachloral, Supprettes) [C-IV] Uses: *Short-term nocturnal & preop sedation* **Action:** Sedative hypnotic; active metabolite trichloroethanol **Dose:** *Adults. Hypnotic:* 500 mg–1 g PO or PR 30 min hs or before procedure. *Sedative:* 250 mg PO or PR tid. *Peds. Hypnotic:* 20–50 mg/kg/24 h PO or PR 30 min hs or before procedure. *Sedative:* 5–15 mg/kg/dose q8h; avoid w/ CrCl <50 mL/min or severe hepatic impair **Caution:** [C, +] Porphyria & neonates **Contra:** Allergy to components; severe renal, hepatic or cardiac Dz **Disp:** Caps 500 mg; syrup 250, 500 mg/5 mL; supp 324, 648 mg **SE:** GI irritation, drowsiness, ataxia, dizziness, nightmares, rash **Notes:** May accumulate; tolerance may develop >2 wk; taper dose; mix syrup in H₂O or fruit juice; avoid EtOH & CNS depressants

Chlorambucil (Leukeran) Uses: *CLL, Hodgkin Dz, Waldenström's macroglobulinemia* **Action:** Alkylating agent **Dose:** 0.1–0.2 mg/kg/d for 3–6 wk or 0.4 mg/kg/dose q2wk (per protocol) **Caution:** [D, ?] Sz disorder & BM suppression; affects human fertility **Contra:** Previous resistance; alkylating agent allergy **Disp:** Tabs 2 mg **SE:** Myelosuppression, CNS stimulation, N/V, drug fever, skin rash, secondary leukemias, alveolar dysplasia, pulmonary fibrosis, hepatotox **Notes:** Monitor LFTs, CBC, plts, serum uric acid; ↓ dose if pt has received radiation

Chlordiazepoxide (Librium, Mitran, Libritabs) [C-IV] Uses: *Anxiety, tension, EtOH withdrawal,* & preop apprehension **Action:** Benzodiazepine; antianxiety agent **Dose:** *Adults. Mild anxiety:* 5–10 mg PO tid–qid or PRN. *Severe anxiety:* 25–50 mg IM, IV, or PO q6–8h or PRN. *EtOH withdrawal:* 50–100 mg IM or IV; repeat in 2–4 h if needed, up to 300 mg in 24 h; gradually taper daily dose. *Peds >6 y,* 0.5 mg/kg/24 h PO or IM ÷ q6–8h; ↓ in renal impair, elderly **Caution:** [D, ?] Resp depression, CNS impair, Hx of drug dependence; avoid in hepatic impair **Contra:** Preexisting CNS depression **Disp:** Caps 5, 10, 25 mg; inj 100 mg **SE:** Drowsiness, CP, rash, fatigue, memory impair, xerostomia, weight gain **Notes:** Erratic IM absorption

Chlorothiazide (Diuril) Uses: *HTN, edema* **Action:** Thiazide diuretic **Dose:** *Adults.* 500 mg–1 g PO daily–bid; 100–500 mg/d IV (for edema only). *Peds >6 mo.* 20–30 mg/kg/24 h PO ÷ bid; 4 mg/kg/d IV; OK w/food **Caution:** [D, +] **Contra:** Cross-sensitivity to thiazides/sulfonamides, anuria **Disp:** Tabs 250, 500 mg; susp 250 mg/5 mL; inj 500 mg/vial **SE:** ↓ K⁺, Na⁺, dizziness, hyperglycemia, hyperuricemia, hyperlipidemia, photosensitivity **Notes:** Do not use IM/SQ; take early in the day to avoid nocturia; use sunblock; monitor electrolytes

Chlorpheniramine (Chlor-Trimeton, others [OTC]) Uses: *Allergic Rxns; common cold* **Action:** Antihistamine **Dose:** *Adults.* 4 mg PO q4–6h or 8–12 mg PO bid of SR **Peds.** 0.35 mg/kg/24 h PO ÷ q4–6h or 0.2 mg/kg/24 h SR **Caution:** [C, ?/–] BOO; NA glaucoma; hepatic insuff **Contra:** Allergy **Disp:** Tabs 4 mg; chew tabs 2 mg; SR tabs 8, 12 mg; syrup 2 mg/5 mL **SE:** Anticholinergic SE & sedation common, postural ↓ BP, QT changes, extrapyramidal Rxns, photosensitivity

Chlorpromazine (Thorazine) Uses: *Psychotic disorders, N/V,* apprehension, intractable hiccups **Action:** Phenothiazine antipsychotic; antiemetic **Dose: Adults.** Psychosis: 10–25 mg PO or PR bid–tid (usual 30–800 mg/d in ÷ doses). *Severe Sxs:* 25 mg IM/IV initial; may repeat in 1–4 h; then 25–50 mg PO or PR tid. *Hiccups:* 25–50 mg PO bid–tid. *Children >6 mo.* Psychosis & N/V: 0.5–1 mg/kg/dose PO q4–6h or IM/IV q6–8h; **Caution:** [C, ?/–] Safety in children <6 mo not established; Szs, avoid w/ hepatic impair, BM suppression **Contra:** Cross-sensitivity w/ phenothiazines; NA glaucoma **Disp:** Tabs 10, 25, 50, 100, 200 mg; conc 100 mg/mL; supp 100 mg; inj 25 mg/mL **SE:** Extrapyramidal SE & sedation; α-adrenergic blocking properties; ↓ BP; ↑ QT interval **Notes:** Do not D/C abruptly; dilute PO conc in 2–4 oz of liq

Chlorpropamide (Diabinese) Uses: *Type 2 DM* **Action:** Sulfonylurea; ↑ pancreatic insulin release; ↑ peripheral insulin sensitivity; ↓ hepatic glucose output **Dose:** 100–500 mg/d; w/ food **Caution:** [C, ?/–] CrCl < 50 mL/min; ↓ in hepatic impair **Contra:** Cross-sensitivity w/ sulfonamides **Disp:** Tabs 100, 250 mg **SE:** HA, dizziness, rash, photosensitivity, hypoglycemia, SIADH **Notes:** Avoid EtOH (disulfiram-like Rxn)

Chlorthalidone (Hygroton, others) Uses: *HTN* **Action:** Thiazide diuretic **Dose: Adults.** 50–100 mg PO daily. **Peds.** (Not approved) 2 mg/kg/dose PO 3X/wk or 1–2 mg/kg/d PO; ↓ in renal impair; OK w/food, milk **Caution:** [D, +] **Contra:** Cross-sensitivity w/ thiazides or sulfonamides; anuria **Disp:** Tabs 15, 25, 50, 100 mg **SE:** ↓ K⁺, dizziness, photosensitivity, hyperglycemia, hyperuricemia, sexual dysfunction

Chlorzoxazone (Paraflex, Parafon Forte DSC, others) Uses: *Adjunct to rest & physical therapy to relieve discomfort associated w/ acute, painful musculoskeletal conditions* **Action:** Centrally acting skeletal muscle relaxant **Dose: Adults.** 250–500 mg PO tid–qid. **Peds.** 20 mg/kg/d in 3–4 ÷ doses **Caution:** [C, ?] Avoid EtOH & CNS depressants **Contra:** Severe liver Dz **Disp:** Tabs 250, 500 mg **SE:** Drowsiness, tachycardia, dizziness, hepatotox, angioedema

Cholecalciferol [Vitamin D₃] (Delta D) Uses: *Dietary suppl to Rx vitamin D deficiency* **Action:** ↑ intestinal Ca²⁺ absorption **Dose:** 400–1000 IU/d PO **Caution:** [A (D doses above the RDA), +] **Contra:** ↑ Ca²⁺, hypervitaminosis, allergy **Disp:** Tabs 400, 1000 IU **SE:** Vitamin D tox (renal failure, HTN, psychosis) **Notes:** 1 mg cholecalciferol = 40,000 IU vitamin D activity

Cholestyramine (Questran, Prevalite) Uses: *Hypercholesterolemia; Rx pruritus associated w/ partial biliary obstruction; diarrhea associated w/ excess fecal bile acids* **Action:** Binds intestinal bile acids, forms insoluble complexes **Dose: Adults.** Individualize: 4 g/d–bid ↑ to max 24 g/d & 6 doses/d. **Peds.** 240 mg/kg/d in 3 ÷ doses **Caution:** [C, ?] Constipation, phenylketonuria **Contra:** Complete biliary obstruction; hypolipoproteinemia types III, IV, V **Disp:** 4 g of cholestyramine resin/9 g powder; w/ aspartame: 4 g resin/5 g powder **SE:** Constipation, abdominal pain, bloating, HA, rash **Notes:** OD may cause GI obstruction; mix 4 gm in 2–6 oz of noncarbonated beverage; take other meds 1–2 h before or 6 h after

Ciclopirox (Loprox, Penlac) Uses: *Tinea pedis, tinea cruris, tinea corporis, cutaneous candidiasis, tinea versicolor, tinea rubrum* Action: Antifungal antibiotic; cellular depletion of essential substrates &/or ions Dose: *Adults & Peds >10 y.* Massage into affected area bid, Onychomycosis:– apply to nails QD, with removal every 7 d Caution: [B, ?] Contra: Component sensitivity Disp: Cream gel, topical sus 0.77%, shampoo 1%, nail lacquer 8% SE: Pruritus, local irritation, burning Notes: D/C w/ irritation; avoid dressings; gel best for athlete's foot

Cidofovir (Vistide) WARNING: Renal Impair is the major tox. Follow administration instructions Uses: *CMV retinitis w/ HIV* Action: Selective inhibition of viral DNA synthesis Dose: *Rx:* 5 mg/kg IV over 1 h once/wk for 2 wk w/ probenecid. *Maint:* 5 mg/kg IV once/2 wk w/ probenecid (2 g PO 3 h prior to cidofovir, then 1 g PO at 2 h & 8 h after cidofovir); ↓ in renal impair Caution: [C, –] SCr >1.5 mg/dL or CrCl = 55 mL/min or urine protein >100 mg/dL; w/ other nephrotoxic drugs Contra: Probenecid or sulfa allergy Disp: Inj 75 mg/mL SE: Renal tox, chills, fever, HA, N/V/D, thrombocytopenia, neutropenia Notes: Hydrate w/ NS prior to each inf

Cilostazol (Pletal) Uses: *Reduce Sxs of intermittent claudication* Action: Phosphodiesterase III inhibitor; ↑'s cAMP in plts & blood vessels, vasodilation & inhibit plt aggregation Dose: 100 mg PO bid, 1/2 h before or 2 h after breakfast & dinner Caution: [C, +/] ↓ dose w/ drugs that inhibit CYP3A4 & CYP2C19 (Table 13) Contra: CHF Disp: Tabs 50, 100 mg SE: HA, palpitation, D

Cimetidine (Tagamet) (Tagamet HB, Tagamet DS OTC) [OTC] Uses: *Duodenal ulcer; ulcer prophylaxis in hypersecretory states, (eg, trauma, burns); & GERD* Action: H2 receptor antagonist Dose: *Adults.* Active ulcer: 2400 mg/d IV cont inf or 300 mg IV q6h; 400 mg PO bid or 800 mg hs. *Maint:* 400 mg PO hs. *GERD:* 300–600 mg PO q6h; maint 800 mg PO hs. *Peds.* Infants: 10–20 mg/kg/24 h PO or IV + q6 12h. *Children:* 20–40 mg/kg/24 h PO or IV + q6h, ↑ interval w/ renal insuff; ↓ dose in the elderly Caution: [B, +] Many drug interactions (P-450 system) Contra: Component sensitivity Disp: Tabs 200, 300, 400, 800 mg; liq 300 mg/5 mL; inj 300 mg/2 mL SE: Dizziness, HA, agitation, thrombocytopenia, gynecomastia Notes: 1 h before or 2 h after antacids; avoid EtOH

Cinacalcet (Sensipar) Uses: *Secondary hyperparathyroidism in CRF; ↑ Ca2+ in parathyroid carcinoma* Action: ↓ PTH by ↑ calcium-sensing receptor sensitivity Dose: *Secondary hyperparathyroidism:* 30 mg PO daily. *Parathyroid carcinoma:* 30 mg PO bid; titrate q2–4wk based on calcium & PTH levels; swallow whole; take w/ food Caution: [C, ?/–] Adjust w/ CYP3A4 inhibitors (Table 13) Disp: Tabs 30, 60, 90 mg SE: N/V/D, myalgia, dizziness, ↓ Ca2+ Notes: Monitor Ca2+, PO4–2, PTH

Ciprofloxacin (Cipro, Proquin XR) Uses: *Rx lower resp tract, sinuses, skin & skin structure, bone/joints, & UT Infxns including prostatitis* Ac-

tion: Quinolone antibiotic; ↓ DNA gyrase. *Spectrum:* Broad-spectrum gram(+) & gram(−) aerobics; little against *Strep*; good *Pseudomonas, E. coli, B. fragilis, P. mirabilis, K. pneumoniae, Campylobacter jejuni,* or *Shigella* **Dose:** *Adults.* 250–750 mg PO q12h; XR 500–1000 mg PO q24h; or 200–400 mg IV q12h; ↓ in renal impair **Caution:** [C, ?/–] Children <18 y **Contra:** Component sensitivity **Disp:** Tabs 100, 250, 500, 750 mg; Tabs XR 500, 1000 mg; susp 5 g/100 mL, 10 g/100 mL; inj 200, 400 mg **SE:** Restlessness, N/V/D, rash, ruptured tendons, ↑ LFTs **Notes:** Avoid antacids; reduce/restrict caffeine intake; interactions w/ theophylline, caffeine, sucralfate, warfarin, antacids

Ciprofloxacin, Ophthalmic (Ciloxan) **Uses:** *Rx & prevention of ocular Infxns (conjunctivitis, blepharitis, corneal abrasions)* **Action:** Quinolone antibiotic; ↓ DNA gyrase **Dose:** 1–2 gtt in eye(s) q2h while awake for 2 d, then 1–2 gtt q4h while awake for 5 d, Oint ½″ ribbon in eye 3 × d × 2 days, then 2 × d × 5 days **Caution:** [C, ?/–] **Contra:** Component sensitivity **Disp:** Soln 3.5 mg/mL; oint 35g **SE:** Local irritation

Ciprofloxacin, Otic (Cipro HC Otic) **Uses:** *Otitis externa* **Action:** Quinolone antibiotic; ↓ DNA gyrase **Dose:** *Adult & Peds >1 mo.* 1–2 gtt in ear(s) bid for 7 d **Caution:** [C, ?/–] **Contra:** Perforated tympanic membrane, viral Infxns of the external canal **Disp:** Susp ciprofloxacin 0.2% & hydrocortisone 1% **SE:** HA, pruritus

Cisplatin (Platinol, Platinol AQ) **Uses:** *Testicular, small-cell & non-small-cell lung, bladder, ovarian, breast, head & neck, & penile CAs; osteosarcoma; ped brain tumors* **Action:** DNA-binding; denatures double helix; intrastrand cross-linking **Dose:** 10–20 mg/m^2/d for 5 d q3wk; 50–120 mg/m^2 q3–4wk; (Per protocols); ↓ w/renal impair **Caution:** [D, –] Cumulative renal tox may be severe; monitor Mg^{2+}, electrolytes before & w/in 48 h after cisplatin **Contra:** Allergy to platinum-containing compounds; myelosuppression, hearing impair, preexisting renal insuff **Disp:** Inj 1 mg/mL **SE:** Allergic Rxns, N/V, nephrotox (worse w/administration of other nephrotoxic drugs; minimize by NS inf & mannitol diuresis), high-frequency hearing loss in 30%, peripheral "stocking glove"-type neuropathy, cardiotox (ST-, T-wave changes), ↓ Mg^{2+}, mild myelosuppression, hepatotox; renal impair dose-related & cumulative **Notes:** Give taxanes before platinum derivatives

Citalopram (Celexa) **WARNING:** Closely monitor for worsening depression or emergence of suicidality, particularly in ped pts **Uses:** *Depression* **Action:** SSRI **Dose:** Initial 20 mg/d, may ↑ to 40 mg/d; ↓ in elderly & hepatic/renal insuff **Caution:** [C, +/–] Hx of mania, Szs & pts at risk for suicide **Contra:** MOAI or w/in 14 d of MAOI use **Disp:** Tabs 10, 20, 40 mg; Soln 10 mg/5 mL **SE:** Somnolence, insomnia, anxiety, xerostomia, diaphoresis, sexual dysfunction **Notes:** May cause ↓ Na$^+$/SIADH

Cladribine (Leustatin) **Uses:** *HCL, CLL, NHLs, progressive MS* **Action:** Induces DNA strand breakage; interferes w/ DNA repair/synthesis; purine nucleoside analog **Dose:** 0.09–0.1 mg/kg/d cont IV inf for 1–7 d (Per protocols)

Caution: [D, ?/–] Causes neutropenia & Infxn **Contra:** Component sensitivity **Disp:** Inj 1 mg/mL **SE:** Myelosuppression, T-lymphocyte ↓may be prolonged (26–34 wk), fever in 46%, tumor lysis synd, Infxns (especially lung & IV sites), rash (50%), HA, fatigue **Notes:** Consider prophylactic allopurinol; monitor CBC

Clarithromycin (Biaxin, Biaxin XL)
Uses: *Upper/lower resp tract, skin/skin structure Infxns, *H. pylori* Infxns, & Infxns caused by nontuberculosis (atypical) *Mycobacterium;* prevention of MAC Infxns in HIV-Infxn* **Action:** Macrolide antibiotic, ↓ protein synthesis. *Spectrum:* H. influenzae, M. catarrhalis, S. pneumoniae, Mycoplasma pneumoniae, & H. pylori **Dose:** *Adults,* 250–500 mg PO bid or 1000 mg (2 × 500 mg XL tab)/d. Mycobacterium: 500–1000 mg PO bid. *Peds >9 mo.* 7.5 mg/kg/dose PO bid; ↓ in renal/hepatic impair **Caution:** [C, ?] Antibiotic-associated colitis; rare QT prolongation & ventricular arrhythmias, including torsades de pointes **Contra:** Macrolide allergy; w/ranitidine in pts w/ Hx of porphyria or CrCl <25 mL/min **Disp:** Tabs 250, 500 mg; susp 125, 250 mg/5 mL; 500 mg XL tab **SE:** ↑QT interval, causes metallic taste, N/D, abdominal pain, HA, rash **Notes:** Multiple drug interactions, ↑ theophylline & carbamazepine levels; do not refrigerate suspension

Clemastine Fumarate (Tavist,Dayhist-1) [OTC]
Uses: *Allergic rhinitis & Sxs of urticaria* **Action:** Antihistamine **Dose:** *Adults & Peds >12 y.* 1.34 mg bid–2.68 mg tid; max 8.04 mg/d *<12 y.* 0.4 mg PO bid **Caution:** [C, M] BOO **Contra:** NA glaucoma **Disp:** Tabs 1.34, 2.68 mg; syrup 0.67 mg/5 mL **SE:** Drowsiness, dyscoordination, epigastric distress, urinary retention **Notes:** Avoid EtOH

Clindamycin (Cleocin, Cleocin-T, others)
Uses: * Rx aerobic & anaerobic Infxns; topical for severe acne & vaginal Infxns* **Action:** Bacteriostatic; interferes w/ protein synthesis. *Spectrum:* Streptococci, pneumococci, staphylococci, & gram(+) & gram(–) anaerobes; no activity against gram(–) aerobes & bacterial vaginosis **Dose:** *Adults.* PO: 150–450 mg PO q6–8h. IV: 300–600 mg IV q6h or 900 mg IV q8h. *Vaginal:* 1 applicator hs for 7 d. *Topical:* Apply 1% gel, lotion, or soln bid. *Peds.* Neonates: (Avoid use; contains benzyl alcohol) 10–15 mg/kg/24 h ÷ q8–12h. *Children >1 mo:* 10–30 mg/kg/24 h ÷ q6–8h, to a max of 1.8 g/d PO or 4.8 g/d IV. *Topical:* Apply 1%, gel, lotion, or soln bid; ↓ in severe hepatic impair **Caution:** [B, +] Can cause fatal colitis **Contra:** Hx pseudomembranous colitis **Disp:** Caps 75, 150, 300 mg, susp 75 mg/5 mL; inj 300 mg/2 mL; vaginal cream 2%, topical sol 1%, gel 1%, lotion 1%, vaginal supp 100 mg **SE:** Diarrhea may be C. difficile pseudomembranous colitis, rash, ↑ LFTs **Notes:** D/C drug w/diarrhea, evaluate for C. difficile

Clofarabine (Clolar DS)
Uses: Rx relapsed/refractory ALL after at least 2 regimens in children 1–21 y **Action:** Antimetabolite; ↓ribonucleotide reductase w/ false nucleotide base-inhibiting DNA synthesis **Dose:** 52 mg/m² IV over 2 h qd × 5 d (repeat q2–6wk); Per protocol **Caution:** [D, –] **Disp:** Inj 20 mg/20 mL **SE:** N/V/D, anemia, leukopenia, thrombocytopenia, neutropenia, Infxn, ↑ AST/ALT

Notes: Monitor for tumor lysis syndrome & systemic inflammatory response syndrome (SIRS)/capillary leak syndrome

Clonazepam (Klonopin) [C-IV] Uses: *Lennox–Gastaut syndrome, akinetic & myoclonic Szs, absence Szs, panic attacks,* *restless legs syndrome, neuralgia, parkinsonian dysarthria, bipolar disorder* **Action:** Benzodiazepine; anticonvulsant **Dose:** *Adults.* 1.5 mg/d PO in 3 ÷ doses; ↑ by 0.5–1 mg/d q3d PRN up to 20 mg/d. *Peds.* 0.01–0.03 mg/kg/24 h PO ÷ tid; ↑ to 0.1–0.2 mg/kg/24 h ÷ tid; avoid abrupt D/C **Caution:** [D, M] Elderly pts, resp Dz, CNS depression, severe hepatic impair, NA glaucoma **Contra:** Severe liver Dz, acute NA glaucoma **Disp:** Tabs 0.5, 1, 2 mg, Oral disintegrating tabs 0.125, 0.25, 0.5, 1, 2 mg **SE:** CNS side effects, including drowsiness, dizziness, ataxia, memory impair **Notes:** Can cause retrograde amnesia; a CYP3A4 substrate

Clonidine, Oral (Catapres) Uses: *HTN*; opioid, EtOH, & tobacco withdrawal **Action:** Centrally acting α-adrenergic stimulant **Dose:** *Adults.* 0.1 mg PO bid, adjust QD by 0.1- to 0.2-mg increments (max 2.4 mg/d). *Peds.* 5–10 mcg/kg/d ÷ q8–12h (max 0.9 mg/d); ↓in renal impair **Caution:** [C, +/–] Avoid w/ β-blocker **Contra:** Component sensitivity **Disp:** Tabs 0.1, 0.2, 0.3 mg **SE:** drowsiness, orthostatic ↓ BP, xerostomia, constipation, bradycardia, dizziness **Notes:** More effective for HTN if combined w/ diuretics; withdraw slowly, rebound HTN w/ abrupt D/C of doses >0.2 mg bid

Clonidine, Transdermal (Catapres TTS) Uses: *HTN* **Action:** Centrally acting α-adrenergic stimulant **Dose:** 1 patch q7d to hairless area (upper arm/torso); titrate to effect; ↓w/ severe renal impair; **Caution:** [C, +/–] Avoid w/ β-blocker, withdraw slowly **Contra:** Component sensitivity **Disp:** TTS-1, TTS-2, TTS-3 (delivers 0.1, 0.2, 0.3 mg, respectively, of clonidine/d for 1 wk) **SE:** Drowsiness, orthostatic ↓ BP, xerostomia, constipation, bradycardia **Notes:** Do not D/C abruptly (rebound HTN) Doses >2 TTS-3 usually not associated w/ ↑ efficacy; steady state in 2–3 d

Clopidogrel (Plavix) Uses: *Reduce atherosclerotic events* **Action:** ↓ Plt aggregation **Dose:** 75 mg/d; 300 mg PO × 1 dose can be used to load pts **Caution:** [B, ?] Active bleeding; risk of bleeding from trauma & other; TTP; liver Dz **Contra:** Active bleeding; intracranial bleeding **Disp:** Tabs 75 mg **SE:** Prolongs bleeding time, GI intolerance, HA, dizziness, rash, thrombocytopenia, ↓ WBC **Notes:** Plt aggregation to baseline ≈ five days after Dlc, plt transfusion to reverse acutely

Clorazepate (Tranxene) [C-IV] Uses: *Acute anxiety disorders, acute EtOH withdrawal Sxs, adjunctive therapy in partial Szs* **Action:** Benzodiazepine; antianxiety agent **Dose:** *Adults.* 15–60 mg/d PO single or ÷ doses. *Elderly & debilitated pts:* Initial 7.5–15 mg/d in ÷ doses. *EtOH withdrawal:* Day 1: Initial 30 mg; then 30–60 mg ÷ doses; Day 2: 45–90 mg ÷ doses; Day 3: 22.5–45 mg ÷ doses; Day 4: 15–30 mg ÷ doses. *Peds.* 3.75–7.5 mg/dose bid to 60 mg/d max ÷ bid–tid **Caution:** [D, ?/–] Elderly; Hx depression **Contra:** NA glaucoma; Not OK <9 y of age **Disp:** Tabs 3.75, 7.5, 15 mg; Tabs-SD (QD) 11.25, 22.5 mg **SE:** CNS depres-

Codeine

63

sant effects (drowsiness, dizziness, ataxia, memory impair), ↓ BP **Notes:** Monitor pts w/ renal/hepatic impair (drug may accumulate); avoid abrupt D/C; may cause dependence

Clotrimazole (Lotrimin, Mycelex, others) [OTC] **Uses:** *Candidiasis & tinea Infxns* **Action:** Antifungal; alters cell wall permeability. *Spectrum:* Oropharyngeal candidiasis, dermatophytes, superficial mycoses, cutaneous candidiasis, & vulvovaginal candidiasis **Dose:** *PO: Prophylaxis:* One troche dissolved in mouth tid *Rx:* One troche dissolved in mouth 5X d for 14 d. *Vaginal 1% Cream:* 1 applicatorful hs for 7 d. *2% Cream:* 1 applicatorful hs for 3 d *Tabs:* 100 mg vaginally hs for 7 d or 200 mg (2 tabs) vaginally hs for 3 d or 500-mg tabs vaginally hs once. *Topical:* Apply bid 10–14 d **Caution:** [B, (C if PO), ?] Not for systemic fungal Infxn; safety in children <3 y not established **Contra:** Component allergy **Disp:** 1% cream; soln; lotion; troche 10 mg; vaginal tabs 100, 500 mg; vaginal cream 1%, 2% **SE:** Topical: Local irritation; PO: N/V, ↑ LFTs **Notes:** PO prophylaxis immunosuppressed pts

Clotrimazole & Betamethasone (Lotrisone) **Uses:** *Fungal skin Infxns* **Action:** Imidazole antifungal & antiinflammatory. *Spectrum:* Tinea pedis, cruris, & corpora **Dose:** *Pts ≥ 17 y.* Apply & massage into area bid for 2–4 wk **Caution:** [C, ?] Varicella Infxn **Contra:** Children <12 y **Disp:** Cream 15, 45 g; lotion 30 mL **SE:** Local irritation, rash **Notes:** Not for diaper dermatitis or under occlusive dressings

Clozapine (Clozaril) **WARNING:** Myocarditis, agranulocytosis, Szs, & orthostatic ↓ BP associated w/ clozapine; ↑ mortality in elderly w/dementia-related psychosis **Uses:** *Refractory severe schizophrenia*; childhood psychosis **Action:** "Atypical" TCA **Dose:** 25 mg daily–bid initial; ↑ to 300–450 mg/d over 2 wk; maint lowest dose possible; do not D/C abruptly **Caution:** [B, +/–] Monitor for psychosis & cholinergic rebound **Contra:** Uncontrolled epilepsy; comatose state; WBC ≤3500 cells/mm³ before Rx or <3000 cells/mm³ during Rx **Disp:** Tabs 25, 100 mg **SE:** Tachycardia, drowsiness, ↑ weight, constipation, incontinence, rash, Szs, CNS stimulation, hyperglycemia **Notes:** Benign temperature ↑ may occur during the 1st 3 wk of Rx, weekly CBC mandatory 1st 6 mo, then qowk

Cocaine [C-II] **Uses:** *Topical anesthetic for mucous membranes* **Action:** Narcotic analgesic, local vasoconstrictor **Dose:** Lowest topical amount that provides relief; 1 mg/kg max **Caution:** [C, ?] **Disp:** Topical soln & viscous preparations 4–10%, powder **SE:** CNS stimulation, nervousness, loss of taste/smell, chronic rhinitis **Notes:** Use only on PO, laryngeal, & nasal mucosa; do not use on extensive areas of broken skin

Codeine [C-II] **Uses:** *Mild–moderate pain; symptomatic relief of cough* **Action:** Narcotic analgesic; depresses cough reflex **Dose:** *Adults. Analgesic:* 15–60 mg PO or IM qid PRN. *Antitussive:* 10–20 mg PO q4h PRN; max 120 mg/d. *Peds. Analgesic:* 0.5–1 mg/kg/dose PO q4–6h PRN. *Antitussive:* 1–1.5 mg/kg/24 h PO ÷ q4h; max 30 mg/24 h; ↓ in renal/hepatic impair **Caution:** [C, (D if prolonged use or high doses at term), +] **Contra:** Component sensitivity **Disp:** Tabs 15, 30,

60 mg; soln 15 mg/5 mL; inj 15, 30 mg/mL **SE:** Drowsiness, constipation **Notes:** Usually combined w/ APAP for pain or w/ agents (eg, terpin hydrate) as an antitussive; 120 mg IM = 10 mg IM morphine

Colchicine **Uses:** *Acute gouty arthritis & prevention of recurrences; familial Mediterranean fever*; primary biliary cirrhosis **Action:** ↓ migration of leukocytes; ↓ leukocyte lactic acid production **Dose:** *Initial:* 0.5–1.2 mg PO, then 0.5–0.6 mg q1–2h until relief or GI SE develop (max 8 mg/d); do not repeat for 3 d. IV: 1–3 mg, then 0.5 mg q6h until relief (max 4 mg/d); do not repeat for 7 d. *Prophylaxis:* PO: 0.5–0.6 mg/d or 3–4 d/wk; ↓ renal impair **Caution:** [D, +] Elderly **Contra:** Serious renal, GI, hepatic, or cardiac disorders; blood dyscrasias **Disp:** Tabs 0.6 mg; inj 1 mg/2 mL **SE:** N/V/D, abdominal pain, BM suppression, hepatotox; local Rxn w/ SQ/IM **Notes:** Colchicine 1–2 mg IV w/in 24–48 h of an acute attack diagnostic/therapeutic in monoarticular arthritis

Colesevelam (WelChol) **Uses:** *Reduction of LDL & total cholesterol alone or in combo w/ an HMG-CoA reductase inhibitor* **Action:** Bile acid sequestrant **Dose:** 3 tabs PO bid w/ meals **Caution:** [B, ?] Severe GI motility disorders; safety & efficacy not established in peds **Contra:** Bowel obstruction **Disp:** Tabs 625 mg **SE:** Constipation, dyspepsia, myalgia, weakness **Notes:** May ↓ absorption of fat-soluble vitamins

Colestipol (Colestid) **Uses:** *Adjunct to ↓ serum cholesterol in primary hypercholesterolemia* **Action:** Binds intestinal bile acids to form insoluble complex **Dose:** Granules: 5–30 g/d ÷ 2–4 doses; tabs: 2–16 g/d daily–bid **Caution:** [C, ?] Avoid w/ high triglycerides, GI dysfunction **Contra:** Bowel obstruction **Disp:** Tabs 1 g; granules 5, 7.5, 300, 450, 500 g **SE:** Constipation, abdominal pain, bloating, HA **Notes:** Do not use dry powder; mix w/ beverages, cereals, etc; may ↓ absorption of other medications and fat-soluble vitamins

Conivaptan HCL (Vaprisol) **Uses:** Euvolemic hyponatremia **Action:** Dual arginine vasopressin V_{1A}/V_2 receptor antagonist **Dose:** 20 mg IV × 1 over 30 min, then 20 mg cont IV inf over 24 h; 20 mg/d cont IV inf for 1–3 more d; may ↑ to 40 mg/d if Na⁺ not responding; 4 d max use; use large vein, change site q 24 h **Caution:** [C; ?/-] Rapid ↑ Na⁺ (>12 mEq/L/24 h) may cause osmotic demyelination syndrome; impaired renal/hepatic fxn; may ↑ digoxin levels; CYP3A4 inhibitor (Table 13) **Contra:** Hypovolemic hyponatremia; w/CYP3A4 inhibitors **Disp:** Ampule 20 mg/4 mL **SE:** Infusion site Rxns, HA, N/V/D, constipation, ↓ K⁺, thirst, dry mouth, pyrexia, pollakiuria, polyuria, Infxn **Notes:** Monitor Na⁺, volume and neurologic status; D/C w/every rapid ↑ Na⁺; mix only w/ 5% dextrose

Cortisone See Steroids (page 175) and Tables 4 & 5

Cromolyn Sodium (Intal, NasalCrom, Opticrom) **Uses:** *Adjunct to the Rx of asthma; prevent exercise-induced asthma; allergic rhinitis; ophth allergic manifestations*; food allergy **Action:** Antiasthmatic; mast cell stabilizer **Dose:** *Adults & Children >12 y.* Inhal: 20 mg (as powder in caps) inhaled qid or met-dose inhaler 2 puffs qid. *PO:* 200 mg qid 15–20 min ac, up to 400 mg qid.

Nasal instillation: Spray once in each nostril 2–6×/d. *Ophth:* 1–2 gtt in each eye 4–6 × d–. **Peds.** Inhal: 2 puffs qid of met-dose inhaler. *PO: Infants <2 y:* (not OK) 20 mg/kg/d in 4 ÷ doses. *2–12 y:* 100 mg qid ac **Caution:** [B, ?] **Contra:** Acute asthmatic attacks **Disp:** PO conc 100 mg/5 mL; soln for neb 20 mg/2 ml .; met-dose inhaler; nasal soln 40 mg/mL; ophth soln 4% **SE:** Unpleasant taste, hoarseness, coughing **Notes:** No benefit in acute Rx; 2–4 wk for maximal effect in perennial allergic disorders

Cyanocobalamin [Vitamin B₁₂]   Uses: *Pernicious anemia & other vitamin B_{12} deficiency states; ↑ requirements due to PRG; thyrotoxicosis; liver or kidney Dz* **Action:** Dietary vitamin B_{12} supl **Dose: *Adults.*** 100 mcg IM or SQ qd for 5–10 d, then 100 mcg IM 2×/wk for 1 mo, then 100 mcg IM monthly. **Peds.** 100 mcg/d IM or SQ for 5–10 d, then 30–50 mcg IM q4wk **Caution:** [A (C if dose exceeds RDA), +] **Contra:** Allergy to cobalt; hereditary optic nerve atrophy; Leber Dz **Disp:** Tabs 50, 100, 250, 500, 1000, 2500 mcg; inj 100, 1000 mcg/mL; gel 500 mcg/0.1 mL **SE:** Itching, D, HA, anxiety **Notes:** PO absorption erratic, altered by many drugs & not recommended; for use w/ hyperalimentation

Cyclobenzaprine (Flexeril)   Uses: *Relief of muscle spasm* **Action:** Centrally acting skeletal muscle relaxant; reduces tonic somatic motor activity **Dose:** 10 mg PO bid–qid (2–3 wk max) Caution: [B, ?] Shares the toxic potential of the TCAs; urinary hesitancy or angle-closure glaucoma **Contra:** Do not use concomitantly or w/in 14 d of MAOIs; hyperthyroidism; heart failure; arrhythmias **Disp:** Tabs 5, 7.5, 10 mg **SE:** Sedation & anticholinergic effects Notes: May inhibit mental alertness or physical coordination

Cyclopentolate ophthalmic (Cyclogyl)   Uses: * Cycloplegia, mydriasis* **Action:** Cycloplegic mydriatic, anticholinergic inhibits iris sphincter and ciliary body **Dose: *Adults.*** 1 gtt in eye 40–50 min preprocedure, may repeat × 1 in 5–10 min **Peds.** As adult, children 0.5–1.0%; infants use 0.5% **Caution:** [C [may cause late-term fetal anoxia/bradycardia, +/–], premature infants HTN, Down synd, elderly, **Contra:** Narrow-angle glaucoma **Disp:** Ophth soln 0.5, 1, 2% **SE:** Tearing, HA, irritation, eye pain, photophobia, arrhythmia, tremor, ↑ IOP, confusion **Note:** Compress lacrimal sac for several min after dose; heavily pigmented irises may require ↑ strength; peak 25–75 min, cycloplegia 6–24 h, mydriasis up to 24 h

Cyclopentolate with Phenylephrine (Cyclomydril)   Uses: * Action: Cycloplegic mydriatic, α-Adrenergic agonist w/ anticholinergic to inhibit iris sphincter **Dose:** 1 gtt in eye q 5–10 min (max 3 doses) 40–50 min preprocedure **Caution:** [C [may cause late-term fetal anoxia/bradycardia, +/–] HTN, w/elderly w/CAD, **Contra:** Narrow-angle glaucoma **Disp:** Ophth soln Cyclopentolate 0.2%/phenlephrine 1% (2, 5 mL) **SE:** Tearing, HA, irritation, eye pain, photophobia, arrhythmia, tremor **Notes:** Compress lacrimal sac for several min after dose; heavily pigmented irises may require ↑ strength; peak 25–75 min, cycloplegia 6–24 h, mydriasis up to 24 h

Cyclophosphamide (Cytoxan, Neosar) Uses: *Hodgkin Dz & NHLs; multiple myeloma; small-cell lung, breast, & ovarian CAs; mycosis fungoides; neuroblastoma; retinoblastoma; acute leukemias; allogeneic & ABMT in high doses; severe rheumatologic disorders* **Action:** Converted to acrolein & phosphoramide mustard, the active alkylating moieties **Dose:** 500–1500 mg/m² single dose at 2- to 4-wk intervals; 1.8 g/m² to 160 mg/kg (or ≅12 g/m² in 75-kg individual) in the BMT setting (per protocols); ↓ renal/hepatic impair **Caution:** [D, ?] w/ BM suppression **Contra:** Component sensitivity **Disp:** Tabs 25, 50 mg; inj 500 mg, 1g, 2g **SE:** Myelosuppression (leukopenia & thrombocytopenia); hemorrhagic cystitis, SIADH, alopecia, anorexia; N/V; hepatotox; rare interstitial pneumonitis; irreversible testicular atrophy possible; cardiotox rare; 2nd malignancies (bladder, ALL), risk 3.5% at 8 y, 10.7% at 12 y **Notes:** Hemorrhagic cystitis prophylaxis: continuous bladder irrigation & mesna uroprotection; encourage hydration, long-term bladder Ca screening

Cyclosporine (Sandimmune, NeOral, Gengraf) Uses: *Organ rejection in kidney, liver, heart, & BMT w/ steroids; RA; psoriasis* **Action:** Immunosuppressant; reversible inhibition of immunocompetent lymphocytes **Dose:** *Adults & Peds.* PO: 15 mg/kg/d 12 h pretransplant; after 2 wk, taper by 5 mg/wk to 5–10 mg/kg/d. IV: If NPO, give 1/3 PO dose IV; ↓ in renal/hepatic impair **Caution:** [C, ?] Dose-related risk of nephrotox/hepatotox; live, attenuated vaccines may be less effective **Contra:** Abnormal renal Fxn; uncontrolled HTN **Disp:** Caps 25, 50, 100 mg; PO soln 100 mg/mL; inj 50 mg/mL **SE:** May ↑ BUN & Cr & mimic transplant rejection; HTN; HA; hirsutism **Notes:** Administer in glass container; many drug interactions; NeOral & Sandimmune not interchangeable; interaction w/ St. John's wort. Follow levels (Table 2)

Cyclosporine ophthalmic (Restasis) Uses: * ↑ Tear production suppressed due to ocular inflammation * **Action:** Immune modulator, anti-inflammatory **Dose:** 1 gtt bid each eye 12 h apart; OK w/ artificial tears, allow 15 min between **Caution:** [C, –] **Contra:** Ocular Infxn, component allergy **Disp:** Single-use vial 0.05% **SE:** Ocular burning/hyperemia **Notes:** Mix vial well

Cyproheptadine (Periactin) Uses: *Allergic Rxns; itching* **Action:** Phenothiazine antihistamine; serotonin antagonist **Dose:** *Adults.* 4–20 mg PO ÷ q8h; max 0.5 mg/kg/d. *Peds.* 2–6 y: 2 mg bid–tid (max 12 mg/24 h). 7–14 y: 4 mg bid–tid; ↓ in hepatic impair **Caution:** [B, ?] BPH **Contra:** Neonates or <2 y; NA glaucoma; BOO; acute asthma; GI obstruction **Disp:** Tabs 4 mg; syrup 2 mg/5 mL **SE:** Anticholinergic, sedation, **Notes:** May stimulate appetite

Cytarabine [ARA-C] (Cytosar-U) Uses: *Acute leukemias, CML, NHL; IT for leukemic meningitis or prophylaxis* **Action:** Antimetabolite; interferes w/ DNA synthesis **Dose:** 100–150 mg/m²/d for 5–10 d (low dose); 3 g/m² q12h for 8–12 doses (high dose); 1 mg/kg 1–2/wk (SQ maint); 5–70 mg/m² up to 3/wk IT (per protocols); ↓ in renal/hepatic impair **Caution:** [D, ?] w/ marked BM suppression, ↓ dosage by ↓ the number of days of administration **Contra:** Component sensitivity **Disp:** Inj 100, 500 mg, 1, 2 g **SE:** Myelosuppression, N/V/D, stomatitis, flulike syndrome, rash on palms/soles, hepatic dysfunction, cerebellar dysfunction, noncardiogenic pulmonary edema, neuropathy **Notes:** Little use in solid tumors; high-dose Rx limited by corticosteroid ophth soln

Cytarabine Liposome (DepoCyt) Uses: *Lymphomatous meningitis* **Action:** Antimetabolite; interferes w/DNA synthesis **Dose:** 50 mg IT q14d for 5 doses, then 50 mg IT q28d × 4 doses; use dexamethasone prophylaxis **Caution:** [D, ?] May cause neurotox; blockage to CSF flow may ↑ the risk of neurotox; use in peds not established **Contra:** Active meningeal Infxn **Disp:** IT inj 50 mg/5 mL **SE:** Neck pain/rigidity, HA, confusion, somnolence, fever, back pain, N/V, edema, neutropenia, thrombocytopenia, anemia **Notes:** Cytarabine liposomes are similar in microscopic appearance to WBCs; caution in interpreting CSF studies

Cytomegalovirus Immune Globulin [CMV-IG IV] (CytoGam) Uses: *Attenuation CMV Dz associated w/ transplantation* **Action:** Exogenous IgG antibodies to CMV **Dose:** 150 mg/kg/dose w/in 72 h of transplant, for 16 wk posttransplant; see insert **Caution:** [C, ?] Anaphylactic Rxns; renal dysfunction **Contra:** Allergy to immunoglobulins; IgA deficiency **Disp:** Inj 50 mg/mL **SE:** Flushing, N/V, muscle cramps, wheezing, HA, fever **Notes:** IV only; administer by separate line; do not shake

Dacarbazine (DTIC) Uses: *Melanoma, Hodgkin Dz, sarcoma* **Action:** Alkylating agent; antimetabolite as a purine precursor; ↓ protein synthesis, RNA, & especially DNA **Dose:** 2–4.5 mg/kg/d or 250 mg/m²/d for 5 d (Per protocols); ↓ in renal impair **Caution:** [C, ?] In BM suppression; renal/hepatic impair **Contra:** Component sensitivity **Disp:** Inj 100, 200 mg **SE:** Myelosuppression, severe N/V, hepatox, flulike syndrome, ↓ BP, photosensitivity, alopecia, facial flushing, facial paresthesias, urticaria, phlebitis at inj site **Notes:** Avoid extravasation

Daclizumab (Zenapax) Uses: *Prevent acute organ rejection* **Action:** IL-2 receptor antagonist **Dose:** 1 mg/kg/dose IV; 1st dose pretransplant, then 4 doses 14 d apart posttransplant **Caution:** [C, ?] **Contra:** Component sensitivity **Disp:** Inj 5 mg/mL **SE:** Hyperglycemia, edema, HTN, ↓ BP, constipation, HA, dizziness, anxiety, nephrotox, pulmonary edema, pain **Notes:** Administer w/in 4 h of preparation

Dactinomycin (Cosmegen) Uses: *Choriocarcinoma, Wilms' tumor, Kaposi's sarcoma, Ewing sarcoma, rhabdomyosarcoma, testicular CA* **Action:** DNA intercalating agent **Dose:** 0.5 mg/d for 5 d; 2 mg/wk for 3 consecutive wk; 15 mcg/kg or 0.45 mg/m²/d (max 0.5 mg) for 5 d q3–8wk in ped sarcoma (Per protocols); ↓ in renal impair **Caution:** [C, ?] **Contra:** concurrent/recent chickenpox or herpes zoster; infants <6 mo **Disp:** Inj 0.5 mg **SE:** Myelo-/immunosuppression, severe N/V, alopecia, acne, hyperpigmentation, radiation recall phenomenon, tissue damage w/ extravasation, hepatotox

Dalteparin (Fragmin) Uses: *Unstable angina, non-Q-wave MI, prevention of ischemic complications due to clot formation in pts on concurrent ASA,

68 Dantrolene

prevent & Rx DVT following surgery* **Action:** LMW heparin Dose: *Angina/MI:* 120 U/kg (max 10,000 IU) SQ q12h w/ ASA. DVT prophylaxis: 2500–5000 IU SC 1–2 h preop, then qd for 5–10 d. *Systemic anticoagulation:* 200 IU/kg/d SQ or 100 IU/kg bid SQ **Caution:** [B, ?] in renal/hepatic impair, active hemorrhage, cerebrovascular Dz, cerebral aneurysm, severe HTN **Contra:** HIT; pork product allergy **Disp:** Inj 2500 IU (16 mg/0.2 mL), 5000 IU (32 mg/0.2 mL), 7,500 IU (48 mg/0.3 mL), 10,000 IU (64 mg/mL) **SE:** Bleeding, pain at site, thrombocytopenia **Notes:** Predictable effects eliminates lab monitoring; not for IM/IV use

Dantrolene (Dantrium) Uses: *Rx spasticity due to upper motor neuron disorders (eg, spinal cord injuries, stroke, CP, MS); malignant hyperthermia* **Action:** Skeletal muscle relaxant **Dose:** *Adults.* Spasticity: 25 mg PO daily; ↑ 25 mg to effect to 100 mg max PO qid PRN. *Peds.* 0.5 mg/kg/dose bid; ↑ by 0.5 mg/kg to effect, to 3 mg/kg/dose max qid PRN. *Adults & Peds.* Malignant hyperthermia: Rx: Continuous rapid IV, start 1 mg/kg until Sxs subside or 10 mg/kg is reached. *Postcrisis F/U:* 4–8 mg/kg/d in 3–4 ÷ doses for 1–3 d to prevent recurrence **Caution:** [C, ?] Impaired cardiac/pulmonary Fxn **Contra:** Active hepatic Dz; where spasticity needed to maintain posture or balance **Disp:** Caps 25, 50, 100 mg; powder for inj 20 mg/vial **SE:** Hepatotox,↑ LFTs, drowsiness, dizziness, rash, muscle weakness, pleural effusion w/ pericarditis, D, blurred vision, hepatitis **Notes:** Monitor LFT; avoid sunlight/EtOH/CNS depressants

Dapsone (Avlosulfon) Uses: *Rx & prevent PCP; toxoplasmosis prophylaxis; leprosy* **Action:** Unknown; bactericidal **Dose:** *Adults.* PCP prophylaxis 50–100 mg/d PO; Rx PCP 100 mg/d PO w/ TMP 15–20 mg/kg/d for 21 d. *Peds.* Prophylaxis of PCP 1–2 mg/kg/24 h PO daily; max 100 mg/d **Caution:** [C, +] G6PD deficiency; severe anemia **Contra:** Component sensitivity **Disp:** Tabs 25, 100 mg **SE:** Hemolysis, methemoglobinemia, agranulocytosis, rash, cholestatic jaundice **Notes:** Absorption ↑ by an acidic environment; for leprosy, combine w/ rifampin & other agents

Daptomycin (Cubicin) Uses: *Complicated skin/skin structure Infxns due to gram(+) organisms* **Action:** Cyclic lipopeptide; rapid membrane depolarization & bacterial death *Spectrum: Staph aureus* (including MRSA), *Streptococcus pyogenes, S. agalactiae, S. dysgalactiae subsp Equisimilis & Enterococcus faecalis* (vancomycin-susceptible strains only) **Dose:** 4 mg/kg IV daily × 7–14 d (over 30 min); w/ CrCl < 30 mL/min/ or dialysis: 4 mg/kg q48h **Caution:** [B, ?] w/HMG-CoA inhibitors **Disp:** Inj 250, 500 mg/10 mL **SE:** Constipation, N/V/D, HA, rash, site Rxn, muscle pain/weakness, edema, cellulitis, hypo/hyperglycemia, ↑ alkaline phosphatase, cough, back pain, abdominal pain, ↓ K+, anxiety, chest pain, sore throat, cardiac failure, confusion, Candida Infxns **Notes:** Monitor CPK weekly; Consider D/C stopping HMG-CoA reductase inhibitors to ↓myopathy risk

Darbepoetin Alfa (Aranesp) Uses: *Anemia associated w/ CRF* **Action:** ↑ Erythropoiesis, recombinant erythropoietin variant **Dose:** 0.45 mcg/kg single IV or SQ qwk; titrate, do not exceed target Hgb of 12 g/dL; see insert to convert from Epogen **Caution:** [C, ?] May ↑ risk of CV &/or neurologic SE in renal failure; HTN; w/ Hx Szs **Contra:** Uncontrolled HTN, component allergy **Disp:** 25, 40, 60, 100 mcg/mL, in polysorbate or albumin excipient **SE:** May ↑ cardiac risk, CP, hypo/hypertension, N/V/D, myalgia, arthralgia, dizziness, edema, fatigue, fever, ↑ risk Infxn **Notes:** Longer ½-life than Epogen; weekly CBC until stable

Darifenacin (Enablex) **Uses:** *OAB* Urinary antispasmodic, **Action:** Muscarinic receptor antagonist **Dose:** 7.5 mg/d PO; 15 mg/d max (7.5 mg/d w/ moderate hepatic impair or w/ CYP3A4 inhibitors) (Table 13); swallow whole **Caution:** [C, ?/–] **Contra:** Urinary/gastric retention, uncontrolled NA glaucoma **Disp:** Tabs ER 7.5 mg, 15 mg **SE:** Xerostomia/eyes, constipation, dyspepsia, abdominal pain, retention, abnormal vision, dizziness, asthenia

Daunorubicin (Daunomycin, Cerubidine) WARNING: Cardiac Fxn should be monitored due to potential risk for cardiac tox & CHF **Uses:** Acute leukemias **Action:** DNA intercalating agent; ↓ topoisomerase II; generates oxygen free radicals **Dose:** 45–60 mg/m²/d for 3 consecutive d; 25 mg/m²/wk (Per protocols); ↓ in renal/hepatic impair **Caution:** [D, ?] **Contra:** Component sensitivity **Disp:** Inj 20, 50 mg **SE:** Myelosuppression, mucositis, N/V, alopecia, radiation recall phenomenon, hepatotox (hyperbilirubinemia), tissue necrosis w/ extravasation, cardiotox (1–2% CHF w/ 550 mg/m² cumulative dose) **Notes:** Prevent cardiotox w/ dexrazoxane (when pt received > 300mg/m² of daunorubicin cum dose), allopurinol prior to ↓ hyperuricemia

Decitabine (Dacogen) **Uses:** *MDS* **Action:** Inhibits DNA methyltransferase **Dose:** 15 mg/m² cont inf over 3 h; repeat q 8 h × 3 days; repeat cycle q 6 wk, min 4 cycles; delay Tx and ↓ dose if inadequate hematologic recovery at 6 wk (see label protocol) **Caution:** [D, ?/-]; avoid pregnancy; males should not father a child during or 2 months after; renal/hepatic impair **Disp:** Powder 50 mg/vial **SE:** Neutropenia, febrile neutropenia, thrombocytopenia, anemia, leukopenia, petechiae, N/V/D, constipation, stomatitis, dyspepsia, cough, fever, fatigue, ↑ LFTs & bili, hyperglycemia, Infxn, HA **Notes:** Check CBC and plt before each cycle and prn; may premedicate w/anti-emetic

Delavirdine (Rescriptor) **Uses:** *HIV Infxn* **Action:** Nonnucleoside RT inhibitor **Dose:** 400 mg PO tid **Caution:** [C, ?] CDC recommends HIV-infected mothers not breast-feed (risk of HIV transmission); w/renal/hepatic impair **Contra:** Use w/ drugs dependent on CYP3A for clearance (Table 13) **Disp:** Tabs 100, 200 mg **SE:** IIA, fatigue, rash, ↑ transaminases, N/V/D **Notes:** Avoid antacids; ↓ cytochrome P-450 enzymes; numerous drug interactions; monitor LFTs

Deferasirox (Exjade) **Uses:** *Chronic iron overload due to transfusion in patients >2 yrs* **Action:** Oral iron chelator **Dose:** Initial: 20 mg/kg PO/d; adjust by 5–10 mg/kg q 3–6 mo based on monthly ferritin; 30 mg/kg max; on empty stomach 30 min before food; dissolve in water, orange, apple juice (< 1 gm/3.5 oz; >1 gm in 7 oz) drink immediately; resuspend residue and swallow; do not chew, swallow whole tabs or take w/ Al-containing antacids **Caution:** [B, ?/–] **Disp:** Tabs for oral susp 125, 250, 500 mg **SE:** N/V/D, abdominal pain, skin rash, HA, fever, cough, ↑ creatinine & LFTs, Infxn, hearing loss, dizziness, cataracts, retinal disorders, ↑ IOP, lens opacities, dizziness **Notes:** Dose to nearest whole tablet; auditory and ophthalmic testing initially and q 12 mo; monthly Cr, urine protein, and LFTs

Demeclocycline (Declomycin)
Uses: SIADH **Action:** Antibiotic, antagonizes ADH action on renal tubules **Dose:** 300–600 mg PO q12h on empty stomach; ↓ in renal failure; avoid antacids **Caution:** [D, +] Avoid in hepatic/renal impair & children **Contra:** Tetracycline allergy **Disp:** Tabs 150, 300 mg **SE:** D, abdominal cramps, photosensitivity, DI **Notes:** Avoid sunlight

Desipramine (Norpramin)
WARNING: Closely monitor for worsening depression or emergence of suicidality **Uses:** *Endogenous depression,* chronic pain, peripheral neuropathy **Action:** TCA; ↑ synaptic serotonin or norepinephrine in CNS **Dose:** 100–200 mg/d single or ÷ dose; usually single hs dose (max 300 mg/d) **Caution:** [C, ?/–] CV Dz, Sz disorder, hypothyroidism **Contra:** MAOIs w/in 14 d; during AMI recovery phase Disp: Tabs 10, 25, 50, 75, 100, 150 mg; caps 25, 50 mg **SE:** Anticholinergic (blurred vision, urinary retention, xerostomia); orthostatic ↓ BP; ↑ QT interval, arrhythmias **Notes:** Numerous drug interactions; blue-green urine; avoid sunlight

Desloratadine (Clarinex)
Uses: *Seasonal & perennial allergic rhinitis; chronic idiopathic urticaria* **Action:** Active metabolite of Claritin, H₁-antihistamine, blocks inflammatory mediators **Dose:** Adults & Peds >12 y. 5 mg PO qd; 5 mg PO qod w/hepatic/renal impair **Caution:** [C, ?/–] RediTabs contain phenylalanine; safety not established for <12 y **Disp:** Tabs & Reditabs (rapid dissolving) 5 mg **SE:** Allergy, anaphylaxis, somnolence, HA, dizziness, fatigue, pharyngitis, xerostomia, nausea, dyspepsia, myalgia

Desmopressin (DDAVP, Stimate)
Uses: *DI (intranasal & parenteral); bleeding due to uremia, hemophilia A, & type I von Willebrand Dz (parenteral), nocturnal enuresis* **Action:** Synthetic analog of vasopressin (human ADH); ↑ factor VIII **Dose:** *DI: Intranasal: Adults.* 0.1–0.4 mL (10–40 mcg/d in 1–3 ÷ doses). *Peds 3 mo–12 y.* 0.05–0.3 mL/d in 1 or 2 doses. *Parenteral: Adults.* 0.5–1 mL (2–4 mcg/d in 2 ÷ doses); converting from nasal to parenteral, use 1/10 nasal dose. *PO: Adults.* 0.05 mg bid; ↑ to max of 1.2 mg. *Hemophilia A & von Willebrand Dz (type I); Adults & Peds >10 kg.* 0.3 mcg/kg in 50 mL NS. inf over 15–30 min. *Peds <10 kg.* As above w/ dilution to 10 mL w/ NS. *Nocturnal enuresis: Peds >6 y.* 20 mcg intranasally hs **Caution:** [B, M] Avoid overhydration **Contra:** Hemophilia B; severe classic von Willebrand Dz; pts w/ factor VIII antibodies **Disp:** Tabs 0.1, 0.2 mg; inj 4, 15 mcg/mL; nasal soln 0.1, 1.5 mg/mL **SE:** Facial flushing, HA, dizziness, vulval pain, nasal congestion, pain at inj site, ↓ Na⁺, H₂O intox **Notes:** In very young & old pts, ↓ fluid intake to prevent H₂O intox & ↓ Na⁺

Dexamethasone, Nasal (Dexacort Phosphate Turbinaire)
Uses: *Chronic nasal inflammation or allergic rhinitis* **Action:** Anti-inflammatory

corticosteroid **Dose:** *Adult & Peds >12 y.* 2 sprays/nostril bid–tid, max 12 sprays/d. *Peds 6–12 y.* 1–2 sprays/nostril bid, max 8 sprays/d **Caution:** [C, ?] **Contra:** Untreated Infxn **Disp:** Aerosol, 84 mcg/activation **SE:** Local irritation

Dexamethasone, Ophthalmic (AK-Dex Ophthalmic, Decadron Ophthalmic) Uses: *Inflammatory or allergic conjunctivitis* **Action:** Anti-inflammatory corticosteroid **Dose:** Instill 1–2 gtt tid–qid **Caution:** [C, ?/–] **Contra:** Active untreated bacterial, viral, & fungal eye Infxns **Disp:** Susp & soln 0.1%; oint 0.05% **SE:** Long-term use associated w/ cataracts

Dexamethasone Systemic, Topical (Decadron) See Steroids, Systemic, page 175, & Tables 4 + 5

Dexpanthenol (Ilopan-Choline PO, Ilopan) Uses: *Minimize paralytic ileus, Rx postop distention* **Action:** Cholinergic agent **Dose:** *Adults. Relief of gas:* 2–3 tabs PO tid. *Prevent postop ileus:* 250–500 mg IM stat, repeat in 2 h, then q6h PRN. *Ileus:* 500 mg IM stat, repeat in 2 h, then q6h, PRN **Caution:** [C, ?] **Contra:** Hemophilia, mechanical obstruction **Disp:** Inj; tabs 50 mg; cream **SE:** GI cramps

Dexrazoxane (Zinecard) Uses: *Prevent anthracycline-induced (eg, doxorubicin) cardiomyopathy* **Action:** Chelates heavy metals; binds intracellular iron & prevents anthracycline-induced free radicals **Dose:** 10:1 ratio dexrazoxane:doxorubicin 30 min prior to each dose **Caution:** [C, ?] **Contra:** Component sensitivity **Disp:** Inj powder 250, 500 mg (10 mg/mL) **SE:** Myelosuppression (especially leukopenia), fever, Infxn, stomatitis, alopecia, N/V/D, mild ↑ transaminase, pain at inj site

Dextran 40 (Rheomacrodex) Uses: *Shock, prophylaxis of DVT & thromboembolism, adjunct in peripheral vascular surgery* **Action:** Expands plasma volume; ↓ blood viscosity **Dose:** *Shock:* 10 mL/kg inf rapidly; 20 mL/kg max 1st 24 h; beyond 24 h 10 mL/kg max; D/C after 5 d. *Prophylaxis of DVT & thromboembolism:* 10 mL/kg IV day of surgery, then 500 mL/d IV for 2–3 d, then 500 mL IV q2–3d based on risk for up to 2 wk **Caution:** [C, ?] Inf Rxns; pts receiving corticosteroids **Contra:** Major hemostatic defects; cardiac decompensation; renal Dz w/ severe oliguria/anuria **Disp:** 10% dextran 40 in 0.9% NaCl or 5% dextrose **SE:** Allergy/anaphylactoid Rxn (observe during 1st min of inf), arthralgia, cutaneous Rxns, ↓ BP, fever **Notes:** Monitor Cr & electrolytes; keep well hydrated

Dextromethorphan (Mediquell, Benylin DM, PediaCare 1, others) [OTC] Uses: *Control nonproductive cough* **Action:** Suppresses medullary cough center **Dose:** *Adults.* 10–30 mg PO q4h PRN (max 120 mg/24 h). *Peds.* 7 mo–1 y: 2–4 mg q6–8h. *2–6 y:* 2.5–7.5 mg q4–8h (max 30 mg/24 h). *7–12 y:* 5–10 mg q4–8h (max 60 mg/24/h) **Caution:** [C, ?/–] Not for persistent or chronic cough **Disp:** Caps 30 mg; lozenges 2.5, 5, 7.5, 15 mg; syrup 15 mg/15 mL, 10 mg/5 mL; liq 10 mg/15 mL, 3.5, 7.5, 15 mg/5 mL; sustained-action liq 30 mg/5 mL **SE:** GI disturbances **Notes:** Found in combo OTC products w/ guaifenesin

Dezocine (Dalgan) Uses: *Moderate–severe pain* Action: Narcotic agonist–antagonist Dose: 5–20 mg IM or 2.5–10 mg IV q2–4h PRN; ↓ in renal impair Caution: [C, ?] Contra: Pts <18 y Disp: Inj 5, 10, 15 mg/mL SE: Sedation, dizziness, vertigo, N/V, inj site Rxn Notes: Withdrawal possible in narcotic dependency

Diazepam (Valium) [C-IV] Uses: *Anxiety, EtOH withdrawal, muscle spasm, status epilepticus, panic disorders, amnesia, preop sedation* Action: Benzodiazepine Dose: *Adults. Status epilepticus:* 5–10 mg q10–20min to 30 mg max in 8-h period. *Anxiety, muscle spasm:* 2–10 mg PO bid–qid or IM/IV q3–4h PRN. *Preop:* 5–10 mg PO or IM 20–30 min or IV just prior to procedure. *EtOH withdrawal:* Initial 2–5 mg IV, then 5–10 mg q5–10min, 100 mg in 1 h max. May require up to 1,000 mg in 24-h period for severe withdrawal. Titrate to agitation; avoid excessive sedation; may lead to aspiration or resp arrest. *Peds. Status epilepticus:* <5 y: 0.05–0.3 mg/kg/dose IV q15–30min up to a max of 5 mg. >5 y: Give up to max of 10 mg. *Sedation, muscle relaxation:* 0.04–0.3 mg/kg/dose q2–4h IM or IV to max of 0.6 mg/kg in 8 h, or 0.12–0.8 mg/kg/24 h PO ÷ tid–qid; ↓ w/hepatic impair Caution: [D, ?/–] Contra: Coma, CNS depression, resp depression, NA glaucoma, severe uncontrolled pain, PRG Disp: Tabs 2, 5, 10 mg; soln 1, 5 mg/mL; inj 5 mg/mL; rectal gel 5 mg/mL SE: Sedation, amnesia, bradycardia, ↓ BP, rash, ↓ resp rate Notes: Do not exceed 5 mg/min IV in adults or 1–2 mg/min in peds (resp arrest possible); IM absorption erratic; avoid abrupt D/C

Diazoxide (Hyperstat, Proglycem) Uses: *Hypoglycemia due to hyperinsulinism (Proglycem); hypertensive crisis (Hyperstat)* Action: ↓ Pancreatic insulin release; antihypertensive Dose: *Hypertensive crisis:* 1–3 mg/kg IV (150 mg max in single inj); repeat in 5–15 min until BP controlled; repeat every 4–24 h; monitor BP closely. *Hypoglycemia:* **Adults & Peds.** 3–8 mg/kg/24 h PO ÷ q8–12h. *Neonates.* 8–15 mg/kg/24 h ÷ in 3 equal doses; maint 8–10 mg/kg/24 h PO in 2–3 equal doses Caution: [C, ?] ↓ effect w/ phenytoin; ↑ effect w/ diuretics, warfarin Contra: Allergy to thiazides or other sulfonamide-containing products; HTN associated w/ aortic coarctation, AV shunt, or pheochromocytoma Disp: Inj 15 mg/mL; caps 50 mg; PO susp 50 mg/mL SE: Hyperglycemia, ↓ BP, dizziness, Na+ & H2O retention, N/V, weakness Notes: Can give false-negative insulin response to glucagons; treat extravasation w/ warm compress

Dibucaine (Nupercainal) Uses: *Hemorrhoids & minor skin conditions* Action: Topical anesthetic Dose: Insert PR w/ applicator bid & after each bowel movement; apply sparingly to skin Caution: [C, ?] Contra: Component sensitivity Disp: 1% Oint w/ rectal applicator; 0.5% cream SE: Local irritation, rash

Diclofenac (Cataflam, Voltaren) WARNING: May ↑risk of cardiovascular events & GI bleeding Uses: *Arthritis & pain* Action: NSAID Dose: 50–75 mg PO bid; w/ food or milk Caution: [B (D 3rd tri or near delivery), ?] CHF, HTN, renal/hepatic dysfunction, & Hx PUD Contra: NSAID/aspirin allergy; porphyria Disp: Tabs 50 mg; tabs DR 25, 50, 75, 100 mg; XR tabs 100 mg; ophthal soln 0.1% **SE:** Abdominal cramps, heartburn, GI ulceration, rash, interstitial nephritis **Notes:** Do not crush; watch for GI bleed

Dicloxacillin (Dynapen, Dycill) **Uses:** *Rx of pneumonia, skin, & soft tissue Infxns, & osteomyelitis caused by penicillinase-producing staphylococci* **Action:** Bactericidal; ↓ cell wall synthesis. *Spectrum: S. aureus & Strep* **Dose:** *Adults.* 250–500 mg qid *Peds <40 kg.* 12.5–25 mg/kg/d ÷ qid; take on empty stomach **Caution:** [B, ?] **Contra:** Component or PCN sensitivity **Disp:** Caps 125, 250, 500 mg; soln 62.5 mg/5 mL **SE:** N/D, abdominal pain **Notes:** Monitor PTT if pt on warfarin

Dicyclomine (Bentyl) **Uses:** *Functional IBS* **Action:** Smooth-muscle relaxant **Dose:** Adults. 20 mg PO qid; ↑ to 160 mg/d max or 20 mg IM q6h *Peds.* Infants >6 mo: 5 mg/dose tid–qid. *Children:* 10 mg/dose tid–qid **Caution:** [B, –] **Contra:** Infants < 6 mo, NA glaucoma, MyG, severe UC, BOO **Disp:** Caps 10, 20 mg; tabs 20 mg; syrup 10 mg/5 mL; inj 10 mg/mL **SE:** Anticholinergic SEs may limit dose **Notes:** Take 30–60 min before meal; avoid EtOH

Didanosine [ddI] (Videx) **WARNING:** Allergy manifested as fever, rash, fatigue, GI/resp Sxs reported; stop drug immediately & do not rechallenge; lactic acidosis & hepatomegaly/steatosis reported **Uses:** *HIV Infxn in zidovudine-intolerant pts* **Action:** Nucleoside antiretroviral agent **Dose:** Adults. >60 kg: 400 mg/d PO or 200 mg PO bid. *<60 kg:* 250 mg/d PO or 125 mg PO bid; adults should take 2 tabs/administration. *Peds.* Dose by following table; ↓ in renal Impair:

Peds Didanosine Dosing

BSA (m²)	Tablets (mg)	Powder (mg)
1.1–1.4	100 bid	125 bid
0.8–1	75 bid	94 bid
0.5–0.7	50 bid	62 bid
<0.4	25 bid	31 bid

Caution: [B, –] CDC recommends HIV-infected mothers not breast-feed (risk of HIV transmission) **Contra:** Component sensitivity **Disp:** Chew tabs 25, 50, 100, 150, 200 mg; powder packets 100, 167, 250, 375 mg; powder for soln 2, 4 g **SE:** Pancreatitis, peripheral neuropathy, D, HA **Notes:** Do not take w/ meals; thoroughly chew tablets, do not mix w/ fruit juice or acidic beverages; reconstitute powder w/ H_2O

Diflunisal (Dolobid) **WARNING:** May ↑risk of cardiovascular events & GI bleeding **Uses:** *Mild–moderate pain; osteoarthritis* **Action:** NSAID **Dose:** *Pain:* 500 mg PO bid. *Osteoarthritis:* 500–1500 mg PO in 2–3 ÷ doses; ↓ in renal impair, take w/ food/milk **Caution:** [C (D 3rd tri or near delivery), ?] CHF, HTN, renal/hepatic dysfunction, & Hx PUD. **Contra:** Allergy to NSAIDs or aspirin, active GI bleed **Disp:** Tabs 250, 500 mg **SE:** May ↑ bleeding time; HA, abdominal cramps, heartburn, GI ulceration, rash, interstitial nephritis, fluid retention

Digoxin (Lanoxin, Lanoxicaps) Uses: *CHF, AF & flutter, & PAT* **Action:** Positive inotrope; ↑ AV node refractory period **Dose:** *Adults.* PO digitalization: 0.5–0.75 mg PO, then 0.25 mg PO q6–8h to total 1–1.5 mg. *IV or IM digitalization:* 0.25–0.5 mg IM or IV, then 0.25 mg q4–6h to total ≅1 mg. *Daily maint:* 0.125–0.5 mg/d PO, IM, or IV (average daily dose 0.125–0.25 mg). *Peds.* Preterm infants: Digitalization: 30 mcg/kg PO or 25 mcg/kg IV; give 1/2 of dose initial, then 1/4 of dose at 8–12-h intervals for 2 doses. *Maint:* 5–7.5 mcg/kg/24 h PO or 4–6 mcg/ kg/24 h IV ÷ q12h. *Term infants: Digitalization:* 25–35 mcg/kg PO or 20–30 mcg/kg IV; give ½ the initial dose , then ⅓ of dose at 8–12 h. *Maint:* 6–10 mcg/kg/24 h PO or 5–8 mcg/kg/24 h ÷ q12h. *1 mo–2 y: Digitalization:* 35–60 mcg/kg PO or 30–50 mcg/kg IV; give 1/2 the initial dose, then 1/3 dose at 8–12-h intervals for 2 doses. *Maint:* 10–15 mcg/kg/24 h PO or 7.5–15 mcg/kg/24 h IV ÷ q12h. *2–10 y: Digitalization:* 30–40 mcg/kg PO or 25 mcg/kg IV; give ½ initial dose, then ⅓ of the dose at 8–12-h intervals for 2 doses. *Maint:* 8–10 mcg/kg/24 h PO or 6–8 mcg/kg/24 h IV ÷ q12h. *7–10 y:* Same as for adults; ↓ in renal impair **Caution:** [C, +] **Contra:** AV block; idiopathic hypertrophic subaortic stenosis; constrictive pericarditis **Disp:** Caps 0.05, 0.1, 0.2 mg; tabs 0.125, 0.25, 0.5 mg; elixir 0.05 mg/mL; inj 0.1, 0.25 mg/mL **SE:** Can cause heart block; ↓ K+ potentiates tox; N/V, HA, fatigue, visual disturbances (yellow-green halos around lights), cardiac arrhythmias **Notes:** Multiple drug interactions; IM inj painful, has erratic absorption & should not be used; follow serum levels (Table 2).

Digoxin Immune Fab (Digibind) Uses: *Life-threatening digoxin intox* **Action:** Antigen-binding fragments bind & inactivate digoxin **Dose:** *Adults & Peds.* Based on serum level & pt's weight; see charts provided w/ drug **Caution:** [C, ?] **Contra:** Sheep product allergy **Disp:** Inj 38,–40 mg/vial **SE:** Worsening of cardiac output or CHF, ↓ K+, facial swelling, & redness **Notes:** Each vial binds ≅0.6 mg of digoxin; renal failure may require redosing in several days

Diltiazem (Cardizem, Cardizem CD, Cardizem SR, Cartia XT, Dilacor XR, Diltia XT, Tiamate, Tiazac) Uses: *Angina, prevention of reinfarction, HTN, AF or flutter, & PAT* **Action:** CCB **Dose:** *PO:* Initial, 30 mg PO qid; ↑ to 180–360 mg/d in 3–4 ÷ doses PRN. SR: 60–120 mg PO bid; ↑ to 360 mg/d max. *CD or XR:* 120–360 mg/d (max 480 mg/d). *IV:* 0.25 mg/kg IV bolus over 2 min; may repeat in 15 min at 0.35 mg/kg; begin inf of 5–15 mg/h **Caution:** [C, +] ↑ effect w/ amiodarone, cimetidine, fentanyl, lithium, cyclosporine, digoxin, β-blockers, cisapride, theophylline **Contra:** SSS, AV block, ↓ BP, AMI, pulmonary congestion **Disp:** *Cardizem CD:* Caps 120, 180, 240, 300, 360 mg; *Cardizem SR:* caps 60, 90, 120 mg; *Cardizem:* Tabs 30, 60, 90, 120 mg; *Cartia XT:* Caps 120, 180, 240, 300 mg; *Dilacor XR:* Caps 180, 240 mg; *Diltia XT:* Caps 120, 180, 240 mg; *Tiazac:* Caps 120, 180, 240, 300, 360, 420 mg; *Tiamate (XR):* Tabs 120, 180, 240 mg; inj 5 mg/mL **SE:** Gingival hyperplasia, bradycardia, AV block, ECG abnormalities, peripheral edema, dizziness, HA **Notes:** Cardizem CD, Dilacor XR, & Tiazac not interchangeable

Dimenhydrinate (Dramamine, others)
Uses: *Prevention & Rx of N/V, dizziness, or vertigo of motion sickness* **Action:** Antiemetic **Dose:** *Adults.* 50–100 mg PO q4–6h, max 400 mg/d; 50 mg IM/IV PRN. *Peds.* 2–6 yrs: 12.5–25 mg Q6–8 h max 75 mg/day, *6–12 yrs:* 25–50 mg q6–8h max 150 mg/d; 1.25 mg/kg or 37.5/mg/m² IM q6h 300 mg/day max **Caution:** [B, ?] **Contra:** Component sensitivity **Disp:** Tabs 50 mg; chew tabs 50 mg; liq 12.5 mg/4 mL, 12.5 mg/5 mL, 15.62 mg/5 mL; inj 50 mg/mL **SE:** Anticholinergic side effects

Dimethyl Sulfoxide [DMSO] (Rimso 50)
Uses: *Interstitial cystitis* **Action:** Unknown **Dose:** Intravesical, 50 mL, retain for 15 min; repeat q2wk until relief **Caution:** [C, ?] **Contra:** Component sensitivity **Disp:** 50% & 100% soln **SE:** Cystitis, eosinophilia, GI, & taste disturbance

Dinoprostone (Cervidil Vaginal Insert, Prepidil Vaginal Gel)
Uses: *Induce labor; terminate PRG (12–20 wk); evacuate uterus in missed abortion or fetal death* **Action:** Prostaglandin, changes consistency, dilatation, & effacement of the cervix; induces uterine contraction **Dose:** *Gel:* 0.5 mg; if no cervical/uterine response, repeat 0.5 mg q6h (max 24-h dose 1.5 mg). *Vaginal insert:* 1 insert (10 mg = 0.3 mg dinoprostone/h over 12 h); remove w/ onset of labor or 12 h after insertion. *Vaginal supp:* 20 mg repeated every 3–5 h; adjust PRN supp: 1 high in vagina, repeat at 3–5-h intervals until abortion (240 mg max) **Caution:** [X, ?] **Contra:** Ruptured membranes, allergy to prostaglandins, placenta previa or unexplained vaginal bleeding, when oxytocic drugs contraindicated or if prolonged uterine contractions are inappropriate (Hx C-section, cephalopelvic disproportion, etc) **Disp:** *Endocervical gel:* 0.5 mg in 3-g syringes (w/10-mm & 20-mm shielded catheter) *Vaginal gel:* 0.5 mg/3 g *Vaginal supp:* 20 mg *Vaginal insert, CR:* 0.3 mg/h **SE:** N/V/D, dizziness, flushing, HA, fever

Diphenhydramine (Benadryl) [OTC]
Uses: *Rx & prevent allergic Rxns, motion sickness, potentiate narcotics, sedation, cough suppression, & Rx of extrapyramidal Rxns* **Action:** Antihistamine, antiemetic **Dose:** *Adults.* 25–50 mg PO, IV, or IM bid–tid. *Peds.* 5 mg/kg/24 h PO or IM ÷ q6h (max 300 mg/d); ↑ dosing interval w/ moderate–severe renal insuff **Caution:** [B, –] **Contra:** in acute asthma attack **Disp:** Tabs & caps 25, 50 mg; chew tabs 12.5 mg; elixir 12.5 mg/5 mL; syrup 12.5 mg/5 mL; liq 6.25 mg/5 mL, 12.5 mg/5 mL; inj 50 mg/mL **SE:** Anticholinergic (xerostomia, urinary retention, sedation)

Diphenoxylate + Atropine (Lomotil) [C-V]
Uses: *D* **Action:** Constipating meperidine congener, ↓ GI motility **Dose:** *Adults.* Initial, 5 mg PO tid–qid until controlled, then 2.5–5 mg PO bid. *Peds >2 y:* 0.3–0.4 mg/kg/24 h (of diphenoxylate) bid–qid **Caution:** [C, +] **Contra:** Obstructive jaundice, diarrhea due to bacterial Infxn; children <2 y **Disp:** Tabs 2.5 mg diphenoxylate/0.025 mg at-

ropine; liq 2.5 mg diphenoxylate/0.025 mg atropine/5 mL **SE:** Drowsiness, dizziness, xerostomia, blurred vision, urinary retention, constipation

Diphtheria, Tetanus Toxoids, & Acellular pertussis adsorbed, Hepatitis B (Recombinant), & Inactivated Poliovirus Vaccine [IPV] combined (Pediarix) **Uses:** *Vaccine against diphtheria, tetanus, pertussis, HBV, polio (types 1, 2, 3) as a 3-dose primary series in infants & children <7, born to HBsAg– mothers* **Actions:** Active immunization **Dose:** *Infants:* Three 0.5-mL doses IM, at 6–8-wk intervals, start at 2 mo; child given 1 dose of hep B vaccine, same; previously vaccinated w/ one or more doses IPV, use to complete series **Caution:** [C, N/A] **Contra:** HbsAG+ mother, adults, children >7 y, immunosuppressed, allergy to yeast, neomycin, polymyxin B,or any component, encephalopathy, or progressive neurologic disorders; caution in bleeding disorders. **Disp:** Single-dose vials 0.5 mL **SE:** Drowsiness, restlessness, fever, fussiness, ↓ appetite, nodule redness, inj site pain/swelling **Notes:** Give IM only

Dipivefrin (Propine) **Uses:** *Open-angle glaucoma* **Action:** α-Adrenergic agonist **Dose:** 1 gtt in eye q12h **Caution:** [B, ?] **Contra:** Closed-angle glaucoma **Disp:** 0.1% soln **SE:** HA, local irritation, blurred vision, photophobia, HTN

Dipyridamole (Persantine) **Uses:** *Prevent postop thromboembolic disorders, often in combo w/ ASA or warfarin (eg, CABG, vascular graft); w/ warfarin after artificial heart valve; chronic angina; w/ ASA to prevent coronary artery thrombosis; dipyridamole IV used in place of exercise stress test for CAD* **Action:** Anti-plt activity; coronary vasodilator **Dose:** *Adults.* 75–100 mg PO tid–qid; stress test 0.14 mg/kg/min (max 60 mg over 4 min). *Peds >12 y.* 3–6 mg/kg/d divided tid (safety/efficacy not established) **Caution:** [B, ?/–] w/ other drugs that affect coagulation **Contra:** Component sensitivity **Disp:** Tabs 25, 50, 75 mg; inj 5 mg/mL **SE:** HA, ↓ BP, nausea, abdominal distress, flushing rash, dyspnea **Notes:** IV use can worsen angina

Dipyridamole & Aspirin (Aggrenox) **Uses:** *↓ Reinfarction after MI; prevent occlusion after CABG; ↓ risk of stroke* **Action:** ↓ Plt aggregation (both agents) **Dose:** 1 cap PO bid **Caution:** [C, ?] **Contra:** Ulcers, bleeding diathesis **Disp:** Dipyridamole (XR) 200 mg/aspirin 25 mg **SE:** ASA component: allergic Rxns, skin Rxns, ulcers/GI bleed, bronchospasm; dipyridamole component: dizziness, HA, nausea **Notes:** Swallow capsule whole

Dirithromycin (Dynabac) **Uses:** *Bronchitis, community-acquired pneumonia, & skin & skin structure Infxns* **Action:** Macrolide antibiotic. *Spectrum: M. catarrhalis, Streptococcus pneumoniae, Legionella, H. influenzae, S. pyogenes, S. aureus* **Dose:** 500 mg/d PO; w/ food; swallow whole **Caution:** [C, M] **Contra:** w/ pimozide **Disp:** Tabs 250 mg **SE:** Abdominal discomfort, HA, rash, ↑ K+

Disopyramide (Norpace, NAPamide) **Uses:** *Suppression & prevention of VT* **Action:** Class 1A antiarrhythmic **Dose:** *Adults.* 400–800 mg/d ÷ q6h for regular & q12h for SR. *Peds.* <1 y: 10–30 mg/kg/24 h PO ÷ qid). *1–4 y:* 10–20 mg/kg/24 h PO (÷ qid). *4–12 y:* 10–15 mg/kg/24 h PO (÷ qid). *12–18 y:*

6–15 mg/kg/24 h PO (÷ qid); ↓ in renal/hepatic impair **Caution:** [C, +] **Contra:** AV block, cardiogenic shock **Disp:** Caps 100, 150 mg; SR caps 100, 150 mg **SE:** Anticholinergic SEs; negative inotrope, may induce CHF **Notes:** Check levels (Table 2).

Dobutamine (Dobutrex) **Uses:** *Short-term in cardiac decompensation secondary to depressed contractility* **Action:** Positive inotrope **Dose:** *Adults & Peds.* Cont IV inf of 2.5–15 mcg/kg/min; rarely, 40 mcg/kg/min required; titrate **Caution:** [C, ?] **Contra:** Sensitivity to sulfites, IHSS **Disp:** Inj 250 mg/20 mL **SE:** Chest pain, HTN, dyspnea **Notes:** Monitor PWP & cardiac output if possible, check ECG for ↑ heart rate, ectopic activity; follow BP

Docetaxel (Taxotere) **Uses:** *Breast (anthracycline-resistant), ovarian, lung, & prostate CA* **Action:** Antimitotic agent; promotes microtubular aggregation; semisynthetic taxoid **Dose:** 100 mg/m² over 1 h IV q3wk (Per protocols); dexamethasone 8 mg bid prior & continue for 3–4 d; ↓ dose w/ ↑ bilirubin levels **Caution:** [D, –] **Contra:** Component sensitivity **Disp:** Inj 20, 40, 80 mg/mL **SE:** Myelosuppression, neuropathy, N/V, alopecia, fluid retention syndrome; cumulative doses of 300–400 mg/m² w/o steroid prep & posttreatment & 600–800 mg/m² w/ steroid prep; allergy possible (rare w/ steroid prep)

Docusate Calcium (Surfak)/Docusate Potassium (Dialose)/ Docusate Sodium (DOSS, Colace) **Uses:** *Constipation; adjunct to painful anorectal conditions (hemorrhoids)* **Action:** Stool softener **Dose:** *Adults.* 50–500 mg PO ÷ daily qid. *Peds.* Infants–3 y: 10–40 mg/24 h ÷ daily–qid. *3–6 y:* 20–60 mg/24 h ÷ daily–qid. *6–12 y:* 40–120 mg/24 h ÷ daily–qid **Caution:** [C, ?] **Contra:** Use w/mineral oil; intestinal obstruction, acute abdominal pain, N/V **Disp:** *Ca:* Caps 50, 240 mg. *K:* Caps 100, 240 mg. *Na:* Caps 50, 100 mg; syrup 50, 60 mg/15 mL; liq 150 mg/15 mL; soln 50 mg/mL **SE:** Rare abdominal cramping, D; **Notes:** Take w/ full glass of H₂O; no laxative action; do not use >1 wk

Dofetilide (Tikosyn) **WARNING:** To minimize the risk of induced arrhythmia, pts initiated or reinitiated on Tikosyn should be placed for a minimum of 3 d in a facility that can provide calculations of CrCl, continuous ECG monitoring, & cardiac resuscitation **Uses:** *Maintain normal sinus rhythm in AF/A flutter after conversion* **Action:** Type III antiarrhythmic **Dose:** 125–500 mcg PO bid based on CrCl & QTc (see insert) **Caution:** [C, –] **Contra:** Baseline QTc is > 440 ms (500 ms w/ ventricular conduction abnormalities) or CrCl < 20 mL/min; w/verapamil, cimetidine, trimethoprim, or ketoconazole **Disp:** Caps 125, 250, 500 mcg **SE:** Ventricular arrhythmias, HA, CP, dizziness **Notes:** Avoid w/ other drugs that ↑ QT interval; hold class I or III antiarrhythmics for at least 3 ½-lives prior to dofetilide; amiodarone level should be <0.3 mg/L prior to dosing

Dolasetron (Anzemet) **Uses:** *Prevent chemo-associated N/V* **Action:** 5-HT₃ receptor antagonist **Dose:** *Adults & Peds.* IV: 1.8 mg/kg IV as single dose 30 min prior to chemo **Adults.** PO: 100 mg PO as a single dose 1 h prior to chemo

Peds. PO: 1.8 mg/kg PO to max 100 mg as single dose **Caution:** [B, ?] **Contra:** Component sensitivity **Disp:** Tabs 50, 100 mg; inj 20 mg/mL **SE:** ↑ QT interval, HTN, HA, abdominal pain, urinary retention, transient ↑ LFTs

Dopamine (Intropin) Uses: *Short-term use in cardiac decompensation secondary to ↓ contractility; ↑ organ perfusion (at low dose)* **Action:** Positive inotropic agent w/ dose response: 2–10 mcg/kg/min β-effects (↑ CO & renal perfusion); 10–20 mcg/kg/min β-effects (peripheral vasoconstriction, pressor); >20 mcg/kg/min peripheral & renal vasoconstriction **Dose:** *Adults & Peds.* 5 mcg/kg/min by cont inf, ↑ by 5 mcg/kg/min to 50 mcg/kg/min max to effect **Caution:** [C, ?] **Contra:** Pheochromocytoma, VF, sulfite sensitivity **Disp:** Inj 40, 80, 160 mg/mL **SE:** Tachycardia, vasoconstriction, ↓ BP, HA, N/V, dyspnea **Notes:** >10 mcg/kg/min may ↓ renal perfusion; monitor urinary output & ECG for ↑ heart rate, BP, ectopy; monitor PCWP & cardiac output if possible

Dornase Alfa (Pulmozyme) Uses: *↓ Frequency of resp Infxns in CF* **Action:** Enzyme that selectively cleaves DNA **Dose:** Inhal 2.5 mg/d, BID dosing w/ FVC >85% w/ recommended nebulizer **Caution:** [B, ?] **Contra:** Chinese hamster product allergy **Disp:** Soln for inhal 1 mg/mL **SE:** Pharyngitis, voice alteration, CP, rash

Dorzolamide (Trusopt) Uses: *Glaucoma* **Action:** Carbonic anhydrase inhibitor **Dose:** 1 gtt in eye(s) tid **Caution:** [C, ?] **Contra:** Component sensitivity **Disp:** 2% soln **SE:** irritation, bitter taste, punctate keratitis, ocular allergic Rxn

Dorzolamide & Timolol (Cosopt) Uses: *Glaucoma* **Action:** Carbonic anhydrase inhibitor w/ β-adrenergic blocker **Dose:** 1 gtt in eye(s) bid **Caution:** [C, ?] **Contra:** Component sensitivity **Disp:** Soln dorzolamide 2% & timolol 0.5% **SE:** irritation, bitter taste, superficial keratitis, ocular allergic Rxn

Doxazosin (Cardura, Cardura XL) Uses: *HTN & symptomatic BPH* **Action:** α₁-Adrenergic blocker; relaxes bladder neck smooth muscle **Dose:** *HTN:* Initial 1 mg/d PO; may be ↑ to 16 mg/d PO. *BPH:* Initial 1 mg/d PO, may ↑ to 8 mg/d; XL 2–8mg Q AM **Caution:** [B, ?] **Contra:** Component sensitivity **Disp:** Tabs 1, 2, 4, 8 mg; XL 4, 8 mg **SE:** Dizziness, HA, drowsiness, sexual dysfunction, doses >4 mg ↑ postural ↓ BP risk **Notes:** First dose hs; syncope may occur w/in 90 mins of initial dose

Doxepin (Sinequan, Adapin) WARNING: Closely monitor for worsening depression or emergence of suicidality Uses: *Depression, anxiety, chronic pain* **Action:** TCA; ↑ synaptic CNS serotonin or norepinephrine **Dose:** 25–150 mg/d PO, usually hs but can ÷ doses; up to 300 mg/day for depression ↓ in hepatic impair **Caution:** [C, ?/–] **Contra:** NA glaucoma **Disp:** Caps 10, 25, 50, 75, 100, 150 mg; PO conc 10 mg/mL **SE:** Anticholinergic SEs, ↓ BP, tachycardia, drowsiness, photosensitivity

Doxepin, Topical (Zonalon) Uses: *Short-term Rx pruritus (atopic dermatitis or lichen simplex chronicus)* **Action:** Antipruritic; H₁- & H₂-receptor antagonism **Dose:** Apply thin coating qid, 8 d max **Caution:** [C, ?/–] **Contra:**

Drotrecogin Alfa

Component sensitivity **Disp:** 5% cream **SE:** ↓ BP, tachycardia, drowsiness, photosensitivity **Notes:** Limit application area to avoid systemic tox

Doxorubicin (Adriamycin, Rubex) Uses: *Acute leukemias; Hodgkin Dz & NHLs; soft tissue, osteo & Ewing's sarcoma; Wilms' tumor; neuroblastoma; bladder, breast, ovarian, gastric, thyroid, & lung CAs* **Action:** Intercalates DNA; ↓ DNA topoisomerases I & II **Dose:** 60–75 mg/m² q3wk; ↓ cardiotox w/ weekly (20 mg/m²/wk) or cont inf (60–90 mg/m² over 96 h); (per protocols) **Caution:** [D, ?] **Contra:** Severe CHF, cardiomyopathy, preexisting myelosuppression, previous Rx w/ complete cumulative doses of doxorubicin, idarubicin, daunorubicin **Disp:** Inj 10, 20, 50, 75, 200 mg **SE:** Myelosuppression, venous streaking & phlebitis, N/V/D, mucositis, radiation recall phenomenon, cardiomyopathy rare(dose-related); limit of 550 mg/m² cumulative dose (400 mg/m² w/prior mediastinal irradiation) **Notes:** Dexrazoxane may limit cardiac tox; tissue damage w/extravasation; discolors urine red/orange

Doxycycline (Vibramycin, Vibra-Tabs) Uses: *Broad-spectrum antibiotic *acne vulgaris, uncomplicated GC, chalymidia, PID, Lyme disease, skin infections, anthrax, malaria prophylaxis **Action:** Tetracycline; bacteriostatic; ↓ protein synthesis. *Spectrum: some gram (+) and (-)Rickettsia* sp, *Chlamydia, M. pneumoniae, B. Anthraxus* **Dose:** *Adults.* 100 mg PO q12h on 1st d, then 100 mg PO daily–bid or 100 mg IV q12h; acne QD dosing, chlamydia 7d, Lyme disease 14-21 d, PID 14 d *Peds >8y.* 5 mg/kg/24 h PO, to a max of 200 mg/d ÷ daily–bid **Caution:** [D, +] hepatic impair **Contra:** Children <8 y, severe hepatic dysfunction **Disp:** Tabs 50, 75, 100, 150 mg; caps 50, 100 mg; syrup 50 mg/5 mL; susp 25 mg/5 mL; inj 100, 200 mg/vial **SE:** D, GI disturbance, photosensitivity **Notes:** ↓ effect w/ antacids; tetracycline of choice w/in renal impair; for inhalational anthrax use w/ 1–2 additional antibiotics, not for CNS anthrax

Dronabinol (Marinol) [C-II] Uses: *N/V associated w/ CA chemo; appetite stimulation* **Action:** Antiemetic; ↓ vomiting center in the medulla **Dose:** *Adults & Peds.* Antiemetic: 5–15 mg/m²/dose q4–6h PRN. *Adults.* Appetite stimulant: 2.5 mg PO before lunch & dinner; max 20mg/day **Caution:** [C, ?] **Contra:** Hx schizophrenia **Disp:** Caps 2.5, 5, 10 mg **SE:** Drowsiness, dizziness, anxiety, mood change, hallucinations, depersonalization, orthostatic ↓ BP, tachycardia **Notes:** Principal psychoactive substance present in marijuana

Droperidol (Inapsine) Uses: *N/V; anesthetic premedication* **Action:** Tranquilizer, sedation, antiemetic **Dose:** *Adults.* Nausea: initial max 2.5 mg IV/IM, may repeat 1.25 mg based on response; *Premed:* 2.5–10 mg IV, 30–60 min preop. *Peds.* Premed: 0.1–0.15 mg/kg/dose **Caution:** [C, ?] **Contra:** Component sensitivity **Disp:** Inj 2.5 mg/mL **SE:** Drowsiness, ↓ BP, occasional tachycardia & extrapyramidal Rxns, ↑ QT interval, arrhythmias **Notes:** Give IVP slowly over 2–5 min

Drotrecogin Alfa (Xigris) Uses: *↓ Mortality in adults w/ severe sepsis (w/ acute organ dysfunction) at high risk of death (eg, determined by APACHE II WWW.NCEMI.ORG)* **Action:** Recombinant human-activated protein C; ? mechanism **Dose:** 24 mcg/kg/h, total of 96 h **Caution:** [C, ?] **Contra:** Active bleeding, recent stroke/CNS surgery, head trauma or CNS lesion W/ herniation risk, epidural catheter **Disp:** 5-, 20-mg vials **SE:** Bleeding **Notes:** W/ single organ dysfunction & recent surgery may not be at high risk of death irrespective of APACHE II score & therefore not indicated. *Percutaneous procedures:* Stop inf 2 h before the procedure & resume 1 h after; major surgery: stop inf 2 h before surgery & resume 12 h after surgery in absence of bleeding

Duloxetine (Cymbalta) WARNING: Antidepressants may ↑ risk of suicidality; consider risks/benefits of use. Closely monitor for clinical worsening, suicidality, or behavior changes **Uses:** *Depression, DM peripheral neuropathic pain* **Action:** Selective serotonin & norepinephrine reuptake inhibitor (SSNRI) **Dose:** *Depression:* 40–60 mg/d PO ÷ bid. *DM neuropathy:* 60 mg/d PO; **Caution:** [C, ?/–]; use in 3rd tri; avoid if CrCl <30 mL/min, NA glaucoma, w/fluvoxamine, inhibitors of CYP2D6 (Table 13), TCAs, phenothiazines, type 1C antiarrhythmics **Contra:** MAOI use w/in 14 d, w/ thioridazine, NA glaucoma, hepatic insuff **Disp:** Caps delayed-release 20, 30, 60 mg **SE:** N, dizziness, somnolence, fatigue, sweating, xerostomia, constipation, decreased appetite, sexual dysfunction, urinary hesitancy, ↑ LFTs, HTN **Notes:** Swallow whole; monitor BP; avoid abrupt D/C

Dutasteride (Avodart) **Uses:** *Symptomatic BPH* **Action:** 5α-Reductase inhibitor **Dose:** 0.5 mg PO daily **Caution:** [X, –] Hepatic impair; pregnant women should not handle pills **Contra:** Women & children **Disp:** Caps 0.5 mg **SE:** ↓ PSA levels, impotence, ↓ libido, gynecomastia **Notes:** No blood donation until 6 mo after stopping

Echothiophate Iodine (Phospholine Ophthalmic) **Uses:** *Glaucoma* **Action:** Cholinesterase inhibitor **Dose:** 1 gtt eye(s) bid w/ one dose hs **Caution:** [C, ?] **Contra:** Active uveal inflammation or any inflammatory Dz of iris/ciliary body, glaucoma iridocyclitis **Disp:** Powder to reconstitute 1.5 mg/0.03%; 3 mg/ 0.06%; 6.25 mg/0.125%; 12.5 mg/0.25% **SE:** Local irritation, myopia, blurred vision, ↓ BP, bradycardia

Econazole (Spectazole) **Uses:** *Tinea, cutaneous Candida, & tinea versicolor Infxns* **Action:** Topical antifungal **Dose:** Apply to areas bid (QD for tinea versicolor) for 2–4 wk **Caution:** [C, ?] **Contra:** Component sensitivity **Disp:** Topical cream 1% **SE:** Local irritation, pruritus, erythema **Notes:** Early symptom/clinical improvement; complete course to avoid recurrence

Edrophonium (Tensilon) **Uses:** *Diagnosis of MyG; acute MyG crisis; curare antagonist* **Action:** Anticholinesterase **Dose:** Adults. Test for MyG: 2 mg IV in 1 min; if tolerated, give 8 mg IV; (+) test is brief ↑ in strength. *Peds.* Test for MyG: Total dose 0.2 mg/kg; 0.04 mg/kg test dose; if no Rxn, give remainder in 1-mg increments to 10 mg max; ↓ in renal impair **Caution:** [C, ?] **Contra:** GI or GU obstruction; allergy to sulfite **Disp:** Inj 10 mg/mL **SE:** N/V/D, excessive salivation, stomach cramps, ↑ aminotransferases **Notes:** Can cause severe cholinergic effects; keep atropine available

Efalizumab (Raptiva) **WARNING:** Associated w/ serious Infxns, malignancy, thrombocytopenia **Uses:** Chronic moderate–severe plaque psoriasis **Action:** MoAb **Dose:** *Adults.* 0.7 mg/kg SQ conditioning dose, followed by 1 mg/kg/wk; single doses should not exceed 200 mg **Caution:** [C, +/–] **Contra:** Admin of most vaccines **Disp:** 125-mg vial **SE:** First-dose Rxn, HA, worsening psoriasis, ↑ LFT, immunosuppressive-related Rxns (see Warning) **Notes:** Minimize 1st-dose Rxn by conditioning dose; plts monthly, then every 3 mo & w/ dose ↑; pts may be trained in self-admin

Efavirenz (Sustiva) **Uses:** *HIV Infxns* **Action:** Antiretroviral; nonnucleoside RTI **Dose:** *Adults.* 600 mg/d PO q hs. *Peds.* See insert; avoid high-fat meals **Caution:** [D,?] CDC recommends HIV-infected mothers not breast-feed (risk of HIV transmission) **Contra:** Component sensitivity **Disp:** Caps 50, 100, 200, 600 mg tab **SE:** Somnolence, vivid dreams, dizziness, rash, N/V/D **Notes:** Monitor LFT, cholesterol

Efavirenz, emtricitabine, tenofovir (Atripla) **WARNING:** Lactic acidosis and severe hepatomegaly with steatosis, including fatal cases, have been reported with the use of nucleoside analogs alone or in combination with other antiretrovirals **Uses:** *HIV Infxns* **Action:** Triple fixed-dose combination antiretroviral **Dose:** *Adults.* 1 tab QD on empty stomach; HS dose may ↓ CNS effects **Caution:** [D, ?] CDC recommends HIV-infected mothers not breast-feed (risk of HIV transmission) **Contra:** <18 yrs, component sensitivity, w/ astemizole, cisapride, midazolam, triazolam or ergot derivatives (competition for CYP3A4 by efavirenz could result in serious and/or life-threatening SE **Disp:** Tab containing efavirenz 600 mg/emtricitabine 200 mg/tenofovir/300 mg **SE:** Somnolence, vivid dreams, HA, dizziness, rash, N/V/D **Notes:** Monitor LFT, cholesterol; see individual agents for additional info

Eletriptan (Relpax) **Uses:** *Acute Rx of migraine* **Action:** Selective serotonin receptor (5-HT$_1$B/$_1$D) agonist **Dose:** 20–40 mg PO, may repeat in 2 h; 80 mg/24h max **Caution:** [C, +] **Contra:** Hx ischemic heart Dz, coronary artery spasm, stroke or TIA, peripheral vascular Dz, IBD, uncontrolled HTN, hemiplegic or basilar migraine, severe hepatic impair, w/in 24 h of another 5-HT$_1$ agonist or ergot, w/in 72 h of CYP3A4 inhibitors **Disp:** Tabs 20, 40 mg **SE:** Dizziness, somnolence, N, asthenia, xerostomia, paresthesias; pain, pressure, or tightness in chest, jaw or neck; serious cardiac events

Emedastine (Emadine) **Uses:** *Allergic conjunctivitis* **Action:** Antihistamine; selective H$_1$-antagonist **Dose:** 1 gtt in eye(s) up to qid **Caution:** [B, ?] **Contra:** Allergy to ingredients (preservatives benzalkonium, tromethamine) **Disp:** 0.05% soln **SE:** HA, blurred vision, burning/stinging, corneal infiltrates/staining, dry eyes, foreign body sensation, hyperemia, keratitis, tearing, pruritus, rhinitis, sinusitis, asthenia, bad taste, dermatitis, discomfort **Notes:** Do not use contact lenses if eyes are red

Emtricitabine (Emtriva) **WARNING:** Class warning for lipodystrophy, lactic acidosis, & severe hepatomegaly **Uses:** HIV-1 Infxn **Action:** Nucleoside RT inhibitor (NRTI) **Dose:** 200 mg cap or 240 mg sol PO daily; ↓ w/in renal impair **Caution:** [B, –] risk of liver dz **Contra:** Component sensitivity **Disp:** Solution: 10 mg/mL, 200 mg caps **SE:** HA, D, N, rash, rare hyperpigmentation of feet & hands, posttreatment exacerbation of hepatitis **Notes:** First one-daily NRTI; caps/sol not equivalent; not rec as monotherapy; screen for HepB

Enalapril (Vasotec) **Uses:** *HTN, CHF, LVD,* DN **Action:** ACE inhibitor **Dose:** *Adults.* 2.5–40 mg/d PO; 1.25 mg IV q6h. *Peds.* 0.05–0.08 mg/kg/dose PO q12–24h; ↓ w/renal impair **Caution:** [C (1st tri; D 2nd & 3rd tri), +] w/NSAIDs, K+ supls **Contra:** Bilateral renal artery stenosis, angioedema **Disp:** Tabs 2.5, 5, 10, 20 mg; IV 1.25 mg/mL (1, 2 mL) **SE:** ↓ BP w/ initial dose (especially w/ diuretics), ↑ K+, nonproductive cough, angioedema **Notes:** Monitor Cr; D/C diuretic for 2–3 d prior to start

Enfuvirtide (Fuzeon) **WARNING:** Rarely causes allergy; never rechallenge **Uses:** *w/ antiretroviral agents for HIV-1 Infxn in treatment-experienced pts with evidence of viral replication despite ongoing antiretroviral therapy* **Action:** Viral fusion inhibitor **Dose:** 90 mg (1 mL) SQ bid in upper arm, anterior thigh, or abdomen; rotate site **Caution:** [B,–] **Contra:** Previous allergy to drug **Disp:** 90 mg/mL reconstituted; pt kit w/ monthly supplies **SE:** Inj site reactions (in most); pneumonia, D, nausea, fatigue, insomnia, peripheral neuropathy **Notes:** Available only via restricted distribution system; use immediately on reconstitution or refrigerate (24 h max)

Enoxaparin (Lovenox) **WARNING:** Recent or anticipated epidural/spinal anesthesia ↑ risk of spinal/epidural hematoma w/ subsequent paralysis **Uses:** *Prevention & Rx of DVT; Rx PE; unstable angina & non-Q-wave MI* **Action:** LMW heparin **Dose:** *Adults.* Prevention: 30 mg SQ bid or 40 mg SQ q24h. *DVT/PE Rx:* 1 mg/kg SQ q12h or 1.5 mg/kg SQ q24h. *Angina:* 1 mg/kg SQ q12h. *Peds.* Prevention: 0.5 mg/kg SQ q12h. *DVT/PE Rx:* 1 mg/kg SQ q12h; ↓ dose w/ CrCl <30 mL/min **Caution:** [B, ?] Not for prophylaxis in prosthetic heart valves **Contra:** Active bleeding, HIT Ab(+) **Disp:** Inj 10 mg/0.1 mL (30-,40-,60- ,80-,100-,120-,150-mg syringes) **SE:** Bleeding, hemorrhage, bruising, thrombocytopenia, pain/hematoma at site, ↑ AST/ALT **Notes:** No effect on bleeding time, plt Fxn, PT, or aPTT; monitor plt (HIT), clinical bleeding; may monitor anti-factor Xa

Entacapone (Comtan) **Uses:** *Parkinson Dz* **Action:** Selective & reversible carboxymethyl transferase inhibitor **Dose:** 200 mg w/ each levodopa/carbidopa dose; max 1600 mg/d; ↓ levodopa/carbidopa dose by 25% if levodopa dose >800 mg **Caution:** [C, ?] Hepatic impair **Contra:** Use w/MAOI **Disp:** Tabs 200 mg **SE:** Dyskinesia, hyperkinesia, N, D, dizziness, hallucinations, orthostatic ↓ BP, brown-orange urine **Notes:** Monitor LFT; do not D/C abruptly

Ephedrine **Uses:** *Acute bronchospasm, bronchial asthma, nasal congestion,* ↓ BP, narcolepsy, enuresis, & MyG **Action:** Sympathomimetic; stimulates α- & β-receptors; bronchodilator **Dose:** *Adults. Congestion:* 25–50 mg PO q6h PRN; ↓ *BP:* 25–50 mg IV q 5-10 min, 150 mg/d max. *Peds.* 0.2–0.3 mg/kg/dose IV q4–6h

PRN **Caution:** [C, ?/–] **Contra:** Arrhythmias; closed-angle glaucoma **Disp:** Nasal solution 0.48%, 0.5%, oral capsule: 25, 37.5, 50 mg Inj 50 mg/mL; nasal spray 0.25% **SE:** CNS stimulation (nervousness, anxiety, trembling), tachycardia, arrhythmia, HTN, xerostomia, painful urination **Notes:** Protect from light; monitor BP, HR, urinary output; can cause false(+) amphetamine EMIT; take last dose 4–6h before hs; abuse potential, OTC sales banned/restricted in most states

Epinephrine (Adrenalin, Sus-Phrine, EpiPen, EpiPen Jr, others) **Uses:** *Cardiac arrest, anaphylactic Rxn, bronchospasm, open-angle glaucoma* **Action:** β-adrenergic agonist, some α-effects **Dose:** *Adults, ACLS:* 0.5–1 mg (5–10 mL of 1:10,000) IV q 5 min to response. *Anaphylaxis:* 0.3–0.5 mL SQ of 1:1000 dilution, may repeat q5–15min to a max of 1 mg/dose & 5 mg/d. *Asthma:* 0.1–0.5 mL SQ of 1:1000 dilution, repeat 20-min to 4-h intervals or 1 inhal (metdose) repeat in 1–2 min or susp 0.1–0.3 mL SQ for extended effect. *Peds.* ACLS: 1st dose 0.1 mL/kg IV of 1:10,000 dilution, then 0.1 mL/kg IV of 1:1000 dilution q3–5min to response. *Anaphylaxis:* 0.15–0.3 mg IM depending on weight (<30kg 0.01 mg/kg *Asthma:* 0.01 mL/kg SQ of 1:1000 dilution q8–12h. **Caution:** [C, ?] ↓ bronchodilation with β-blockers **Contra:** Cardiac arrhythmias, closed-angle glaucoma **Disp:** Inj 1:1000, 1:2000, 1:10,000, 1:100,000; susp for inj 1:200; aerosol 220 mcg/spray; 1% inhal soln; EpiPen Autoinjector one dose 0.30 mg; EpiPen Jr 0.15 mg **SE:** CV (tachycardia, HTN, vasoconstriction), CNS stimulation (nervousness, anxiety, trembling), ↓ renal blood flow **Notes:** Can give via ET tube if no central line (use 2–2.5 × IV dose); EpiPen for pt self-use (www.EpiPen.com)

Epinastine (Elestat) **Uses:** Itching w/ allergic conjunctivitis **Action:** Antihistamine **Dose:** 1 gtt bid **Caution:** [C, ?/–] **Disp:** Soln 0.05% **SE:** Burning, folliculosis, hyperemia, pruritus, URI, HA, rhinitis, sinusitis, cough, pharyngitis **Notes:** Remove contacts before, reinsert in 10 min

Epirubicin (Ellence) **Uses:** *Adjuvant therapy for + axillary nodes after resection of primary breast CA* **Actions:** Anthracycline cytotoxic agent **Dose:** Per protocols; ↓ dose w/ hepatic impair. **Caution:** [D, –] **Contra:** Baseline neutrophil count <1500 cells/mm³, severe myocardial insuff, recent MI, severe arrhythmias, severe hepatic dysfunction, previous anthracyclines Rx to max cumulative dose **Disp:** Inj 50 mg/25 mL, 200 mg/100 mL **SE:** Mucositis, N/V/D, alopecia, myelosuppression, cardiotox, secondary AML, tissue necrosis w/ extravasation

Eplerenone (Inspra) **Uses:** *HTN* **Action:** Selective aldosterone antagonist **Dose:** *Adults:* 50 mg PO daily–bid, doses >100 mg/d no benefit w/ ↑ K⁺; ↓ to 25 mg PO qd if giving w/ CYP3A4 inhibitors **Caution:** [B, +/–] Use of CYP3A4 inhibitors (Table 13); monitor K⁺ with ACE inhibitor, ARBs, NSAIDs, K⁺-sparing diuretics; grapefruit juice, St. John's wort **Contra:** K⁺ >5.5 mEq/L; NIDDM w/ microalbuminuria; SCr >2 mg/dL (males), >1.8 mg/dL (females); CrCl <50 mL/min; w/ K⁺ supls/K⁺-sparing diuretics **Disp:** Tabs 25, 50, 100 mg **SE:** Hypertriglyceridemia, ↑ K⁺, HA, dizziness, gynecomastia, ↑ Cholesterol, D, orthostatic ↓ BP **Notes:** May take 4 wk for full effect

Epoetin Alfa [Erythropoietin, EPO] (Epogen, Procrit) Uses: *CRF associated anemia* zidovudine Rx in HIV-infected pts, CA chemo; ↓ transfusions associated w/surgery **Action:** Induces erythropoiesis **Dose:** *Adults & Peds.* 50–150 units/kg IV/SQ 3×/wk; adjust dose q4–6wk PRN. *Surgery:* 300 units/kg/d × 10 d prior to surgery to 4 d after; ↓ dose if Hct approaches 36% or Hgb, ↑ >4 points in 2-wk period **Caution:** [C, +] **Contra:** Uncontrolled HTN **Disp:** Inj 2000, 3000, 4000, 10,000, 20,000, 40,000 units/mL **SE:** HTN, HA, fatigue, fever, tachycardia, N/V **Notes:** Refrigerate; monitor baseline & posttreatment Hct/Hgb, BP, ferritin

Epoprostenol (Flolan) Uses: *Pulmonary HTN* **Action:** Dilates pulmonary/systemic arterial vascular beds; ↓ plt aggregation **Dose:** Initial 2 ng/kg/min; ↑ by 2 ng/kg/min q15min until dose-limiting SE (CP, dizziness, N/V, HA, ↓ BP, flushing); IV cont inf 4 ng/kg/min < maximum-tolerated rate; adjust based on response; see package insert **Caution:** [B, ?] ↑ tox w/diuretics, vasodilators, acetate in dialysis fluids, anticoagulants **Contra:** Chronic use in CHF 2nd-deg severe LVSD **Disp:** Inj 0.5, 1.5 mg **SE:** Flushing, tachycardia, CHF, fever, chills, nervousness, HA, N/V/D, jaw pain, flulike Sxs **Notes:** Abrupt D/C can cause rebound pulmonary HTN; monitor bleeding w/ other antiplatelet/anticoagulants; watch ↓ BP w/ other vasodilators/diuretics

Eprosartan (Teveten) Uses: *HTN,* DN, CHF **Action:** ARB **Dose:** 400–800 mg/d single dose or bid **Caution:** [C (1st tri); D (2nd & 3rd tri), –] Lithium; ↑ K+ with K+-sparing diuretics/supls/high-dose trimethoprim **Contra:** Bilateral renal artery stenosis, 1st-deg aldosteronism **Disp:** Tabs 400, 600 mg **SE:** Fatigue, depression, hypertriglyceridemia, URI, UTI, abdominal pain, rhinitis/pharyngitis/cough

Eptifibatide (Integrilin) Uses: *ACS, PCI* **Action:** Glycoprotein IIb/IIIa inhibitor **Dose:** 180 mcg/kg IV bolus, then 2 mcg/kg/min cont inf; ↓ in renal impair (SCr >2 mg/dL, <4 mg/dL: 135 mcg/kg bolus & 0.5 mcg/kg/min inf) **Caution:** [B, ?] Monitor bleeding with other anticoagulants **Contra:** Other GPIIb/IIIa inhibitors, Hx abnormal bleeding, hemorrhagic stroke (within 30 d), severe HTN, major surgery (within 6 wk), plt count <100,000 cells/mm³, renal dialysis **Disp:** Inj 0.75, 2 mg/mL **SE:** Bleeding, ↓ BP, inj site Rxn, thrombocytopenia **Notes:** Monitor bleeding, coags, plts, SCr, activated coagulation time (ACT) with prothrombin consumption index (maintain ACT between 200–300 s)

Erlotinib (Tarceva) Uses: *NSCLC after 1 chemo agent fails* **Action:** HER1/EGFR tyrosine kinase inhibitor **Dose:** 150 mg/d PO 1 h ac or 2 h pc; ↓ (in 50-mg decrements) w/severe Rxn or w/ CYP3A4 inhibitors (Table 13); per protocols **Caution:** [D, ?/–]; use w/ CYP3A4 (Table 13) inhibitors **Disp:** Tabs 25, 100, 150 mg **SE:** Rash, N/V/D, anorexia, abdominal pain, fatigue, cough, dyspnea, stomatitis, conjunctivitis, pruritus, dry skin, Infxn, ↑ LFT, interstitial lung disease **Notes:** May ↑ INR w/warfarin, monitor INR

Ertapenem (Invanz) Uses: *Complicated intra-abdominal, acute pelvic, & skin Infxns, pyelonephritis, community-acquired pneumonia* **Action:** A carbapenem; β-lactam antibiotic, ↓ cell wall synthesis. Spectrum: Good gram(+/–) & anaerobic coverage, not *Pseudomonas,* PCN-resistant pneumococci, MRSA, *Enterococcus,* β-lactamase(+) *H. influenza, Mycoplasma, Chlamydia* **Dose:** *Adults.* 1 g IM/IV qd; 500 mg/d in CrCl <30 mL/min **Caution:** [C, ?/–] Probenecid ↓ renal clearance **Contra:** <18 y, PCN allergy **Disp:** Inj 1 g/vial **SE:** HA, N/V/D, inj site Rxns, thrombocytosis, ↑ LFTs **Notes:** Can give IM × 7 d, IV × 14 d; 137 mg Na⁺ (6 mEq)/g ertapenem

Erythromycin (E-Mycin, E.E.S., Ery-Tab, EryPed, Ilotycin)
Uses: *Bacterial Infxns; bowel prep*; *↑GI motility (prokinetic); *acne vulgaris* **Action:** Bacteriostatic; interferes w/ protein synthesis. *Spectrum:* Group A streptococci (*S. pyogenes*), *S. pneumoniae, N. meningitides, N. gonorrhea* (if PCN allergic) Legionella, M. pneumonia **Dose:** *Adults.* Base 250–500 mg PO q6–12h or ethylsuccinate 400–800 mg q6–12h; 500 mg–1 g IV q6h. *Prokinetic:* 250 mg PO tid 30 mins ac. *Peds.* 30–50 mg/kg/d PO ÷ q6–8h or 20–40 mg/kg/d IV ÷ q6h, max 2 g/d **Caution:** [B, +] ↑ tox of carbamazepine, cyclosporine, digoxin, methylprednisolone, theophylline, felodipine, warfarin, simvastatin/lovastatin; ↓ sildenafil dose w/ use **Contra:** Hepatic impair, preexisting liver Dz (estolate), use with pimozide **Disp:** *lactobionate (Ilotycin): Powder for inj* 500 mg, 1 g. *Base:* Tabs 250, 333, 500 mg; caps 250 mg. *Estolate (Ilosone):* Susp 125, 250 mg/5 mL. *Stearate (Erythrocin):* Tabs 250, 500 mg. *Ethylsuccinate (EES, EryPed):* Chew tabs 200 mg; tabs 400 mg; susp 200, 400 mg/5 mL **SE:** HA, abdominal pain, N/V/D; [QT prolongation, torsades de pointes, ventricular arrhythmias/tachycardias (rarely)]; cholestatic jaundice (estolate) **Notes:** 400 mg ethylsuccinate = 250 mg base/estolate; w/ food minimizes GI upset; lactobionate contains benzyl alcohol (caution in neonates)

Erythromycin & Benzoyl Peroxide (Benzamycin) **Uses:** *Topical for acne vulgaris* **Action:** Macrolide antibiotic w/ keratolytic **Dose:** Apply bid (AM & PM) **Caution:** [C, ?] **Contra:** Component sensitivity **Disp:** Gel erythromycin 30 mg/benzoyl peroxide 50 mg/g **SE:** Local irritation, dryness

Erythromycin & Sulfisoxazole (Eryzole, Pediazole) **Uses:** *Upper & lower resp tract; bacterial Infxns; H. influenzae otitis media in children*; Infxns in PCN-allergic pts **Action:** Macrolide antibiotic w/ sulfonamide **Dose:** *Adults.* Based on erythromycin content; 400 mg erythromycin/1200 mg sulfisoxazole PO q6h. *Peds >2 mo.* 40–50 mg/kg/d erythromycin & 150 mg/kg/d sulfisoxazole PO ÷ q6h; max 2 g/d erythromycin or 6 g/d sulfisoxazole × 10 d; ↓ in renal impair **Caution:** [C (D if near term), +] w/PO anticoagulants, MRX, hypoglycemics, phenytoin, cyclosporine **Contra:** Infants <2 mo **Disp:** Susp erythromycin ethylsuccinate 200 mg/sulfisoxazole 600 mg/5 mL (100, 150, 200 mL) **SE:** GI disturbance

Erythromycin, Ophthalmic (Ilotycin Ophthalmic) **Uses:** *Conjunctival/corneal Infxns* **Action:** Macrolide antibiotic **Dose:** ½ in. 2–6 X/d **Caution:** [B, +] **Contra:** Erythromycin hypersensitivity **Disp:** 0.5% oint **SE:** Local irritation

Erythromycin, Topical (A/T/S, Eryderm, Erycette, T-Stat)
Uses: *Acne vulgaris* Action: Macrolide antibiotic Dose: Wash & dry area, apply 2% product over area bid Caution: [B, +] Contra: Component sensitivity Disp: Soln 1.5%, 2%; gel 2%; pads & swabs 2% SE: Local irritation

Escitalopram (Lexapro) WARNING: Closely monitor for worsening depression or emergence of suicidality, particularly in ped pts Uses: Depression, anxiety Action: SSRI Dose: *Adults.* 10–20 mg PO qd; 10 mg/d in elderly & hepatic impair Caution: [C, +/–] Risk of serotonin syndrome (Table 14) Contra: W/ or w/in 14 d of MAOI Disp: Tabs 5, 10, 20 mg; soln 1 mg/mL SE: N/V/D, sweating, insomnia, dizziness, xerostomia, sexual dysfunction Notes: Full effects may take 3 wk

Esmolol (Brevibloc) Uses: *SVT & noncompensatory sinus tachycardia, AF/flutter* Action: β₁-Adrenergic blocker; class II antiarrhythmic Dose: *Adults & Peds.* Initial 500 mcg/kg load over 1 min, then 50 mcg/kg/min × 4 min; if inadequate response, repeat load & maint inf of 100 mcg/kg/min × 4 min; titrate by repeating load, then incremental ↑ in the maint dose of 50 mcg/kg/min for 4 min until desired heart rate reached or ↓ BP; average dose 100 mcg/kg/min Caution: [C (1st tri; D 2nd or 3rd tri), ?] Contra: Sinus bradycardia, heart block, uncompensated CHF, cardiogenic shock, ↓ BP Disp: Inj 10, 20, 250 mg/mL; premix inf 10 mg/mL SE: ↓ BP; bradycardia, diaphoresis, dizziness, pain on inj Notes: Hemodynamic effects back to baseline w/in 30 mins after D/C inf

Esomeprazole (Nexium) Uses: *Short-term (4–8 wk) for erosive esophagitis/GERD; H. pylori Infxn in combo with antibiotics* Action: Proton pump inhibitor, ↓ gastric acid Dose: *Adults.* GERD/erosive gastritis: 20–40 mg/d PO × 4–8 wk; 20-40 mg IV 10–30 min inf or >3 min IV push, 10 d max; *Maint:* 20 mg/d PO. H. pylori Infxn: 40 mg/d PO, plus clarithromycin 500 mg PO bid & amoxicillin 1000 mg/bid for 10 d; Caution: [B, ?/–] Contra: Component sensitivity Disp: Caps 20, 40 mg; IV 20, 40 mg SE: HA, D, abdominal pain Notes: Do not chew; may open capsule & sprinkle on applesauce

Estazolam (ProSom) [C-IV] Uses: *Short-term management of insomnia* Action: Benzodiazepine Dose: 1–2 mg PO qhs PRN; ↓ in hepatic impair/elderly/debilitated Caution: [X, –] ↑ effects w/ CNS depressants Contra: PRG Disp: Tabs 1, 2 mg SE: Somnolence, weakness, palpitations Notes: May cause psychological/physical dependence; avoid abrupt D/C after prolonged use

Esterified Estrogens (Estratab, Menest) WARNING: Do not use in the prevention of CV Dz Uses: *Vasomotor Sxs or vulvar/vaginal atrophy w/ menopause*; female hypogonadism Action: Estrogen supl Dose: *Menopause:* 0.3–1.25 mg/d, cyclically 3 wk on, 1 wk off. *Hypogonadism:* 2.5–7.5 mg/d PO × 20 d, off × 10 d Caution: [X, –] Contra: Genital bleeding of unknown cause, breast CA, estrogen-dependent tumors, thromboembolic disorders, thrombophlebitis, recent MI, PRG, severe hepatic Dz Disp: Tabs 0.3, 0.625, 1.25, 2.5 mg SE: N, HA, bloating, breast enlargement/tenderness, edema, venous thromboembolism, hypertriglyceridemia, gallbladder Dz **Notes:** Use lowest dose for shortest time (see Women's Health Initiatives (WHI) data www.whi.org)

Esterified Estrogens + Methyltestosterone (Estratest, Estratest HS) **Uses:** *Vasomotor Sxs*; postpartum breast engorgement **Action:** Estrogen & androgen supl **Dose:** 1 tab/d × 3 wk, 1 wk off **Caution:** [X, –] **Contra:** Genital bleeding of unknown cause, breast CA, estrogen-dependent tumors, thromboembolic disorders, thrombophlebitis, recent MI, PRG **Disp:** Tabs (estrogen/methyltestosterone) 0.625 mg/1.25 mg (hs), 1.25 mg/2.5 mg **SE:** Nausea, HA, bloating, breast enlargement/tenderness, edema, ↑ triglycerides, venous thromboembolism, gallbladder Dz **Notes:** Use lowest dose for shortest time; (see Women's Health Initiatives (WHI) data www.whi.org)

Estradiol (Estrace) **Uses:** *Atrophic vaginitis, vasomotor Sxs associated w/ menopause, osteoporosis* **Action:** Estrogen supl **Dose:** *PO:* 1–2 mg/d, adjust PRN to control Sxs. *Vaginal cream:* 2–4 g/d × 2 wk, then 1 g 1–3×/wk **Caution:** [X, –] **Contra:** Genital bleeding of unknown cause, breast CA, estrogen-dependent tumors, thromboembolic disorders, thrombophlebitis; recent MI; hepatic impair **Disp:** Tabs 0.5, 1, 2 mg; vaginal cream 0.1 mg/g **SE:** Nausea, HA, bloating, breast enlargement/tenderness, edema, ↑ triglycerides, venous thromboembolism, gallbladder Dz

Estradiol Cypionate & Medroxyprogesterone Acetate (Lunelle) **WARNING:** Cigarette smoking ↑ risk of serious CV side effects from contraceptives containing estrogen. This risk ↑ with age & with heavy smoking (>15 cigarettes/d) & is quite marked in women >35 y. Women who use Lunelle should be strongly advised not to smoke **Uses:** *Contraceptive* **Action:** Estrogen & progestin **Dose:** 0.5 mL IM (deltoid, ant thigh, buttock) monthly, do not exceed 33 d **Caution:** [X, M] HTN, gallbladder Dz, ↑ lipids, migraines, sudden HA, valvular heart Dz with complications **Contra:** PRG, heavy smokers >35 y, DVT, PE, cerebro/CV Dz, estrogen-dependent neoplasm, undiagnosed abnormal uterine bleeding, hepatic tumors, cholestatic jaundice **Disp:** Estradiol cypionate (5 mg), medroxyprogesterone acetate (25 mg) single-dose vial or syringe (0.5 mL) **SE:** Arterial thromboembolism, HTN, cerebral hemorrhage, MI, amenorrhea, acne, breast tenderness **Notes:** Start w/in 5 d of menstruation

Estradiol, Transdermal (Estraderm, Climara, Vivelle) **Uses:** *Severe menopausal vasomotor Sxs; female hypogonadism* **Action:** Estrogen supl **Dose:** 0.1 mg/d patch 1–2 × wk based on product; adjust PRN to control Sxs **Caution:** [X, –] (See estradiol) **Contra:** PRG, undiagnosed genital bleeding, carcinoma of breast, estrogen-dependent tumors, Hx thrombophlebitis, thrombosis, **Disp:** TD patches (deliver mg/24 h) 0.025, 0.0375, 0.05, 0.075, 0.1 **SE:** Nausea, bloating, breast enlargement/tenderness, edema, HA, hypertriglyceridemia, gallbladder Dz **Notes:** Do not apply to breasts, place on trunk & rotate sites

Estramustine Phosphate (Estracyt, Emcyt) **Uses:** *Advanced CAP* **Action:** Antimicrotubule agent; weak estrogenic & antiandrogenic activity

Dose: 14 mg/kg/d in 3–4 ÷ doses on empty stomach, not w/ dairy products **Caution:** [NA, not used in females] **Contra:** Active thrombophlebitis or thromboembolic disorders **Disp:** Caps 140 mg **SE:** N/V, exacerbation of preexisting CHF, thrombophlebitis, MI, PE, gynecomastia in 20–100%

Estrogen, Conjugated (Premarin)   WARNING: Should not be used for the prevention of CV Dz. The WHI reported ↑ risk of MI, stroke, breast CA, PE, & DVT when combined with methoxyprogesterone over 5 y of Rx; ↑ risk of endometrial CA **Uses:** *Moderate–severe menopausal vasomotor Sxs; atrophic vaginitis; palliative advanced CAP; prevent & Tx of estrogen-deficiency osteoporosis* **Action:** Estrogen hormonal replacement **Dose:** 0.3–1.25 mg/d PO cyclically; prostatic CA 1.25–2.5 mg PO tid; **Caution:** [X, –] **Contra:** Severe hepatic impair, genital bleeding of unknown cause, breast CA, estrogen-dependent tumors, thromboembolic disorders, thrombosis, thrombophlebitis, recent MI **Disp:** Tabs 0.3, 0.625, 0.9, 1.25, 2.5 mg; inj 25 mg/mL, vag cream 0.625 mg/gm **SE:** ↑ Risk of endometrial CA, gallbladder Dz, thromboembolism, HA, & possibly breast CA; generic products not equivalent

Estrogen, Conjugated-Synthetic (Cenestin) **Uses:** *Rx of moderate–severe vasomotor menopausal Sxs* **Action:** Hormonal replacement **Dose:** –initial 0.45 mg – 1.25 mg PO daily daily Caution: [X, –] **Contra:** See estrogen, conjugated **Disp:** Tabs 0.3, 0.45, 0.625, 0.9, 1.25 mg **SE:** Associated with an ↑ risk of endometrial CA, gallbladder Dz, thromboembolism, & possibly breast CA

Estrogen, Conjugated + Medroxyprogesterone (Prempro, Premphase)   WARNING: Should not be used for the prevention of CV Dz; the WHI study reported ↑ risk of MI, stroke, breast CA, PE, & DVT over 5 y of Rx **Uses:** *Moderate–severe menopausal vasomotor Sxs; atrophic vaginitis; prevent postmenopausal osteoporosis* **Action:** Hormonal replacement **Dose:** Prempro 1 tab PO daily; Premphase 1 tab PO daily **Caution:** [X, –] **Contra:** Severe hepatic impair, genital bleeding of unknown cause, breast CA, estrogen-dependent tumors, thromboembolic disorders, thrombosis, thrombophlebitis **Disp:** (expressed as estrogen/medroxyprogesterone) *Prempro:* Tabs 0.625/2.5, 0.625/5 mg *Premphase:* Tabs 0.625/0 (days 1–14) & 0.625/5 mg (days 15–28) **SE:** Gallbladder Dz, thromboembolism, HA, breast tenderness **Notes:** See www.whi.org

Estrogen, Conjugated + Methylprogesterone (Premarin + Methylprogesterone) **Uses:** *Menopausal vasomotor Sxs; osteoporosis* **Action:** Estrogen & androgen combo **Dose:** 1 tab/d **Caution:** [X, –] **Contra:** Severe hepatic impair, vaginal bleeding of unknown cause, breast CA, estrogen-dependent tumors, thromboembolic disorders, thrombosis, thrombophlebitis **Disp:** Tabs 0.625 mg estrogen, conjugated, & 2.5 or 5 mg of methylprogesterone **SE:** N, bloating, breast enlargement/tenderness, edema, HA, hypertriglyceridemia, gallbladder Dz

Estrogen, Conjugated + Methyltestosterone (Premarin + Methyltestosterone) **Uses:** *Moderate–severe menopausal vasomotor

Sxs*; postpartum breast engorgement **Action:** Estrogen & androgen combo **Dose:** 1 tab/d × 3 wk, then 1 wk off **Caution:** [X, –] **Contra:** Severe hepatic impair, genital bleeding of unknown cause, breast CA, estrogen-dependent tumors, thromboembolic disorders, thrombophlebitis **Disp:** Tabs (estrogen/ methyltestosterone) 0.625 mg/5 mg, 1.25 mg/10 mg **SE:** N, bloating, breast enlargement/tenderness, edema, HA, hypertriglyceridemia, gallbladder Dz

Eszopiclone (Lunesta) [C-IV] **Uses:** *Insomnia* **Action:** Nonbenzodiazepine hypnotic **Dose:** 2–3 mg/d hs *Elderly:* 1–2 mg/d hs; hepatic impair/use w/ CYP3A4 inhibitor (Table 13): 1 mg/d hs **Caution:** [C, ?/–] **Disp:** Tabs 1, 2, 3 mg **SE:** HA, xerostomia, dizziness, somnolence, hallucinations, rash, Infxn, unpleasant taste **Notes:** High-fat meals ↓ absorption

Etanercept (Enbrel) **Uses:** *Reduces Sxs of RA in pts who fail other DMARD,* Crohn Dz **Action:** Binds TNF **Dose:** *Adults.* RA 50 mg sc weekly or 25 mg sc 2×/wk (separated by at least 72–96 h). *Peds 4–17 y.* 0.8 mg/kg/week (max 50 mg/week) 72–96 h apart **Caution:** [B, ?] w/ predisposition to Infxn (ie, DM) **Contra:** Active Infxn; **Disp:** Inj 25 mg/vial **SE:** HA, rhinitis, inj site Rxn, URI, rhinitis **Notes:** Rotate inj sites

Ethambutol (Myambutol) **Uses:** *Pulmonary TB* & other mycobacterial Infxns, MAC **Action:** ↓ RNA synthesis **Dose:** *Adults & Peds >12 y.* 15–25 mg/kg/d PO single dose; ↓ in renal impair, take w/ food, avoid antacids **Caution:** [B, +] **Contra:** Optic neuritis **Disp:** Tabs 100, 400 mg **SE:** HA, hyperuricemia, acute gout, abdominal pain, ↑ LFTs, optic neuritis, GI upset

Ethinyl Estradiol (Estinyl, Feminone) **Uses:** *Menopausal vasomotor Sxs; female hypogonadism* **Action:** Estrogen supl **Dose:** 0.02–1.5 mg/d ÷ daily–tid **Caution:** [X, –] **Contra:** Severe hepatic impair; genital bleeding of unknown cause, breast CA, estrogen-dependent tumors, thromboembolic disorders, thrombophlebitis **Disp:** Tabs 0.02, 0.05, 0.5 mg **SE:** Nausea, bloating, breast enlargement/tenderness, edema, HA, hypertriglyceridemia, gallbladder Dz

Ethinyl Estradiol & Levonorgestrel (Preven) **Uses:** *Emergency contraceptive* ("morning-after pill"); prevent PRG (contraceptive failure, unprotected intercourse) **Actions:** Estrogen & progestin; interferes with implantation **Dose:** 4 tabs, take 2 tabs q12h × 2 (w/in 72 h of intercourse) **Caution:** [X, M] **Contra:** Known/suspected PRG, abnormal uterine bleeding **Disp:** Kit: ethinyl estradiol (0.05), levonorgestrel (0.25) blister pack with 4 pills & urine PRG test **SE:** Peripheral edema, N/V/D, bloating, abdominal pain, fatigue, HA, & menstrual changes **Notes:** Will not induce abortion; may ↑ risk of ectopic PRG

Ethinyl Estradiol & Norelgestromin (Ortho Evra) **Uses:** *Contraceptive patch* **Action:** Estrogen & progestin **Dose:** Apply patch to abdomen, buttocks, upper torso (not breasts), or upper outer arm at the beginning of the menstrual cycle; new patch is applied weekly for 3 wk; week 4 is patch-free **Caution:** [X, M] **Contra:** Thrombophlebitis, undiagnosed vaginal bleeding, PRG, carcinoma of breast, estrogen-dependent tumor **Disp:** 20 cm^2 patch (6 mg norelgestromin (active metabolite norgestimate) & 0.75 mg of ethinyl estradiol) **SE:** Breast discomfort, HA, site Rxns, nausea, menstrual cramps; thrombosis risks similar to OCP **Notes:** Less effective in women >90 kg; instruct patient does not protect against STD/HIV

Ethosuximide (Zarontin) **Uses:** *Absence (petit mal) Szs* **Action:** Anticonvulsant; ↑ Sz threshold **Dose:** *Adults.* Initial, 250 mg PO ÷ bid; ↑ by 250 mg/d q4–7d PRN (max 1500 mg/d) usual maint 20–30 mg/kg. *Peds 3–6 y.* Initial: 15 mg/kg/d PO ÷ bid. Maint: 15–40 mg/kg/d ÷ bid, max 1500 mg/d **Caution:** [C, +] in renal/hepatic impair **Contra:** Component sensitivity **Disp:** Caps 250 mg; syrup 250 mg/5 mL **SE:** Blood dyscrasias, GI upset, drowsiness, dizziness, irritability

Etidronate Disodium (Didronel) **Uses:** *↑ Ca^{2+} of malignancy, Paget Dz, & heterotopic ossification* **Action:** ↓ Nl & abnormal bone resorption **Dose:** *Paget Dz:* 5–10 mg/kg/d PO ÷ doses (for 3–6 mo). *↑ Ca^{2+}:* 7.5 mg/kg/d IV inf over 2 h × 3 d, then 20 mg/kg/d PO on last day of inf × 1–3 mo **Caution:** [B PO (C parenteral), ?] **Contra:** SCr >5 mg/dL **Disp:** Tabs 200, 400 mg; inj 50 mg/mL **SE:** GI intolerance (↓ by ÷ daily doses); hypophosphatemia, hypomagnesemia, bone pain, abnormal taste, fever, convulsions, nephrotox **Notes:** Take PO on empty stomach 2 h before any med

Etodolac (Lodine) WARNING: May ↑ risk of cardiovascular events & GI bleeding **Uses:** *Osteoarthritis & pain,* RA **Action:** NSAID **Dose:** 200–400 mg PO bid–qid (max 1200 mg/d) **Caution:** [C (D 3rd tri), ?] ↑ bleeding risk w/aspirin, warfarin; ↑ nephrotox w/ cyclosporine; Hx CHF, HTN, renal/hepatic impair, PUD **Contra:** Active GI ulcer **Disp:** Tabs 400, 500 mg; ER tabs 400, 500, 600 mg; caps 200, 300 mg **SE:** N/V/D, gastritis, abdominal cramps, dizziness, HA, depression, edema, renal impair **Notes:** Do not crush tabs

Etonogestrel/Ethinyl Estradiol (NuvaRing) **Uses:** *Contraceptive* **Action:** Estrogen & progestin combo **Dose:** Rule out PRG first; insert ring vaginally for 3 wk, remove for 1 wk; insert new ring 7 d after last removed (even if bleeding) at same time of day ring removed. First day of menses is day 1, insert prior to day 5 even if still bleeding. Use other contraception for first 7 d of starting therapy. See insert if converting from other contraceptive; after delivery or 2nd tri abortion, insert 4 wk postpartum (if not breast-feeding) **Caution:** [X, ?/–] HTN, gallbladder Dz, ↑ lipids, migraines, sudden HA **Contra:** PRG, heavy smokers >35 y, DVT, PE, cerebro-/CV Dz, estrogen-dependent neoplasm, undiagnosed abnormal genital bleeding, hepatic tumors, cholestatic jaundice **Disp:** Intravaginal ring: ethinyl estradiol 0.015 mg/d & etonogestrel 0.12 mg/d **Notes:** If ring removed, rinse w/cool/lukewarm H_2O (not hot) & reinsert ASAP; if not reinserted w/in 3 h, effectiveness ↓; do not use with diaphragm

Etoposide [VP-16] (VePesid, Toposar) **Uses:** *Testicular, non-small-cell lung CA, Hodgkin Dz & NHLs, peds ALL, & allogeneic/autologous BMT in high doses* **Action:** Topoisomerase II inhibitor **Dose:** 50 mg/m²/d IV for 3–5 d; 50 mg/m²/d PO for 21 d (PO availability = 50% of IV); 2–6 g/m² or 25–70 mg/kg in BMT (Per protocols); ↓ in renal/hepatic impair **Caution:** [D, –] **Contra:** IT administration **Disp:** Caps 50 mg; inj 20 mg/mL **SE:** N/V (Emesis in 10–30%), myelosuppression, alopecia, ↓ BP w/rapid IV, anorexia, anemia, leukopenia, ↑risk secondary leukemias

Exemestane (Aromasin) Uses: *Advanced breast CA in post-menopausal women w/progression after tamoxifen* **Action:** Irreversible, steroidal aromatase inhibitor; ↓estrogens **Dose:** 25 mg PO QD after a meal **Caution:** [D, ?/–] **Contra:** Component sensitivity **Disp:** Tabs 25 mg **SE:** Hot flashes, N, fatigue

Exenatide (Byetta) Uses: Type 2 DM combined w/ metformin &/or sulfonylurea **Action:** An incretin mimetic: ↑ insulin release, ↓ glucagon secretion, ↓ gastric emptying, promotes satiety **Dose:** 5 mcg SQ bid w/in 60 min before AM & PM meals; ↑ to 10 mcg SQ bid after 1 mo PRN; do not give pc **Caution:** [C, ?/–] may ↓ absorption of other drugs (take antibiotics/contraceptives 1 h before) **Contra:** CrCl < 30 mL/min **Disp:** Soln 5, 10 mcg/dose in prefilled pen **SE:** Hypoglycemia, N/V/D, dizziness, HA, dyspepsia, ↓ appetite, jittery **Notes:** Consider ↓ sulfonylurea to ↓ risk of hypoglycemia; discard pen 30 d after 1st use

Ezetimibe (Zetia) Uses: *Hypercholesterolemia alone or w/a HMG-CoA reductase inhibitor* **Action:** ↓ cholesterol & phytosterols absorption **Dose:** Adults & Peds >10 y. 10 mg/d PO **Caution:** [C, +/–] Bile acid sequestrants ↓ bioavailability **Contra:** Hepatic impair **Disp:** Tabs 10 mg **SE:** HA, D, abdominal pain, ↑ transaminases w/ HMG-CoA reductase inhibitor

Ezetimibe/Simvastatin (Vytorin) Uses: *Hypercholesterolemia* **Action:** ↓ absorption of cholesterol & phytosterols w/HMG-CoA-reductase inhibitor **Dose:** 10/10–10/80 mg/d PO; w/cyclosporine or danazol:10/10 mg/d max: w/ amiodarone or verapamil: 10/20 mg/d max; w/severe renal insuff **Caution:** [X, –]; w/ CYP3A4 inhibitors (Table 13), gemfibrozil, niacin >1 g/d, danazol, amiodarone, verapamil **Contra:** PRG/lactation; liver Dz, ↑ LFTs **Disp:** Tabs (ezetimibe/simvastatin) 10/10, 10/20, 10/40, 10/80 mg **SE:** HA, GI upset, myalgia, myopathy (muscle pain, weakness, or tenderness w/ creatine kinase 10 × ULN, rhabdomyolysis), hepatitis, Infxn **Notes:** Monitor LFTs

Famciclovir (Famvir) Uses: *Acute herpes zoster (shingles) & genital herpes* **Action:** ↓ viral DNA synthesis **Dose:** Zoster: 500 mg PO q8h ×7 d. Simplex: 125–250 mg PO bid;↓ W/renal impair **Caution:** [B, –] **Contra:** Component sensitivity **Disp:** Tabs 125, 250, 500 mg **SE:** Fatigue, dizziness, HA, pruritus, N/D **Notes:** Best w/in 72 h of initial lesion

Famotidine (Pepcid) Uses: *Short-term Tx of duodenal ulcer & benign gastric ulcer; maint for duodenal ulcer, hypersecretory conditions, GERD, & heartburn* **Action:** H_2-antagonist; ↓ gastric acid **Dose:** Adults. Ulcer: 20 mg IV q12h or 20–40 mg PO qhs × 4–8 wk. Hypersecretion: 20–160 mg PO q6h. GERD: 20 mg PO bid × 6 wk; maint: 20 mg PO hs. Heartburn: 10 mg PO PRN q12h. Peds. 0.5–1 mg/kg/d; ↓ in severe renal insuff **Caution:** [B, M] **Contra:** Component sensitivity **Disp:** Tabs 10, 20, 40 mg; chew tabs 10 mg; susp 40 mg/5 mL; gelatin cap 10 mg, inj 10 mg/2 mL **SE:** Dizziness, HA, constipation, D, thrombocytopenia **Notes:** Chew tabs contain phenylalanine

Felodipine (Plendil) **Uses:** *HTN & CHF* **Action:** CCB **Dose:** 2.5–10 mg PO daily; swallow whole;↓ in hepatic impair **Caution:** [C, ?] ↑ effect with azole antifungals, erythromycin, grapefruit juice **Contra:** Component sensitivity **Disp:** ER tabs 2.5, 5, 10 mg **SE:** Peripheral edema, flushing, tachycardia, HA, gingival hyperplasia **Notes:** Follow BP in elderly & w/ hepatic impair

Fenofibrate (Tricor) **Uses:** *Hypertriglyceridemia* **Action:** ↓ Triglyceride synthesis **Dose:** 48–145 mg daily; ↓ in renal impair, take w/ meals **Caution:** [C, ?] **Contra:** Hepatic/severe renal insuff, primary biliary cirrhosis, unexplained ↑ LFTs, gallbladder Dz **Disp:** Tabs 48, 145 mg **SE:** GI disturbances, cholecystitis, arthralgia, myalgia, dizziness **Notes:** Monitor LFTs

Fenoldopam (Corlopam) **Uses:** *Hypertensive emergency* **Action:** Rapid vasodilator **Dose:** Initial 0.03–0.1 mcg/kg/min IV inf, titrate q 15 min by 0.05–0.1 mcg/kg/min **Caution:** [B, ?] ↓ BP w/ β-blockers **Contra:** Allergy to sulfites **Disp:** Inj 10 mg/mL **SE:** ↓ BP, edema, facial flushing, N/V/D, atrial flutter/fibrillation, ↑ intraocular pressure **Notes:** Avoid concurrent β-blockers

Fenoprofen (Nalfon) **WARNING:** May ↑risk of cardiovascular events and GI bleeding **Uses:** *Arthritis & pain* **Action:** NSAID **Dose:** 200–600 mg q4–8h, to 3200 mg/d max; w/ food **Caution:** [B (D 3rd tri), +/–] CHF, HTN, renal/hepatic impair, Hx PUD **Contra:** NSAID sensitivity **Disp:** Caps 200, 300 mg **SE:** GI disturbance, dizziness, HA, rash, edema, renal impair, hepatitis **Notes:** Swallow whole

Fentanyl (Sublimaze) [C-II] **Uses:** *Short-acting analgesic* in anesthesia & PCA **Action:** Narcotic analgesic **Dose:** *Adults.* 25–100 mcg/kg/dose IV/IM titrated. *Peds.* 1–2 mcg/kg IV/IM q1–4h titrate; ↓ in renal impair **Caution:** [B, +] **Contra:** ↑ ICP, resp depression, severe renal/hepatic impair **Disp:** Inj 0.05 mg/mL **SE:** Sedation, ↓ BP, bradycardia, constipation, N, resp depression, miosis **Notes:** 0.1 mg fentanyl = 10 mg morphine IM

Fentanyl, Transdermal (Duragesic) [C-II] **WARNING:** Potential for abuse and fatal overdose. **Uses:** *Persistent moderate–severe chronic pain in patients already tolerant to opioids* **Action:** Narcotic **Dose:** Apply patch to upper torso q72h; dose based on narcotic requirements in previous 24 h; start 25 mcg/h patch q 72h; ↓ in renal impair **Caution:** [B, +] Cyp3A4 inhibitors (Table 13) may ↑ fentanyl effect, in pts w/ Hx substance abuse **Contra:** Not opioid tolerant, short-term pain management, postop pain in outpatient surgery, mild pain, PRN use ↑ ICP, resp depression, severe renal/hepatic impair, peds <2 yr **Disp:** Patches 12.5, 25, 50, 75, 100 mcg/h **SE:** Resp depression (fatal), sedation, ↓ BP, bradycardia, constipation, N, miosis **Notes:** 0.1 mg fentanyl = 10 mg morphine IM; do not cut patch; peak level 24–72 h

Fentanyl, Transmucosal System (Actiq) [C-II] **Uses:** *Induction of anesthesia; breakthrough CA pain* **Action:** Narcotic analgesic **Dose:** *Adults.*

Anesthesia: 5–15 mcg/kg. *Pain:* 200 mcg over 15 min, titrate to effect; ↓ in renal impair **Caution:** [B, +] **Contra:** ↑ ICP, resp depression, severe renal/hepatic impair **Disp:** Lozenges on stick 200, 400, 600, 800, 1200, 1600 mcg **SE:** Sedation, ↓ BP, bradycardia, constipation, nausea, resp depression, miosis **Notes:** 0.1 mg fentanyl = 10 mg IM morphine

Ferrous Gluconate (Fergon) **Uses:** *Iron deficiency anemia* & Fe supl **Action:** Dietary supl **Dose:** *Adults.* 100–200 mg of elemental Fe/d ÷ doses. *Peds.* 4–6 mg/kg/d ÷ doses; on empty stomach (OK w/ meals if GI upset occurs); avoid antacids **Caution:** [A, ?] **Contra:** Hemochromatosis, hemolytic anemia **Disp:** Tabs 300 (34 mg Fe), 325 mg (36 mg Fe) **SE:** GI upset, constipation, dark stools, discoloration of urine, may stain teeth **Notes:** 12% elemental Fe; false + stool guaiac

Ferrous Gluconate Complex (Ferrlecit) **Uses:** *Iron deficiency anemia or supl to erythropoietin therapy* **Action:** Fe Supl **Dose:** Test dose: 2 mL (25 mg Fe) IV over 1 h, if OK, 125 mg (10 mL) IV over 1 h. Usual cumulative dose 1 g Fe over 8 sessions (until favorable Hct) **Caution:** [B, ?] **Contra:** non-Fe-deficiency anemia; CHF; Fe overload **Disp:** Inj 12.5 mg/mL Fe **SE:** ↓ BP, serious allergic Rxns, GI disturbance, inj site Rxn **Notes:** Dose expressed as mg Fe; may infuse during dialysis

Ferrous Sulfate **Uses:** *Fe deficiency anemia & Fe supl* **Action:** Dietary supl **Dose:** *Adults.* 100–200 mg elemental Fe/d in ÷ doses. *Peds.* 1–6 mg/kg/d ÷ daily–tid; on empty stomach (OK w/ meals if GI upset occurs); avoid antacids **Caution:** [A, ?] ↑ absorption w/ vitamin C; ↓ absorption w/ tetracycline, fluoroquinolones, antacids, H_2-blockers, proton pump inhibitors **Contra:** Hemochromatosis, hemolytic anemia **Disp:** Tabs 187 (60 mg Fe), 200 (65 mg Fe), 324 (65 mg Fe), 325 mg (65 mg Fe), SR caplets & tabs 160 mg (50 mg Fe), 200 mg (65 mg Fe), gtt 75 mg/0.6 mL (15 mg Fe/0.6 mL), elixir 220 mg/5 mL (44 mg Fe/5 mL), syrup 90 mg/5 mL (18 mg Fe/5 mL) **SE:** GI upset, constipation, dark stools, discolored urine

Fexofenadine (Allegra, Allegra-D) **Uses:** *Allergic rhinitis* **Action:** Antihistamine **Dose:** *Adults & Peds >12 y.* 60 mg PO bid or 180 mg/d; ↓ in renal impair **Caution:** [C, ?] **Contra:** Component sensitivity **Disp:** Caps 60 mg; tabs 30, 60, 180 mg; Allegra-D (60 mg fexofenadine/120 mg pseudoephedrine) **SE:** Drowsiness rare

Filgrastim [G-CSF] (Neupogen) **Uses:** *↓ incidence of Infxn in febrile neutropenic pts; Rx chronic neutropenia* **Action:** Recombinant G-CSF **Dose:** *Adults & Peds.* 5 mcg/kg/d SQ or IV single daily dose; D/C when ANC >10,000 **Caution:** [C, ?] w/ drugs that potentiate release of neutrophils (eg, lithium) **Contra:** Allergy to *E. coli*-derived proteins or G-CSF **Disp:** Inj 300 mcg/mL **SE:** Fever, alopecia, N/V/D, splenomegaly, bone pain, HA, rash **Notes:** Monitor CBC & plt; monitor for cardiac events; no benefit w/ ANC >10,000/mm³

Finasteride (Proscar, Propecia) **Uses:** *BPH & androgenetic alopecia* **Action:** ↓ 5α-Reductase **Dose:** *BPH:* 5 mg/d PO. *Alopecia:* 1 mg/d PO; food may ↓ absorption **Caution:** [X, –] Hepatic impair **Contra:** Pregnant women should avoid handling pills **Disp:** Tabs 1 mg (Propecia), 5 mg (Proscar) **SE:** ↓ PSA by ~50%; **Notes:** Reestablish PSA baseline 6 mo; 3–6 mo for effect on urinary Sxs; continue to maintain new hair

Flavoxate (Urispas) **Uses:** *Relief of Sx of dysuria, urgency, nocturia, suprapubic pain, urinary frequency, incontinence* **Action:** Antispasmotic **Dose:** 100–200 mg PO tid–qid **Caution:** [B, ?] **Contra:** Pyloric/duodenal obstruction, GI hemorrhage, GI obstruction, ileus, achalasia, BPH **Disp:** Tabs 100 mg **SE:** Drowsiness, blurred vision, xerostomia

Flecainide (Tambocor) **Uses:** Prevent AF/flutter & PSVT, *prevent/suppress life-threatening ventricular arrhythmias* **Action:** Class 1C antiarrhythmic **Dose:** *Adults.* 100 mg PO q12h; ↑ by 50 mg q12h q4d to max 400 mg/d. *Peds.* 3–6 mg/kg/d in 3 ÷ doses; ↓ in renal impair, **Caution:** [C, +] monitor in hepatic impair, ↑ conc with amiodarone, digoxin, quinidine, ritonavir/amprenavir, BB, verapamil **Contra:** 2nd-/3rd-degree AV block, RBBB w/ bifascicular or trifascicular block, cardiogenic shock, CAD, ritonavir/amprenavir, alkalinizing agents **Disp:** Tabs 50, 100, 150 mg **SE:** Dizziness, visual disturbances, dyspnea, palpitations, edema, tachycardia, CHF, HA, fatigue, rash, N **Notes:** May cause new/worsened arrhythmias; initiate Rx in hospital; dose q8h if pt is intolerant/uncontrolled at 12-h intervals

Floxuridine (FUDR) **Uses:** *GI adenoma, liver, renal cancers*; colon & pancreatic CAs **Action:** Inhibits thymidylate synthase; ↓ DNA synthesis (S-phase specific) **Dose:** 0.1–0.6 mg/kg/d for 1–6 wk (per protocols) **Caution:** [D, –] Interaction w/ live & rotavirus vaccine **Contra:** BM suppression, poor nutritional status, potentially serious Infxn **Disp:** Inj 500 mg **SE:** Myelosuppression, anorexia, abdominal cramps, N/V/D, mucositis, alopecia, skin rash, & hyperpigmentation; rare neurotox (blurred vision, depression, nystagmus, vertigo, & lethargy); intra-arterial catheter-related problems (ischemia, thrombosis, bleeding, & Infxn) **Notes:** Need effective birth control; palliative Rx for inoperable/incurable pts

Fluconazole (Diflucan) **Uses:** *Candidiasis (esophageal, oropharyngeal, urinary tract, vaginal, prophylaxis); cryptococcal meningitis* **Action:** Antifungal; ↓ cytochrome P-450 sterol demethylation. *Spectrum:* All *Candida* sp except *C. krusei* **Dose:** *Adults.* 100–400 mg/d PO or IV. *Vaginitis:* 150 mg PO qd. Crypto: 400 mg day 1, then 200 mg × 10–12wk after CSF (–). *Peds.* 3–6 mg/kg/d PO or IV; 12 mg/kg/d/systemic Infxn; ↓ in renal impair **Caution:** [C, –] **Contra:** w/ terfenadine **Disp:** Tabs 50, 100, 150, 200 mg; susp 10, 40 mg/mL; inj 2 mg/mL **SE:** HA, rash, GI upset, ↓ K+, ↑ LFTs **Notes:** PO (preferred) = IV levels

Fludarabine Phosphate (Flamp, Fludara) **Uses:** *Autoimmune hemolytic anemia, CLL, cold agglutinin hemolysis,* low-grade lymphoma, mycosis fungoides **Action:** ↓ Ribonucleotide reductase; blocks DNA polymerase-induced DNA repair **Dose:** 18–30 mg/m²/d for 5 d, as a 30-min inf (per protocols) **Caution:** [D, –] Give cytarabine before fludarabine (↓ its metabolism) **Contra:**

Severe Infxns; CrCl <30 mL/min **Disp:** Inj 50 mg **SE:** Myelosuppression, N/V/D, ↑ LFT, edema, CHF, fever, chills, fatigue, dyspnea, nonproductive cough, pneumonitis, severe CNS tox rare in leukemia

Fludrocortisone Acetate (Florinef) **Uses:** *Adrenocortical insuff, Addison Dz, salt-wasting syndrome* **Action:** Mineralocorticoid **Dose:** *Adults.* 0.1–0.2 mg/d PO. *Peds.* 0.05–0.1 mg/d PO **Caution:** [C, ?] **Contra:** Systemic fungal Infxns; known allergy **Disp:** Tabs 0.1 mg **SE:** HTN, edema, CHF, HA, dizziness, convulsions, acne, rash, bruising, hyperglycemia, HPA suppression, cataracts **Notes:** For adrenal insuff, use w/ glucocorticoid; dose changes based on plasma renin activity

Flumazenil (Romazicon) **Uses:** *Reverse sedative effects of benzodiazepines & general anesthesia* **Action:** Benzodiazepine receptor antagonist **Dose:** *Adults.* 0.2 mg IV over 15 s; repeat PRN, to 1 mg max (3 mg max in benzodiazepine OD). *Peds.* 0.01 mg/kg (0.2 mg/dose max) IV over 15 s; repeat 0.005 mg/kg at 1 min intervals to max 1 mg total; ↓ in hepatic impair **Caution:** [C, ?] **Contra:** TCA OD; if pts given benzodiazepines to control life-threatening conditions (ICP/status epilepticus) **Disp:** Inj 0.1 mg/mL **SE:** N/V, palpitations, HA, anxiety, nervousness, hot flashes, tremor, blurred vision, dyspnea, hyperventilation, withdrawal syndrome **Notes:** Does not reverse narcotic Sx or amnesia

Flunisolide (AeroBid, Nasarel) **Uses:** *Asthma in pts requiring chronic steroid therapy; relieve seasonal/perennial allergic rhinitis* **Action:** Topical steroid **Dose:** *Adults.* Met-dose inhal: 2 inhal bid (max 8/d). *Nasal:* 2 sprays/nostril bid (max 8/d). *Peds >6 y.* Met-dose inhal: 2 inhal bid (max 4/d). *Nasal:* 1–2 sprays/nostril bid (max 4/d) **Caution:** [C, ?] **Contra:** Status asthmaticus **Disp:** Aerobid—0.25 mg/inh; Nasarel 29 mcg/spray **SE:** Tachycardia, bitter taste, local effects, oral candidiasis **Notes:** Not for acute asthma

Fluorouracil [5-FU] (Adrucil) **Uses:** *Colorectal, gastric, pancreatic, breast, basal cell,* head, neck, bladder, CAs **Action:** Inhibitor of thymidylate synthetase (interferes with DNA synthesis, S phase specific) **Dose:** 370–1000 mg/m²/d for 1–5 d IV push to 24-h cont inf; protracted venous inf of 200–300 mg/m²/d (Per protocol);800 mg/d max **Caution:** [D, ?] ↑ tox w/ allopurinol; do not give MRX before 5-FU **Contra:** Poor nutritional status, depressed BM Fxn, thrombocytopenia, major surgery w/in past mo, G6PD enzyme deficiency, PRG, serious Infxn, bilirubin >5 mg/dL **Disp:** Inj 50 mg/mL **SE:** Stomatitis, esophagopharyngitis, N/V/D, anorexia, myelosuppression, rash/dry skin/photosensitivity, tingling in hands/feet w/pain (palmar–plantar erythrodysesthesia), phlebitis/discoloration at inj sites **Notes:** ↑ thiamine intake; contraception recommended

Fluorouracil, Topical [5-FU] (Efudex) **Uses:** *Basal cell carcinoma; actinic/solar keratosis* **Action:** Inhibits thymidylate synthetase (↓ DNA synthesis, S-phase specific) **Dose:** 5% cream bid × 3–6 wk **Caution:** [D, ?] Irritant chemo **Contra:** Component sensitivity **Disp:** Cream 0.5, 1, 5%; soln 1, 2, 5% **SE:** Rash, dry skin, photosensitivity **Notes:** Healing may not be evident for 1–2 mo; wash hands thoroughly; avoid occlusive dressings; do not overuse

Fluoxetine (Prozac, Sarafem) **WARNING:** Closely monitor for worsening depression or emergence of suicidality, particularly in ped pts **Uses:** *Depression, OCD, panic disorder, bulimia* *PMDD (Sarafem)* **Action:** SSRI **Dose:** 20 mg/d PO (max 80 mg/d ÷dose); weekly 90 mg/wk after 1–2 wk of standard dose. *Bulimia:* 60 mg q AM. *Panic disorder:* 20 mg/d. OCD: 20–80 mg/d. *PMDD:* 20 mg/d or 20 mg intermittently, start 14 d prior to menses, repeat with each cycle; ↓ in hepatic failure **Caution:** [B, ?/–] Serotonin syndrome with MAOI, SSRI, serotonin agonists, linezolid; QT prolongation w/ phenothiazines **Contra:** MAOI/thioridazine (wait 5 wk after D/C before MAOI) **Disp:** *Prozac:* Caps 10, 20, 40 mg; scored tabs 10 mg; SR cap 90 mg; soln 20 mg/5 mL. *Sarafem:* Caps 10, 20 mg **SE:** Nausea, nervousness, weight loss, HA, insomnia

Fluoxymesterone (Halotestin) **Uses:** Androgen-responsive metastatic *breast CA, hypogonadism* **Action:** ↓ Secretion of LH & FSH (feedback inhibition) **Dose:** *Breast CA:* 10–40 mg/d ÷ × 1–3 mo. *Hypogonadism:* 5–20 mg/d **Caution:** [X, ?/–] ↑ effect w/ anticoagulants, cyclosporine, insulin, lithium, narcotics **Contra:** Serious cardiac, liver, or kidney Dz; PRG **Disp:** Tabs 2, 5, 10 mg **SE:** Virilization, amenorrhea & menstrual irregularities, hirsutism, alopecia, acne, nausea, & cholestasis; suppression of factors II, V, VII, & X & polycythemia; ↑ libido, HA, anxiety **Notes:** Radiographic exam of hand/wrist q6mo in prepubertal children; ↓ total T₄ levels

Fluphenazine (Prolixin, Permitil) **Uses:** *Schizophrenia* **Action:** Phenothiazine antipsychotic; blocks postsynaptic mesolimbic dopaminergic brain receptors **Dose:** 0.5–10 mg/d in ÷ doses PO q6–8h, average maint 5 mg/d; or 1.25 mg IM, then 2.5–10 mg/d in ÷ doses q6–8h PRN; ↓ in elderly **Caution:** [C, ?/–] **Contra:** Severe CNS depression, coma, subcortical brain damage, blood dyscrasias, hepatic Dz, w/ caffeine, tannic acid, or pectin-containing products **Disp:** Tabs 1, 2.5, 5, 10 mg; conc 5 mg/mL; elixir 2.5 mg/5 mL; inj 2.5 mg/mL; depot inj 25 mg/mL **SE:** Drowsiness, extrapyramidal effects **Notes:** Monitor LFTs; less sedative/hypotensive than chlorpromazine

Flurazepam (Dalmane) [C-IV] **Uses:** *Insomnia* **Action:** Benzodiazepine **Dose:** *Adults & Peds >15 y.* 15–30 mg PO qhs PRN; ↓ in elderly **Caution:** [X, ?/–] Elderly, low albumin, hepatic impair **Contra:** NA glaucoma; PRG **Disp:** Caps 15, 30 mg **SE:** "Hangover" due to accumulation of metabolites, apnea **Notes:** May cause dependency

Flurbiprofen (Ansaid) **WARNING:** May ↑risk of cardiovascular events and GI bleeding **Uses:** *Arthritis* **Action:** NSAID **Dose:** 50–300 mg/d ÷ bid–qid, max 300 mg/d w/ food **Caution:** [B (D in 3rd tri), +] **Contra:** PRG (3rd tri); aspirin allergy **Disp:** Tabs 50, 100 mg **SE:** Dizziness, GI upset, peptic ulcer Dz

Flutamide (Eulexin) **WARNING:** Liver failure & death reported. Measure LFT before, monthly, & periodically after; D/C immediately if ALT 2 × upper limits of nl or jaundice develops **Uses:** Advanced *CAP* (in combo with LHRH agonists, eg, leuprolide or goserelin); w/ radiation & GnRH for localized CAP **Action:**

Nonsteroidal antiandrogen **Dose:** 250 mg PO tid (750 mg total) **Caution:** [D, ?] **Contra:** Severe hepatic impair **Disp:** Caps 125 mg **SE:** Hot flashes, loss of libido, impotence, N/V/D, gynecomastia **Notes:** follow LFT, avoid EtOH

Fluticasone, Nasal (Flonase) Uses: *Seasonal allergic rhinitis* **Action:** Topical steroid **Dose:** *Adults & Adolescents.* Nasal: 2 sprays/nostril/d. *Peds 4–11 y.* Nasal: 1–2 sprays/nostril/d **Caution:** [C, M] **Contra:** Primary Rx of status asthmaticus **Disp:** Nasal spray 50 mcg/actuation **SE:** HA, dysphonia, oral candidiasis

Fluticasone, Oral (Flovent, Flovent Rotadisk) Uses: Chronic *asthma* **Action:** Topical steroid **Dose:** *Adults & Adolescents.* 2–4 puffs bid. *Peds 4–11 y.* 50 mcg bid **Caution:** [C, M] **Contra:** Primary Rx of status asthmaticus **Disp:** Met-dose inhal 44, 110, 220 mcg/activation; Rotadisk dry powder: 50, 100, 250 mcg/activation **SE:** HA, dysphonia, oral candidiasis **Notes:** Risk of thrush, rinse mouth after; counsel on use of device

Fluticasone Propionate & Salmeterol Xinafoate (Advair Diskus) Uses: *Maint therapy for asthma* **Action:** Corticosteroid w/ long-acting bronchodilator **Dose:** *Adults & Peds >12 y.* 1 inhal bid q 12 h **Caution:** [C, M] **Contra:** Not for acute attack or conversion from PO steroids or status asthmaticus **Disp:** Met-dose inhal powder (fluticasone/salmeterol in mcg) 100/50, 250/50, 500/50 **SE:** Upper resp Infxn, pharyngitis, HA **Notes:** Combo of Flovent & Serevent; do not use with spacer, do not wash mouthpiece, do not exhale into device

Fluvastatin (Lescol) Uses: *Atherosclerosis, primary hypercholesterolemia, hypertriglyceridemia* **Action:** HMG-CoA reductase inhibitor **Dose:** 20–80 mg PO qhs; ↓ w/ hepatic impair **Caution:** [X, –] **Contra:** Active liver Dz, ↑ LFTs, PRG, breast-feeding **Disp:** Caps 20, 40 mg; XL 80 mg **SE:** HA, dyspepsia, N/D, abdominal pain

Fluvoxamine (Luvox) WARNING: Closely monitor for worsening depression or emergence of suicidality, particularly in ped pts Uses: *OCD* **Action:** SSRI **Dose:** Initial 50 mg single qhs dose, ↑ to 300 mg/d in ÷ doses; ↓ in elderly/hepatic impair, titrate slowly; ÷ doses >100 mg **Caution:** [C, ?/–] Interactions (MAOIs, phenothiazines, SSRIs, serotonin agonists, others) **Contra:** MAOI w/in 14 days **Disp:** Tabs 25, 50, 100 mg **SE:** HA, N/D, somnolence, insomnia

Folic Acid Uses: *Megaloblastic anemia; folate deficiency* **Action:** Dietary supl **Dose:** *Adults.* Supl: 0.4 mg/d PO. *PRG:* 0.8 mg/d PO. *Folate deficiency:* 1 mg PO qd–tid. *Peds.* Supl: 0.04–0.4 mg/24 h PO, IM, IV, or SQ. *Folate deficiency:* 0.5–1 mg/24 h PO, IM, IV, or SQ **Caution:** [A, +] **Contra:** Pernicious, aplastic, normocytic anemias **Disp:** Tabs 0.4, 0.8, 1 mg; inj 5 mg/mL **SE:** Well tolerated **Notes:** OK for all women of child-bearing age; ↓ fetal neural tube defects by 50%; no effect on normocytic anemias

Fondaparinux (Arixtra) WARNING: When epidural/spinal anesthesia or spinal puncture is used, pts anticoagulated or scheduled to be anticoagulated with LMW heparins, heparinoids, or fondaparinux for prevention of thromboembolic complications are at risk for epidural or spinal hematoma, which can result in long-term or permanent paralysis **Uses:** *DVT prophylaxis* in hip fracture or replacement or knee replacement; w/ DVT or PE in combo w/ warfarin **Action:** Synthetic inhibitor of activated factor X; a LMW heparin **Dose:** 2.5 mg SQ qd, up to 5–9 d; start at least 6 h postop **Caution:** [B, ?] ↑ bleeding risk w/ anticoagulants, antiplatelets, drotrecogin alfa, NSAIDs **Contra:** Wt <50 kg, CrCl <30 mL/min, active bleeding, SBE, ↓ plt w/ antiplatelet Ab **Disp:** Prefilled syringes 2.5 /0.5, 10/0.8 5/0.4, 7.5 /0.6 mg/mL **SE:** Thrombocytopenia, anemia, fever, N **Notes:** D/C if plts <100,000 mm³; only give SQ; may monitor anti-factor Xa levels

Formoterol (Foradil Aerolizer) **Uses:** Maint Rx of *asthma & prevent bronchospasm* w/ reversible obstructive airway Dz; exercise-induced bronchospasm **Action:** Long-acting β_2-adrenergic agonist, bronchodilator **Dose:** *Adults & Peds >5 y.* Asthma: Inhale one 12-mcg cap q12h w/ aerolizer, 24 mcg/d max. *Adults & Peds > 12 y.* Exercise-induced bronchospasm: 1 inhal 12-mcg cap 15 min before exercise **Caution:** [C, ?] **Contra:** Need for acute bronchodilation; use w/in 2 wk of MAOI **Disp:** 12-mcg powder for inhal (as caps) for use in Aerolizer **SE:** Paradoxical bronchospasm; URI, pharyngitis, back pain **Notes:** Do not swallow caps; only use w/ inhaler; do not start w/ worsening or acutely deteriorating asthma

Fosamprenavir (Lexiva) **WARNING:** Do not use with severe liver dysfunction, reduce dose with mild–moderate liver impair (fosamprenavir 700 mg bid w/o ritonavir) **Uses:** HIV Infxn **Action:** Protease inhibitor **Dose:** 1400 mg bid w/o ritonavir; if w/ritonavir, fosamprenavir 1400 mg + ritonavir 200 mg qd or fosamprenavir 700 mg + ritonavir 100 mg bid. If w/ efavirenz & ritonavir: fosamprenavir 1400 mg + ritonavir 300 mg qd **Caution:** [C, ?/–]; **Contra:** w/ergot alkaloids, midazolam, triazolam, or pimozide; sulfa allergy **Disp:** Tabs 700 mg **SE:** N/V/D, HA, fatigue, rash **Notes:** Numerous drug interactions because of hepatic metabolism

Foscarnet (Foscavir) **Uses:** *CMV retinitis*; acyclovir-resistant *herpes Infxns* **Action:** ↓ Viral DNA polymerase & RT **Dose:** *CMV retinitis: Induction:* 60 mg/kg IV q8h or 100 mg/kg q12h × 14–21 d. *Maint:* 90–120 mg/kg/d IV (Monday–Friday). *Acyclovir-resistant HSV induction:* 40 mg/kg IV q8–12h × 14–21 d; use central line; ↓ with renal impair **Caution:** [C, –] ↑ Sz potential w/ fluoroquinolones; avoid nephrotoxic Rx (cyclosporine, aminoglycosides, ampho B, protease inhibitors) **Contra:** CrCl <0.4 mL/min/kg **Disp:** Inj 24 mg/mL **SE:** Nephrotox, electrolyte abnormalities **Notes:** Sodium loading (500 mL 0.9% NaCl) before & after helps minimize nephrotox; monitor ionized Ca

Fosfomycin (Monurol) **Uses:** *Uncomplicated UTI* **Action:** ↓cell wall synthesis. *Spectrum:* Gram(+) (staph, pneumococci); gram(–) (*E. coli, Enterococcus, Salmonella, Shigella, H. influenzae, Neisseria,* indole-negative *Proteus, Providencia*); *B. fragilis* & anaerobic gram(–) cocci are resistant **Dose:** 3 g PO in 90–120 mL of H_2O single dose; ↓ in renal impair **Caution:** [B, ?] ↓ absorption w/

antacids/Ca salts **Contra:** Component sensitivity **Disp:** Granule packets 3 g **SE:** HA, GI upset **Notes:** May take 2–3 d for Sxs to improve

Fosinopril (Monopril) Uses: *HTN, CHF,* DN **Action:** ACE inhibitor **Dose:** 10 mg/d PO initial; max 40 mg/d PO; ↓ in elderly; ↓ in renal impair **Caution:** [D, +] ↑ K+ w/ K+ supls, ARBs, K+ sparing diuretics; ↑ renal AE w/ NSAIDs, diuretics, hypovolemia **Contra:** Hereditary/idiopathic angioedema or angioedema w/ ACE inhibitor, bilateral renal artery stenosis **Disp:** Tabs 10, 20, 40 mg **SE:** Cough, dizziness, angioedema, ↑ K+

Fosphenytoin (Cerebyx) Uses: *Status epilepticus* **Action:** ↓ Sz spread in motor cortex **Dose:** As phenytoin equivalents (PE). Load: 15–20 mg PF/kg *Maint:* 4–6 mg PF/kg/d; ↓ dosage, monitor levels in hepatic impair **Caution:** [D, +] May ↑ phenobarbital **Contra:** Sinus bradycardia, SA block, 2nd-/3rd-degree AV block, Adams–Stokes syndrome, rash during Rx **Disp:** Inj 75 mg/mL **SE:** ↓ BP, dizziness, ataxia, pruritus, nystagmus **Notes:** 15 min to convert fosphenytoin to phenytoin; admin <150 mg PE/min to prevent ↓ BP; administer with BP monitoring

Frovatriptan (Frova) Table 11

Fulvestrant (Faslodex) Uses: *Hormone receptor(+) metastatic breast CA in postmenopausal women with Dz progression following antiestrogen therapy* **Action:** Estrogen receptor antagonist **Dose:** 250 mg IM monthly, either a single 5-mL inj or two concurrent 2.5-mL IM inj into buttocks **Caution:** [X, ?/–] ↑ effects w/ CYP3A4 inhibitors (Table 13) w/ hepatic impair **Contra:** PRG **Disp:** Prefilled syringes 50 mg/mL (single 5 mL, dual 2.5 mL) **SE:** N/V/D, constipation, abdominal pain, HA, back pain, hot flushes, pharyngitis, inj site Rxns **Notes:** Only use IM

Furosemide (Lasix) Uses: *CHF, HTN, edema,* ascites **Action:** Loop diuretic; ↓ Na & Cl reabsorption in ascending loop of Henle & distal tubule **Dose:** Adults. 20–80 mg PO or IV bid. **Peds.** 1 mg/kg/dose IV q6–12h; 2 mg/kg/dose PO q12–24h (max 6 mg/kg/dose) **Caution:** [C, +] ↓ K+ ↑ risk of digoxin tox; ↑ risk of ototox w/ aminoglycosides, cisplatinum (esp in renal dysfunction) **Contra:** Allergy to sulfonylureas; anuria; hepatic coma/severe electrolyte depletion **Disp:** Tabs 20, 40, 80 mg; soln 10 mg/mL, 40 mg/5 mL; inj 10 mg/mL **SE:** ↓ BP, hyperglycemia, ↓ K+ **Notes:** Monitor electrolytes, renal Fxn; high doses IV may cause ototox

Gabapentin (Neurontin) Uses: Adjunct in *partial Szs;* postherpetic neuralgia (PHN)*; chronic pain syndromes **Action:** Anticonvulsant **Dose:** *Anticonvulsant:* 300–1200 mg PO tid (max 3600 mg/d). *PHN:* 300 mg day 1, 300 mg bid day 2, 300 mg tid day 3, titrate (1800–3600 mg/d); ↓ in renal impair **Caution:** [C, ?] **Contra:** Component sensitivity **Disp:** Caps 100, 300, 400, 800 mg; soln 250 mg/5 mL; tab 600, 800 mg **SE:** Somnolence, dizziness, ataxia, fatigue **Notes:** Not necessary to monitor levels

Galantamine (Reminyl) Uses: *Alzheimer Dz* **Action:** Acetylcholinesterase inhibitor **Dose:** 4 mg PO bid, ↑ to 8 mg bid after 4 wk; may ↑ to 12 mg bid in 4 wk **Caution:** [B, ?] ↑ effect w/ succinylcholine, amiodarone, diltiazem, verapamil, NSAIDs, digoxin; ↓ effect w/ anticholinergics **Contra:** Severe renal/hepatic impair **Disp:** Tabs 4, 8, 12 mg; soln 4 mg/mL **SE:** GI disturbances, weight loss, sleep disturbances, dizziness, HA **Notes:** Caution w/ urinary outflow obstruction, Parkinson Dz, severe asthma/COPD, severe heart Dz or ↓ BP

Gallium Nitrate (Ganite) Uses: *↑ Ca^{2+} of malignancy*; bladder CA **Action:** ↓ bone resorption of Ca^{2+} **Dose:** ↑ Ca^{2+}: 200 mg/m²/day × 5 d. *CA:* 350 mg/m² cont inf × 5 d to 700 mg/m² rapid IV inf q2wk in antineoplastic settings (per protocols) **Caution:** [C, ?] Do not give w/ live or rotavirus vaccine **Contra:** SCr >2.5 mg/dL **Disp:** Inj 25 mg/mL **SE:** Renal insuff, ↓ Ca^{2+}, hypophosphatemia, ↓ bicarb, <1% acute optic neuritis **Notes:** Bladder CA, use in combo w/ vinblastine & ifosfamide

Ganciclovir (Cytovene, Vitrasert) Uses: *Rx & prevent CMV retinitis, prevent CMV Dz* in transplant recipients **Action:** ↓ viral DNA synthesis **Dose:** Adults & Peds. IV: 5 mg/kg IV q12h for 14–21 d, then maint 5 mg/kg/d IV × 7 d/wk or 6 mg/kg/d IV × 5 d/wk. *Ocular implant:* One implant q5–8mo. *Adults.* PO: Following induction, 1,000 mg PO tid. *Prevention:* 1,000 mg PO tid; with food; ↓ in renal impair **Caution:** [C, –] ↑ effect w/ immunosuppressives, imipenem/cilastatin, zidovudine, didanosine, other nephrotoxic Rx **Contra:** ANC <500, plt <25,000, intravitreal implant **Disp:** Caps 250, 500 mg; inj 500 mg, ocular implant 4.5 mg **SE:** Granulocytopenia & thrombocytopenia, fever, rash, GI upset **Notes:** Not a cure for CMV; handle inj w/ cytotox cautions; no systemic benefit w/implant

Gatifloxacin (Tequin, Zymar Ophthalmic) Uses: *Bronchitis, sinusitis, community-acquired pneumonia, UTI, uncomplicated skin/soft tissue Infxn* **Action:** Quinolone antibiotic, ↓ DNA-gyrase. *Spectrum:* Gram(+) (except MRSA, *Listeria*), gram(–) (not *Pseudomonas*), atypicals, some anaerobes (*Clostridium*, not *C. difficile*) **Dose:** 400 mg/d PO or IV; *Ophth:* Day 1 & 2 one gtt q2h in eye while awake (8 × day max) day 3–7, one gtt 4Xd while awake; (↓ in renal impair) **Caution:** [C, M] **Contra:** Prolonged QT interval, w/ other Rx that prolong QT interval (Class Ia & III antiarrhythmics, erythromycin, antipsychotics, TCA); uncorrected ↓ K^+, children <18 y or in PRG/lactating women **Disp:** Oral susp 200 mg/5 mL; tabs 200, 400 mg; inj 10 mg/mL; premixed infuse D_5W 200 mg, 400 mg; ophth soln 0.3% **SE:** ↑ QT interval, HA, N/D, tendon rupture, photosensitivity **Notes:** Reliable activity against *S. pneumoniae*; take 4 h after antacids containing Mg, Al, Fe, or Zn; drink plenty of fluids; avoid sunlight

Gefitinib (Iressa) Uses: *Rx locally advanced or metastatic non-small-cell lung CA after failure of platinum-based & docetaxel chemo* **Action:** ↓ phosphorylation of tyrosine kinases **Dose:** 250 mg/d PO **Caution:** [D, –] **Disp:** Tabs 250 mg **SE:** D, rash, acne, dry skin, N/V, interstitial lung Dz, ↑ transaminases **Notes:** Follow LFTs

Gemcitabine (Gemzar) Uses: *Pancreatic CA, brain mets, NSCLC,* *gastric CA **Action:** Antimetabolite; ↓ ribonucleotide reductase; produces false nucleotide base-inhibiting DNA synthesis **Dose:** 1,000 mg/m² over 30 min–1 h IV inf/wk × 3–4 wk or 6–8 wk; modify dose based on hematologic Fxn (per protocol) **Caution:** [D, ?/–] **Contra:** PRG **Disp:** Inj 200 mg, 1 g **SE:** Myelosuppression, N/V/D, drug fever, skin rash **Notes:** Reconstituted soln concn 38 mg/mL (not 40 mg/mL as earlier labeling); monitor hepatic/renal Fxn

Gemfibrozil (Lopid) **Uses:** *Hypertriglyceridemia, coronary heart Dz* **Action:** Fibric acid **Dose:** 1200 mg/d PO ÷ bid 30 min ac AM & PM **Caution:** [C, ?] ↑ warfarin effect, sulfonylureas; ↑ risk of myopathy w/ HMG-CoA reductase inhibitors; ↓ effects w/ cyclosporine **Contra:** Renal/hepatic impair (SCr >2.0 mg/dL), gallbladder Dz, primary biliary cirrhosis **Disp:** Tabs 600 mg **SE:** Cholelithiasis, GI upset **Notes:** Avoid use w/HMG-CoA reductase inhibitors; monitor LFTs & serum lipids

Gemifloxacin (Factive) **Uses:** Community-acquired pneumonia, acute exacerbation of chronic bronchitis **Action:** ↓ DNA gyrase & topoisomerase IV; *Spectrum: S. pneumoniae* (including MDR strains), *H. influenzae, H. parainfluenzae, M. catarrhalis, M. pneumoniae, Chlamydia pneumoniae, K. pneumoniae* **Dose:** 320 mg PO qd; CrCl < 40 mL/min: 160 mg PO qd **Caution:** [C, ?/–]; children < 18 y; Hx of ↑ QTc interval, electrolyte disorders, w/ Class IA/III antiarrhythmics, erythromycin, TCAs, antipsychotics **Contra:** Fluoroquinolone allergy **Disp:** Tab 320 mg **SE:** Rash, N/V/D, abdominal pain, dizziness, xerostomia, arthralgia, allergy/anaphylactic reactions, peripheral neuropathy, tendon rupture **Notes:** Take 3 h before or 2 h after: Al/Mg antacids, Fe, Z or other metal cations

Gemtuzumab Ozogamicin (Mylotarg) **WARNING:** Can cause severe allergic Rxns & other infusion-related reactions including severe pulmonary events; hepatotox, including severe hepatic venoocclusive Dz (VOD), reported **Uses:** *Relapsed CD33+ AML in pts > 60 who are poor candidates for chemo* **Action:** MoAb linked to calicheamicin; selective for myeloid cells **Dose:** Per protocol **Caution:** [D,?/–] **Contra:** Component sensitivity **Disp:** 5 mg/20 mL vial **SE:** Myelosuppression, allergy (including anaphylaxis), inf Rxns (chills, fever, N/V, HA), pulmonary events, hepatotox **Notes:** Single-agent use only, not in combo; premedicate w/ diphenhydramine & acetaminophen

Gentamicin (Garamycin, G-Mycitin, others) **Uses:** *Serious Infxns* caused by *Pseudomonas, Proteus, E. coli, Klebsiella, Enterobacter, & Serratia* & initial Rx of gram(–) sepsis **Action:** Bactericidal; ↓ protein synthesis. *Spectrum:* Synergy w/ PCNs; gram(–) (not *Neisseria, Legionella, Acinetobacter*) **Dose:** *Adults.* 3–7 mg/kg/24h IV ÷ q8–24h. *Synergy:* 1 mg/kg q8h. *Peds. Infants <7 d <1200 g:* 2.5 mg/kg/dose q18–24h. *Infants >1200 g:* 2.5 mg/kg/dose q12–18h. *Infants >7 d:* 2.5 mg/kg/dose q8–12h. *Children:* 2.5 mg/kg/d IV q8h; ↓ w/renal insuff **Caution:** [C, +/–] Avoid other nephrotoxic Rxs **Contra:** Aminoglycoside sensitivity **Disp:** Premixed infus 40, 60, 70, 80, 90, 100, 120 mg; ADD-Vantage inj vials 10 mg/mL; inj 40 mg/mL; IT preservative-free 2 mg/mL **SE:** Nephrotox/ototox/neurotox **Notes:** Follow CrCl, SCr & serum conc for dose adjustments (Table 2); QD dosing popular; use IBW to dose (use adjusted if obese >30% IBW)

Gentamicin & Prednisolone, Ophthalmic (Pred-G Ophthalmic) Uses: *Steroid-responsive ocular & conjunctival Infxns* sensitive to gentamicin **Action:** Bactericidal; ↓ protein synthesis w/anti-inflammatory. *Spectrum: Staph, E. coli, H. influenzae, Klebsiella, Neisseria, Pseudomonas, Proteus, & Serratia* sp **Dose:** *Oint:* ½ in. in conjunctival sac daily–tid. *Susp:* 1 gtt bid–qid, up to 1 gtt/h for severe Infxns **Contra:** Aminoglycoside sensitivity **Caution:** [C, ?] **Disp:** *Oint, ophth:* Prednisolone acetate 0.6% & gentamicin sulfate 0.3% (3.5 g). *Susp, ophth:* Prednisolone acetate 1% & gentamicin sulfate 0.3% (2, 5, 10 mL) **SE:** Local irritation

Gentamicin, Ophthalmic (Garamycin, Genoptic, Gentacidin, Gentak, others) Uses: *Conjunctival Infxns* **Action:** Bactericidal; ↓ protein synthesis **Dose:** *Oint:* Apply in. bid–tid. *Soln:* 1–2 gtt q2–4h, up to 2 gtt/h for severe Infxn **Caution:** [C, ?] **Contra:** Aminoglycoside sensitivity **Disp:** Soln & oint 0.3% **SE:** Local irritation **Notes:** Do not use other eye drops w/in 5–10 mins; do not touch dropper to eye

Gentamicin, Topical (Garamycin, G-Mycitin) Uses: *Skin Infxns* caused by susceptible organisms **Action:** Bactericidal; ↓ protein synthesis **Dose:** *Adults & Peds >1 y.* Apply tid–qid **Caution:** [C, ?] **Contra:** Aminoglycoside sensitivity **Disp:** Cream & oint 0.1% **SE:** Irritation

Glimepiride (Amaryl) Uses: *Type 2 DM* **Action:** Sulfonylurea; ↑ pancreatic insulin release; ↑ peripheral insulin sensitivity; ↓ hepatic glucose output/production **Dose:** 1–4 mg/d, max 8 mg **Caution:** [C, –] **Contra:** DKA **Disp:** Tabs 1, 2, 4 mg **SE:** HA, nausea, hypoglycemia **Notes:** Give w/ 1st meal of day

Glipizide (Glucotrol, Glucotrol XL) Uses: *Type 2 DM* **Action:** Sulfonylurea; ↑ pancreatic insulin release; ↑ peripheral insulin sensitivity; ↓ hepatic glucose output/production; ↓ intestinal glucose absorption **Dose:** 5 mg initial, ↑ by 2.5–5 mg/d, max 40 mg/d; XL max 20 mg; 30 min ac; hold if pt NPO **Caution:** [C, ?/–] Severe liver Dz **Contra:** DKA, Type 1 DM, sulfonamide sensitivity **Disp:** Tabs 5, 10 mg; XL tabs 2.5, 5, 10 mg **SE:** HA, anorexia, N/V/D, constipation, fullness, rash, urticaria, photosensitivity **Notes:** Counsel about DM management; wait several days before adjusting dose; monitor glucose

Glucagon Uses: Severe *hypoglycemic* Rxns in DM with sufficient liver glycogen stores or β-blocker OD **Action:** Accelerates liver gluconeogenesis **Dose:** *Adults.* 0.5–1 mg SQ, IM, or IV; repeat in 20 min PRN. β-*Blocker OD:* 3–10 mg IV; repeat in 10 min PRN; may give cont infus 1–5 mg/h. *Peds. Neonates:* 0.3 mg/kg/dose SQ, IM, or IV q4h PRN. *Children:* 0.025–0.1 mg/kg/dose SQ, IM, or IV; repeat in 20 min PRN **Caution:** [B, M] **Contra:** Pheochromocytoma **Disp:** Inj 1 mg **SE:** N/V, ↓ BP **Notes:** Administration of glucose IV necessary; ineffective in starvation, adrenal insuff, or chronic hypoglycemia

Glyburide (DiaBeta, Micronase, Glynase) Uses: *Type 2 DM* **Action:** Sulfonylurea; ↑ pancreatic insulin release; ↑ peripheral insulin sensitivity;

↓ hepatic glucose output/production; ↓ intestinal glucose absorption **Dose:** 1.25–10 mg qd–bid, max 20 mg/d. *Micronized:* 0.75–6 mg qd–bid, max 12 mg/d **Caution:** [C, ?] Renal impair **Contra:** DKA, Type I DM **Disp:** Tabs 1.25, 2.5, 5 mg; micronized tabs 1.5, 3, 6 mg **SE:** HA, hypoglycemia **Notes:** Not OK for CrCl <50 mL/min; hold dose if NPO

Glyburide/Metformin (Glucovance) Uses: *Type 2 DM* **Action:** *Sulfonylurea:* ↑ Pancreatic insulin release. *Metformin:* Peripheral insulin sensitivity; ↓ hepatic glucose output/production; ↓ intestinal glucose absorption **Dose:** 1st line (naive pts), 1.25/250 mg PO daily–bid; 2nd line, 2.5/500 mg or 5/500 mg bid (max 20/2000 mg); take w/ meals, slowly ↑ dose; hold before & 48 h after ionic contrast media **Caution:** [C, –] **Contra:** SCr >1.4 in females or >1.5 in males; hypoxemic conditions (CHF, sepsis, recent MI); alcoholism; metabolic acidosis; liver Dz; **Disp:** Tabs 1.25/250 mg, 2.5/500 mg, 5/500 mg **SE:** HA, hypoglycemia, lactic acidosis, anorexia, N/V, rash **Notes:** Avoid EtOH; hold dose if NPO; monitor folate levels (megaloblastic anemia)

Glycerin Suppository Uses: *Constipation* **Action:** Hyperosmolar laxative **Dose:** *Adults.* 1 adult supp PR PRN. *Peds.* 1 infant supp PR daily–bid PRN **Caution:** [C, ?] **Disp:** Supp (adult, infant); liq 4 mL/applicatorful **SE:** D

Gonadorelin (Lutrepulse) Uses: *Primary hypothalamic amenorrhea* **Action:** Stimulates pituitary release of LH & FSH **Dose:** 5 mcg IV q 90 min × 21 d using Lutrepulse pump kit **Caution:** [B, M] ↑ levels w/ androgens, estrogens, progestins, glucocorticoids, spironolactone, levodopa; ↓ levels with OCP, digoxin, dopamine antagonists **Contra:** Condition exacerbated by PRG or reproductive hormones, ovarian cysts, causes of anovulation other than hypothalamic, hormonally dependent tumor **Disp:** Inj 100 mcg **SE:** Multiple pregnancy risk; inj site pain **Notes:** Monitor LH, FSH

Goserelin (Zoladex) Uses: Advanced *CAP* & w/ radiation for localized high-risk CAP, *endometriosis, breast CA* **Action:** LHRH agonist, transient ↑ then ↓ in LH, w/ ↓ testosterone **Dose:** 3.6 mg SQ (implant) q 28d or 10.8 mg SQ q3mo; usually lower abdominal wall **Caution:** [X, –] **Contra:** PRG, breast-feeding, 10.8-mg implant not for women **Disp:** SQ implant 3.6 (1 mo), 10.8 mg (3 mo) **SE:** Hot flashes, ↓ libido, gynecomastia, & transient exacerbation of CA-related bone pain ("flare reaction" 7–10 d after 1st dose) **Notes:** Inject SQ into fat in abdominal wall; do not aspirate; females must use contraception

Granisetron (Kytril) Uses: *Prevention of N/V* **Action:** Serotonin receptor antagonist **Dose:** *Adults & Peds.* 10 mcg/kg/dose IV 30 min prior to chemo *Adults.* Inj 0.1, 1 mg/mL 2 mg PO 1 h prior to chemo, then 12 h later. *Postop N/V:* 1 mg IV before end of OR case **Caution:** [B, +/–] St. John's wort ↓ levels **Contra:** Liver Dz, children <2 y **Disp:** Tabs 1 mg; inj 0.1, 1 mg/mL; soln 2 mg/10 mL **SE:** HA, constipation

Guaifenesin (Robitussin, others) Uses: *Relief of dry, nonproductive cough* **Action:** Expectorant **Dose:** *Adults.* 200–400 mg (10–20 mL) PO q4h (max

2.4 g/d). *Peds.* <2 y: 12 mg/kg/d in 6 ÷ doses. *2–5 y:* 50–100 mg (2.5–5 mL) PO q4h (max 600 mg/d). *6–11 y:* 100–200 mg (5–10 mL) PO q4h (max 1.2 g/d) **Caution:** [C, ?] **Disp:** Tabs 100, 200; SR tabs 600, 1200 mg; caps 200 mg; SR caps 300 mg; liq 100 mg/5 mL **SE:** GI upset **Notes** Give w/ large amount of H_2O; some dosage forms contain EtOH

Guaifenesin & Codeine (Robitussin AC, Brontex, others) [C-V]

Uses: *Relief of dry cough* **Action:** Antitussive w/ expectorant **Dose:** *Adults.* 5–10 mL or 1 tab PO q6–8h (max 60 mL/24 h). *Peds.* 2–6 y: 1–1.5 mg/kg codeine/d ÷ dose q4–6h (max 30 mg/24 h). *6–12 y:* 5 mL q4h (max 30 mL/24 h) **Caution:** [C, +] **Disp:** Brontex tab 10 mg codeine/300 mg guaifenesin; liq 2.5 mg codeine/75 mg guaifenesin/5 mL; others 10 mg codeine/100 mg guaifenesin/5 mL **SE:** Somnolence

Guaifenesin & Dextromethorphan (many OTC brands)

Uses: *Cough* due to upper resp tract irritation **Action:** Antitussive w/ expectorant **Dose:** *Adults & Peds >12 y.* 10 mL PO q6–8h (max 40 mL/24 h). *Peds.* 2–6 y: Dextromethorphan 1–2 mg/kg/24 h ÷ 3–4 × d (max 10 mL/d). *6–12 y:* 5 mL q6–8h (max 20 mL/d) **Caution:** [C, +] **Contra:** Administration w/ MAOI **Disp:** Many OTC formulations **SE:** Somnolence **Notes:** Give with plenty of fluids

Haemophilus B Conjugate Vaccine (ActHIB, HibTITER, PedvaxHIB, Prohibit, others)

Uses: Routine *immunization* of children against *H. influenzae* type B Dzs **Action:** Active immunization against *Haemophilus* B Dose: *Peds.* 0.5 mL (25 mg) IM in deltoid or vastus lateralis **Caution:** [C, +] **Contra:** Febrile illness, immunosuppression, allergy to thimerosal **Disp:** Inj 7.5, 10, 15, 25 mcg/0.5 mL **SE:** Observe for anaphylaxis; edema, ↑ risk of *Haemophilus* B Infxn the week after vaccination **Notes:** Booster not required; report SAE to VAERS: 1-800-822-7967

Haloperidol (Haldol)

Uses: *Psychotic disorders, agitation, Tourette disorders, hyperactivity in children* **Action:** Antipsychotic, neuroleptic **Dose:** *Adults.* Moderate Sxs: 0.5–2 mg PO bid–tid. *Severe Sxs/agitation:* 3–5 mg PO bid–tid or 1–5 mg IM q4h PRN (max 100 mg/d). Peds. 3–6 y: 0.01–0.03 mg/kg/24 h PO qd. *6–12 y:* Initial, 0.5–1.5 mg/24 h PO; ↑ by 0.5 mg/24 h to maintenance of 2–4 mg/24 h (0.05–0.1 mg/kg/24 h) or 1–3 mg/dose IM q4–8h to 0.1 mg/kg/24 h max; Tourette Dz may require up to 15 mg/24 h PO; ↓ in elderly **Caution:** [C, ?] ↑ effects w/ SSRIs, CNS depressants, TCA, indomethacin, metoclopramide; avoid levodopa (↓ antiparkinsonian effects) **Contra:** NA glaucoma, severe CNS depression, coma, Parkinson Dz, BM suppression, severe cardiac/hepatic Dz **Disp:** Tabs 0.5, 1, 2, 5, 10, 20 mg; conc liq 2 mg/mL; inj 5 mg/mL; decanoate inj 50, 100 mg/mL **SE:** Extrapyramidal Sxs (EPS), ↓ BP, anxiety, dystonias **Notes:** Do not give decanoate IV; dilute PO conc liq w/ H_2O/juice; monitor for EPS

Haloprogin (Halotex)

Uses: *Topical Rx of tinea pedis, tinea cruris, tinea corporis, tinea manus* **Action:** Topical antifungal **Dose:** *Adults.* Apply bid for ≤2 wk; intertriginous may require ≤4 wk **Caution:** [B, ?] **Contra:** Component sensitivity **Disp:** 1% cream; soln **SE:** Local irritation **Notes:** Avoid contact w/ eyes; improvement w/in 4 wk

Heparin **Uses:** *Rx & prevention of DVT & PE,* unstable angina, AF w/ emboli, & acute arterial occlusion **Action:** Acts w/ antithrombin III to inactivate thrombin & ↓ thromboplastin formation **Dose:** *Adults.* Prophylaxis: 3000–5000 units SQ q8–12h. *Thrombosis Rx:* Load 50–80 units/kg IV, then 10–20 units/kg IV qh (adjust based on PTT). *Peds.* Infants: Load 50 units/kg IV bolus, then 20 units/kg/h IV by cont inf. *Children:* Load 50 units/kg IV, then 15–25 units/kg cont inf or 100 units/kg/dose q4h IV intermittent bolus (adjust based on PTT) **Caution:** [B, +] ↑ risk of hemorrhage w/ anticoagulants, aspirin, antiplatelets, cephalosporins w/ MTT side chain **Contra:** Uncontrolled bleeding, severe thrombocytopenia, suspected ICH **Disp:** Inj 10, 100, 1000, 2000, 2500, 5000, 7500, 10,000, 20,000, 40,000 units/mL **SE:** Bruising, bleeding, thrombocytopenia **Notes:** Follow PTT, thrombin time, or activated clotting time; little PT effect; therapeutic PTT 1.5–2 × control for most conditions; monitor for HIT w/plt counts

Hepatitis A Vaccine (Havrix, Vaqta) **Uses:** *Prevent hepatitis A* in high-risk individuals (eg. travelers, certain professions, or high-risk behaviors) **Action:** Active immunity (Expressed as ELISA units [EL.U.]) Havrix: *Adults.* 1440 EL.U. single IM dose. *Peds >2 y.* 720 EL.U. single IM dose. *Vaqta: Adults.* 50 units single IM dose. *Peds.* 25 units single IM dose **Caution:** [C, +] **Contra:** Component allergy **Disp:** Inj 720 EL.U./0.5 mL, 1440 EL.U./1 mL; 50 units/mL **SE:** Fever, fatigue, HA, inj site pain **Notes:** Booster OK 6–12 mo after primary; report SAE to VAERS: 1-800-822-7967

Hepatitis A (Inactivated) & Hepatitis B (Recombinant) Vaccine (Twinrix) **Uses:** *Active immunization against hepatitis A/B* **Action:** Active immunity **Dose:** 1 mL IM at 0, 1, & 6 mo **Caution:** [C, +] **Contra:** Component sensitivity **Disp:** Single-dose vials, syringes **SE:** Fever, fatigue, pain at site, HA **Notes:** Booster OK 6–12 mo after vaccination; report SAE to VAERS: 1-800-822-7967

Hepatitis B Immune Globulin (HyperHep, H-BIG) **Uses:** *Exposure to HBsAg(+) material* * (eg. blood, plasma, or serum, accidental needlestick, mucous membrane contact, PO) **Action:** Passive immunization **Dose:** *Adults & Peds.* 0.06 mL/kg IM 5 mL max; w/in 24 h of exposure; w/in 14 d of sexual contact; repeat 1 & 6 mo after exposure **Caution:** [C, ?] **Contra:** Allergies to γ-globulin or anti-immunoglobulin Ab; allergies to thimerosal; IgA deficiency **Disp:** Inj **SE:** Inj site pain, dizziness **Notes:** IM in gluteal or deltoid; w/continued exposure, give hepatitis B vaccine

Hepatitis B Vaccine (Engerix-B, Recombivax HB) **Uses:** *Prevent hepatitis B* **Action:** Active immunization; recombinant DNA **Dose:** *Adults.* 3 IM doses 1 mL each; 1st 2 doses 1 mo apart; the 3rd 6 mo after the 1st. *Peds.* 0.5 mL IM adult schedule **Caution:** [C, +] ↓ effect w/ immunosuppressives **Contra:** Yeast allergy **Disp:** Engerix-B: Inj 20 mcg/mL; peds inj 10 mcg/0.5 mL. Recombivax HB: Inj 10 & 40 mcg/mL; peds inj 5 mcg/0.5 mL **SE:** Fever, inj site pain **Notes:** Deltoid IM inj adults/older peds; younger peds, use anterolateral thigh

Hetastarch (Hespan) **Uses:** *Plasma volume expansion* adjunct in shock & leukapheresis **Action:** Synthetic colloid; acts similar to albumin **Dose:** *Volume expansion:* 500–1000 mL (1500 mL/d max) IV (20 mL/kg/h max rate). *Leukapheresis:* 250–700 mL; ↓ in renal failure **Caution:** [C, +] **Contra:** Severe bleeding disorders, CHF, oliguric/anuric renal failure **Disp:** Inj 6 g/100 mL **SE:** Bleeding (↑ PT, PTT, bleed time) **Notes:** Not blood or plasma substitute

Human Papillomavirus (Types 6,11,16,18) Recombinant Vaccine (Gardasil) **Uses:** *Prevent cervical CA, precancerous genital lesions, and genital warts due to HPV types 6, 11, 16, 18 in females 9–26 yrs* **Action:** Recombinant vaccine, passive humoral immunity **Dose:** 0.5 mL IM initial, then 2 and 6 mo **Caution:** [B, ?/-] **Disp:** Single-dose vial and prefilled syringe: 0.5 ml **SE:** Site Rxn (pain, erythema, swelling, pruritus), fever **Notes:** First approved cancer vaccine; report adverse events to VAERS 1-800-822-7967.

Hydralazine (Apresoline, others) **Uses:** *Moderate–severe HTN; CHF* (w/ Isordil) **Action:** Peripheral vasodilator **Dose:** *Adults.* Initial 10 mg PO qid, ↑ to 25 mg qid 300 mg/d max. *Peds.* 0.75–3 mg/kg/24 h PO ÷ q6–12h; ↓ in renal impair; check CBC & ANA before **Caution:** [C, +] ↓ hepatic Fxn & CAD; ↑ tox w/ MAOI, indomethacin, β-blockers **Contra:** Dissecting aortic aneurysm, mitral valve/rheumatic heart Dz **Disp:** Tabs 10, 25, 50, 100 mg; inj 20 mg/mL **SE:** SLE-like syndrome w/ chronic high doses; SVT following IM route, peripheral neuropathy **Notes:** Compensatory sinus tachycardia eliminated w/ β-blocker

Hydrochlorothiazide (HydroDIURIL, Esidrix, others) **Uses:** *Edema, HTN* **Action:** Thiazide diuretic; ↓ distal tubule Na reabsorption **Dose:** *Adults.* 25–100 mg/d PO single or + doses. *Peds.* <6 mo: 2–3 mg/kg/d in 2 ÷ doses. >6 mo: 2 mg/kg/d in 2 ÷ doses **Caution:** [D, +] **Contra:** Anuria, sulfonamide allergy, renal insuff **Disp:** Tabs 25, 50, 100 mg; caps 12.5 mg; PO soln 50 mg/5 mL **SE:** ↓ K⁺, hyperglycemia, hyperuricemia, ↓ Na⁺; sun sensitivity

Hydrochlorothiazide & Amiloride (Moduretic) **Uses:** *HTN* **Action:** Combined thiazide & a K⁺-sparing diuretic **Dose:** 1–2 tabs/d PO **Caution:** [D, ?] **Contra:** Renal failure, sulfonamide allergy **Disp:** Tabs (amiloride/HCTZ) 5 mg/50 mg **SE:** ↓ BP, photosensitivity, ↑ K⁺/↓ K⁺, hyperglycemia, ↓ Na⁺, hyperlipidemia, hyperuricemia

Hydrochlorothiazide & Spironolactone (Aldactazide) **Uses:** *Edema, HTN* **Action:** Thiazide & K⁺-sparing diuretic **Dose:** 25–200 mg each component/d, ÷ doses **Caution:** [D, +] **Contra:** Sulfonamide allergy **Disp:** Tabs (HCTZ/spironolactone) 25 mg/25 mg, 50 mg/50 mg **SE:** Photosensitivity, ↓ BP, ↑ or ↓ K⁺, ↓ Na⁺, hyperglycemia, hyperlipidemia, hyperuricemia

Hydrochlorothiazide & Triamterene (Dyazide, Maxzide) **Uses:** *Edema & HTN* **Action:** Combo thiazide & K⁺-sparing diuretic **Dose:** *Dyazide:* 1–2 caps PO qd–bid. *Maxzide:* 1 tab/d PO **Caution:** [D, +/–] **Contra:**

Sulfonamide allergy **Disp:** (Triamterene/HCTZ) 37.5 mg/25 mg, 75 mg/50 mg **SE:** Photosensitivity, ↓ BP, ↑ or ↓ K⁺, ↓ Na⁺, hyperglycemia, hyperlipidemia, hyperuricemia **Notes:** HCTZ component in Maxzide more bioavailable than in Dyazide

Hydrocodone & Acetaminophen (Lorcet, Vicodin, others) [C-III]
Uses: *Moderate–severe pain* **Action:** Narcotic analgesic w/ nonnarcotic analgesic; hydrocodone is antitussive **Dose:** 1–2 caps or tabs PO q4–6h PRN **Caution:** [C, M] **Contra:** CNS depression, severe resp depression **Disp:** Many formulations; specify hydrocodone/APAP dose; caps 5/500; tabs 2.5/500, 5/400, 5/500, 7.5/400, 10/400, 7.5/500, 7.5/650, 7.5/750, 10/325, 10/400, 10/500, 10/650; elixir & soln (fruit punch) 2.5 mg hydrocodone/167 mg APAP/5 mL **SE:** GI upset, sedation, fatigue **Notes:** Do not exceed >4 g APAP/d

Hydrocodone & Aspirin (Lortab ASA, others) [C-III]
Uses: *Moderate–severe pain* **Action:** Narcotic analgesic with NSAID **Dose:** 1–2 PO q4–6h PRN, w/ food/milk **Caution:** [C, M] ↓renal Fxn, gastritis/PUD, **Contra:** Component sensitivity; children w/chickenpox (Reye's syndrome) **Disp:** 5 mg hydrocodone/500 mg ASA/tab **SE:** GI upset, sedation, fatigue **Notes:** Monitor for GI bleed

Hydrocodone & Guaifenesin (Hycotuss Expectorant, others) [C-III]
Uses: *Nonproductive cough* associated with Infxn **Action:** Expectorant w/ cough suppressant **Dose:** *Adults & Peds >12 y.* 5 mL q4h pc & hs. *Peds.* < 2 y: 0.3 mg/kg/d ÷ qid. *2–12 y:* 2.5 mL q4h pc & hs **Caution:** [C, M] **Contra:** Component sensitivity **Disp:** Hydrocodone 5 mg/guaifenesin 100 mg/5 mL **SE:** GI upset, sedation, fatigue

Hydrocodone & Homatropine (Hycodan, Hydromet, others) [C-III]
Uses: *Relief of cough* **Action:** Combo antitussive **Dose:** (Based on hydrocodone) *Adults.* 5–10 mg q4–6h. *Peds.* 0.6 mg/kg/d ÷ tid–qid **Caution:** [C, M] **Contra:** NA glaucoma, ↑ ICP, depressed ventilation **Disp:** Syrup 5 mg hydrocodone/5 mL; tabs 5 mg hydrocodone **SE:** Sedation, fatigue, GI upset **Notes:** Do not give >q4h; see individual drugs

Hydrocodone & Ibuprofen (Vicoprofen) [C-III]
Uses: *Moderate–severe pain (<10 d)* **Action:** Narcotic w/ NSAID **Dose:** 1–2 tabs q4–6h PRN **Caution:** [C, M] Renal insuff; ↓ effect w/ ACE inhibitors & diuretics; ↑ effect w/ CNS depressants, EtOH, MAOI, aspirin, TCA, anticoagulants **Contra:** Component sensitivity **Disp:** Tabs 7.5 mg hydrocodone/200 mg ibuprofen **SE:** Sedation, fatigue, GI upset

Hydrocodone & Pseudoephedrine (Detussin, Histussin-D, others) [C-III]
Uses: *Cough & nasal congestion* **Action:** Narcotic cough suppressant with decongestant **Dose:** 5 mL qid, PRN **Caution:** [C, M] **Contra:** MAOIs **Disp:** 5 mg hydrocodone/60 mg pseudoephedrine/5 mL **SE:** ↑ BP, GI upset, sedation, fatigue

Hydrocodone, Chlorpheniramine, Phenylephrine, Acetaminophen, & Caffeine (Hycomine Compound)[C-III]
Uses: *Cough & Sxs of URI* **Action:** Narcotic cough suppressant w/ decongestants &

analgesic **Dose:** 1 tab PO q4h PRN **Caution:** [C, M] **Contra:** NA glaucoma **Disp:** Hydrocodone 5 mg/chlorpheniramine 2 mg/phenylephrine 10 mg/APAP 250 mg/caffeine 30 mg/tab **SE:** ↑BP, GI upset, sedation, fatigue

Hydrocortisone, Rectal (Anusol-HC Suppository, Cortifoam Rectal, Proctocort, others) Uses: *Painful anorectal conditions,* radiation proctitis, ulcerative colitis **Action:** Anti-inflammatory steroid **Dose:** *Adults.* Ulcerative colitis: 10–100 mg PR qd–bid for 2–3 wk **Caution:** [B, ?/–] **Contra:** Component sensitivity **Disp:** *Hydrocortisone acetate:* Rectal aerosol 90 mg/applicator; supp 25 mg. *Hydrocortisone base:* Rectal 1%; rectal susp 100 mg/60 mL **SE:** Minimal systemic effect

Hydrocortisone, Topical & Systemic (Cortef, Solu-Cortef) See Steroids page 175 and Tables 4 & 5 **Caution:** [B, –] **Contra:** Viral, fungal, or tubercular skin lesions; serious Infxns (except septic shock or TB meningitis) **SE:** Systemic: ↑ appetite, insomnia, hyperglycemia, bruising **Notes:** May cause HPA axis suppression

Hydromorphone (Dilaudid) [C–II] Uses: *Moderate/severe pain* **Action:** Narcotic analgesic **Dose:** 1–4 mg PO, IM, IV, or PR q4–6h PRN; 3 mg PR q6–8h PRN; ↓ w/ hepatic failure **Caution:** [B (D if prolonged use or high doses near term), ?] **↑** effects w/ CNS depressants, phenothiazines, TCA **Contra:** Component sensitivity **Disp:** Tabs 2, 4 mg, 8 mg; liq 5 mg/5 mL or 1 mg/mL; inj 1, 2, 4, 10 mg/mL; supp 3 mg **SE:** Sedation, dizziness, GI upset **Notes:** Morphine 10 mg IM = hydromorphone 1.5 mg IM

Hydroxyurea (Hydrea, Droxia) Uses: *CML, head & neck, ovarian & colon CA, melanoma, acute leukemia, sickle cell anemia, polycythemia vera, HIV* **Action:** ↓ ribonucleotide reductase system **Dose:** (per protocol) 50–75 mg/kg for WBC >100,000 cells/mL2; 20–30 mg/kg in refractory CML. HIV: 1000–1500 mg/d in single or ÷ doses; ↓ in renal insuff **Caution:** [D, –] ↑ effects w/ zidovudine, zalcitabine, didanosine, stavudine, fluorouracil **Contra:** Severe anemia, BM suppression, WBC <2500 or plt <100,000, PRG **Disp:** Caps 200, 300, 400, 500 mg, tabs 1000 mg **SE:** Myelosuppression (primarily leukopenia), N/V, rashes, facial erythema, radiation recall Rxns, & renal dysfunction **Notes:** Open and empty capsules into H$_2$O

Hydroxyzine (Atarax, Vistaril) Uses: *Anxiety, sedation, itching* **Action:** Antihistamine, antianxiety **Dose:** *Adults.* Anxiety or sedation: 50–100 mg PO or IM qid or PRN (max 600 mg/d). *Itching:* 25–50 mg PO or IM tid–qid. *Peds.* 0.5–1.0 mg/kg/24 h PO or IM q6h; ↓ in hepatic failure **Caution:** [C, +/–] ↑ effects w/ CNS depressants, anticholinergics, EtOH **Contra:** Component sensitivity **Disp:** Tabs 10, 25, 50, 100 mg; caps 25, 50, 100 mg; syrup 10 mg/5 mL; susp 25 mg/5 mL; inj 25, 50 mg/mL **SE:** Drowsiness & anticholinergic effects **Notes:** Useful to potentiate narcotics effects; not for IV/SQ (thrombosis & digital gangrene)

Hyoscyamine (Anaspaz, Cystospaz, Levsin, others) Uses: *Spasm w/ GI & bladder disorders* **Action:** Anticholinergic **Dose:** *Adults.*

0.125–0.25 mg (1–2 tabs) SL/PO tid-qid, ac & hs; 1 SR cap q12h **Caution:** [C, +] ↑ effects w/ amantadine, antihistamines, antimuscarinics, haloperidol, phenothiazines, TCA, MAOI **Contra:** BOO, GI obstruction, glaucoma, MyG, paralytic ileus, ulcerative colitis, MI **Disp:** (Cystospaz-M, Levsinex): time release caps 0.375 mg; elixir (EtOH); soln 0.125 mg/5 mL; inj 0.5 mg/mL; tab 0.125 mg; tab (Cystospaz) 0.15 mg; XR tab (Levbid): 0.375 mg; SL (Levsin SL) 0.125 mg **SE:** Dry skin, xerostomia, constipation, anticholinergic SE, heat prostration w/hot weather **Notes:** Administer tabs before meals/food

Hyoscyamine, Atropine, Scopolamine, & Phenobarbital (Donnatal, others)
Uses: *Irritable bowel, spastic colitis, peptic ulcer, spastic bladder* **Action:** Anticholinergic, antispasmodic **Dose:** 0.125–0.25 mg (1–2 tabs) tid-qid, 1 cap q12h (SR), elixir tid-qid or q8h **Caution:** [D, M] **Contra:** NA glaucoma **Disp:** Many combos/manufacturers; *Cap* (Donnatal, others): Hyosc. 0.1037 mg/atropine 0.0194 mg/scop 0.0065 mg/phenobarbital 16.2 mg. *Tabs* (Donnatal, others): Hyosc. 0.1037 mg/atropine 0.0194 mg/scop 0.0065 mg/phenobarbital 16.2 mg. *Long-acting* (Donnatal): Hyosc. 0.311 mg/atropine 0.0582 mg/scop 0.0195 mg/phenobarbital 48.6 mg. *Flixirs* (Donnatal, others): Hyosc. 0.1037 mg/atropine 0.0194 mg/scop 0.0065 mg/phenobarbital 16.2 mg/5 mL **SE:** Sedation, xerostomia, constipation

Ibandronate (Boniva)
Uses: *Rx & prevent osteoporosis in postmenopausal women* **Action:** Bisphosphonate, ↓ osteoclast-mediated bone-resorption **Dose:** 2.5 mg PO qd or 150 mg once/month on same day (do not lie down for 60 min after); 3 mg IV over 15–30 sec q 3 mo **Caution:** [C, ?/–] avoid w/ CrCl < 30 mL/min **Contra:** Uncorrected ↓ Ca²⁺; inability to stand/sit upright for 60 min (PO) **Disp:** Tabs 2.5, 150 mg, inj IV 3mg/3mL **SE:** N/D, HA, dizziness, asthenia, HTN, Infxn, dysphagia, esophagitis, esophageal/gastric ulcer, musculoskeletal pain, jaw osteonecrosis (avoid extensive dental procedures) **Notes:** Take 1st thing in AM w/ H₂O (6–8 oz) > 60 min before 1st food/beverage & any meds containing multivalent cations; adequate Ca²⁺ & vit D supls necessary

Ibuprofen (Motrin, Rufen, Advil, others) [OTC]
WARNING: May ↑ risk of cardiovascular events & GI bleeding **Uses:** *Arthritis, pain, fever* **Action:** NSAID **Dose:** *Adults.* 200–800 mg PO bid-qid (max 2.4 g/d). *Peds.* 30–40 mg/kg/d in 3–4 ÷ doses (max 40 mg/kg/d); w/ food **Caution:** [B, +] **Contra:** 3rd tri PRG, severe hepatic impair, allergy & use w/ other NSAIDs, UGI bleed, ulcers **Disp:** Tabs 100, 200, 400, 600, 800 mg; chew tabs 50, 100 mg; caps 200 mg; susp 100 mg/2.5 mL, 100 mg/5 mL, 40 mg/mL (200 mg is OTC preparation) **SE:** Dizziness, peptic ulcer, plt inhibition, worsening of renal insuff

Ibutilide (Convert)
Uses: *Rapid conversion of AF/flutter* **Action:** Class III antiarrhythmic **Dose:** 0.01 mg/kg (max 1 mg) IV inf over 10 min; may repeat once; w/ECG monitoring **Caution:** [C, –] Do not use w/ class I or III antiarrhythmics or w/in 4 h of ibutilide **Contra:** QTc > 440 ms **Disp:** Inj 0.1 mg/mL **SE:** Arrhythmias, HA

Idarubicin (Idamycin) Uses: *Acute leukemias* (AML, ALL, ANLL), *CML in blast crisis, breast CA* Action: DNA intercalating agent; ↓ DNA topoisomerases I & II Dose: (per protocol) 10–12 mg/m²/d for 3–4 d; ↓ in renal/hepatic impairment Caution: [D, –] Contra: Bilirubin >5 mg/dL, PRG Disp: Inj 1 mg/mL (5-, 10-, 20-mg vials) SE: Myelosuppression, cardiotox, N/V, mucositis, alopecia, & IV site Rxns, rare changes in renal/hepatic Fxn Notes: Avoid extravasation, potent vesicant; only given IV

Ifosfamide (Ifex, Holoxan) Uses: *Lung, breast, pancreatic & gastric CA, HL/NHL, soft tissue sarcoma* Action: Alkylating agent Dose: (per protocol) 1.2 g/m²/d for 5 d bolus or cont inf; 2.4 g/m²/d for 3 d; w/ mesna uroprotection; ↓ in renal/hepatic impair Caution: [D, M] ↑ effect w/ phenobarbital, carbamazepine, phenytoin; St. John's wort may ↓ levels Contra: ↓ BM Fxn, PRG Disp: Inj 1, 3 g SE: Hemorrhagic cystitis, nephrotox, N/V, mild–moderate leukopenia, lethargy & confusion, alopecia, & ↑ hepatic enzyme Notes: Administer w/ mesna to prevent hemorrhagic cystitis

Iloprost (Ventavis) WARNING: Associated with syncope; may require dosage adjustment Uses: NYHA Class III/IV pulmonary arterial HTN * Action: Prostaglandin analog Dose: Initial 2.5 mcg; if tolerated, ↑ to 5 mcg inh 6–9 X/d (at least 2 h apart) while awake Caution: [C, ?/–] Antiplatelet effects, ↑ bleeding risk w/ anticoagulants; additive hypotensive effects Contra: SBP <85 mm Hg Disp: Inh soln 10 mcg/mL SE: Syncope, ↓ BP, vasodilation, cough, HA, trismus Notes: Requires Pro-Dose AAD nebulizer; counsel on syncope risk

Imatinib (Gleevec) Uses: *Rx of CML, blast crisis, gastrointestinal stromal tumors (GIST)* Action: ↓ BCL-ABL tyrosine kinase (signal transduction) Dose: Chronic phase CML: 400–600 mg PO qd. Accelerated/blast crisis: 600–800 mg PO qd. GIST: 400–600 mg PO qd Caution: [D, ?/–] w/CYP3A4 meds (Table 13), warfarin Contra: Component sensitivity Disp: Tab 100, 400 mg SE: GI upset, fluid retention, muscle cramps, musculoskeletal pain, arthralgia, rash, HA, neutropenia, thrombocytopenia Notes: Follow CBCs & LFTs baseline & monthly; w/ large glass of H₂O & food to ↓ GI irritation

Imipenem–Cilastatin (Primaxin) Uses: *Serious Infxns* due to susceptible bacteria Action: Bactericidal; ↓ cell wall synthesis. Spectrum: Gram(+) (not S. aureus, group A & B streptococci), gram(–) (not Legionella), anaerobes Dose: Adults. 250–1000 mg (imipenem) IV q6–8h. Peds. 60–100 mg/kg/24 h IV ÷ q6h; ↓if CrCl is <70 mL/min Caution: [C, +/–] Probenecid ↑ tox Contra: Ped pts w/ CNS Infxn (↑Sz risk) & <30 kg w/ renal impair Disp: Inj (imipenem/cilastatin) 250/250 mg, 500/500, 750/750 mg SE: Szs if drug accumulates, GI upset, thrombocytopenia

Imipramine (Tofranil) Uses: *Depression, enuresis,* panic attack, chronic pain Action: TCA; ↑ CNS synaptic serotonin or norepinephrine Dose: Adults. Hospitalized: Initial 100 mg/24 h PO in ÷ doses; ↑ over several wks 300 mg/d max. Outpatient: Maint 50–150 mg PO hs, 300 mg/24 h max. Peds. Antidepressant: 1.5–5 mg/kg/24 h ÷ qd–qid. *Enuresis:>6 y:* 10–25 mg PO qhs; ↑ by 10–25 mg at 1–2-wk intervals (max 50 mg for 6–12 y, 75 mg for >12 y); treat for 2–3 mo, then taper **Caution:** [D, ?/–] **Contra:** Use with MAOIs, NA glaucoma, acute recovery from MI, PRG, CHF, angina, CVD, arrhythmias **Disp:** Tabs 10, 25, 50 mg; caps 75, 100, 125, 150 mg **SE:** CV Sxs, dizziness, xerostomia, discolored urine **Notes:** Less sedation than amitriptyline

Imiquimod Cream, 5% (Aldara) **Uses:** *Anogenital warts, HPV, condylomata acuminata* **Action:** Unknown; ? cytokine induction **Dose:** Apply 3×/wk, leave on 6–10 h & wash off w/soap & water, continue 16 wk max **Caution:** [B, ?] **Contra:** Component sensitivity **Disp:** Single-dose packets 5% (250 mg cream) **SE:** Local skin reactions **Notes:** Not a cure; may weaken condoms/vaginal diaphragms, wash hands before & after use

Immune Globulin, IV (Gamimune N, Sandoglobulin, Gammar IV) **Uses:** *IgG Ab deficiency Dz states, (eg, congenital agammaglobulinemia, CVH, & BMT), HIV, hepatitis A prophylaxis, ITP* **Action:** IgG supl **Dose:** *Adults & Peds.* Immunodeficiency: 100–200 mg/kg/mo IV at 0.01–0.04 mL/kg/min to 400 mg/kg/dose max. *ITP:* 400 mg/kg/dose IV qd × 5 d, *BMT:* 500 mg/kg/wk; ↓ in renal insuff **Caution:** [C, ?] Separate administration of live vaccines by 3 mo **Contra:** IgA deficiency w/ Abs to IgA, severe thrombocytopenia or coagulation disorders **Disp:** Inj **SE:** Associated mostly w/inf rate; GI upset

Inamrinone [Amrinone] (Inocor) **Uses:** *Acute CHF, ischemic cardiomyopathy* **Action:** Inotrope w/ vasodilator **Dose:** IV Bolus 0.75 mg/kg over 2–3 min; maint 5–10 mcg/kg/min, 10 mg/kg/d max; ↓ if ClCr <10 mL/min **Caution:** [C, ?] **Contra:** Bisulfite allergy **Disp:** Inj 5 mg/mL **SE:** Monitor fluid, electrolyte, & renal changes **Notes:** Incompatible w/ dextrose solns

Indapamide (Lozol) **Uses:** *HTN, edema, CHF* **Action:** Thiazide diuretic; ↑ Na, Cl, & H₂O excretion in proximal segment of distal tubule **Dose:** 1.25–5 mg/d PO **Caution:** [D, ?] ↑ effect w/ loop diuretics, ACE inhibitors, cyclosporine, digoxin, Li **Contra:** Anuria, thiazide/sulfonamide allergy, renal insuff, PRG **Disp:** Tabs 1.25, 2.5 mg **SE:** ↓ BP, dizziness, photosensitivity **Notes:** No additional effects w/ doses >5 mg; take early to avoid nocturia; use sunscreen; OK w/ food/milk

Indinavir (Crixivan) **Uses:** *HIV Infxn* **Action:** Protease inhibitor; ↓ maturation of immature noninfectious virions to mature infectious virus **Dose:** 800 mg PO q8h; in combo w/ other antiretrovirals; on empty stomach; ↓ in hepatic impair **Caution:** [C, ?] Numerous drug interactions **Contra:** w/ triazolam, midazolam, pimozide, ergot alkaloids, simvastatin, lovastatin, sildenafil, St. John's wort **Disp:** Caps 100, 200, 333, 400 mg **SE:** Nephrolithiasis, dyslipidemia, lipodystrophy, GI effects **Notes:** Drink six 8-oz glasses of H₂O/d

Indomethacin (Indocin) **WARNING:** May ↑risk of cardiovascular events & GI bleeding **Uses:** *Arthritis; close ductus arteriosus; ankylosing spondylitis* **Action:** ↓ prostaglandins **Dose:** *Adults.* 25–50 mg PO bid–tid, max 200 mg/d. Infants: 0.2–0.25 mg/kg/dose IV; may repeat in 12–24 h up to 3 doses;

w/ food **Caution:** [B, +] **Contra:** ASA/NSAID sensitivity, peptic ulcer/active GI bleed, precipitation of asthma/urticaria/rhinitis by NSAIDs/aspirin, premature neonates w/ NEC, ↓ renal Fxn, active bleeding, thrombocytopenia, 3rd tri PRG **Disp:** Inj 1 mg/vial; caps 25, 50 mg; SR caps 75 mg; susp 25 mg/5 mL **SE:** GI bleeding or upset, dizziness, edema **Notes:** Monitor renal Fxn

Infliximab (Remicade) **WARNING:** TB, invasive fungal Infxns, & other opportunistic Infxns reported, some fatal; perform TB skin testing prior to therapy **Uses:** *Moderate–severe Crohn Dz; fistulizing Crohn Dz; ulcerative colitis; RA (w/ MTX),* **Action:** IgG1K neutralizes TNFα **Dose:** *Crohn Dz:* Induction: 5 mg/kg IV inf, w/doses 2 & 6 wk after. *Maint:* 5 mg/kg IV inf q8wk. *RA:* 3 mg/kg IV inf at 0, 2, 6 wk, then q8wk **Caution:** [B, ?/–] Active Infxn, hepatic impairment **Contra:** Murine allergy, moderate–severe CHF **Disp:** 100 mg Inj **SE:** Allergic Rxns; pts predisposed to Infxn (especially TB); HA, fatigue, GI upset, infusion Rxns; hepatotoxicity; reactivation hepatitis B, pneumonia, BM suppression, systemic vasculitis, pericardial effusion **Notes:** Monitor LFTs

Influenza Vaccine (Fluzone, FluShield, Fluvirin) **Uses:** *Prevent influenza* in all adults >50 y, children 6–23 mo, pregnant women (2nd/3rd tri during flu season), nursing home residents, chronic Dzs, health-care workers, household contacts of high-risk pts, children < 9 y receiving vaccine for the first time **Action:** Active immunization **Dose:** *Adults.* 0.5 mL/dose IM. *Peds.>* 3 y: 0.5 mL IM; 6–35 mo 0.25 mL IM; *6 mo to < 9 y* (first-time vaccination): 2 doses > 4 wk apart, 2nd dose before Dec if possible **Caution:** [C, +] **Contra:** Egg, gentamicin, or thimerosal allergy, Infxn at site, high risk of influenza complications, Hx of Guillain–Barré, asthma, children 5–17 y on aspirin **Disp:** Based on specific manufacturer, 0.25- & 0.5-mL prefilled syringes **SE:** Inj site soreness, fever, myalgia, malaise, Guillain–Barré syndrome (controversial) **Notes:** Optimal in US: Oct–Nov, protection begins 1–2 wk after, lasts up to 6 mo; each yr, vaccines based on predictions of flu active in flu season (December–Spring in US); whole or split virus for adults; Peds <13 y either whole or purified surface antigen to ↓ febrile Rxns

Influenza Virus Vaccine Live, Intranasal (FluMist) **Uses:** *Prevent influenza* **Action:** Live-attenuated vaccine **Dose:** *Adults 9–49 y.* 1 dose (0.5 mL)/season **Caution:** [C,?/–] **Contra:** Egg allergy, PRG, Hx Guillain–Barré syndrome, known/suspected immune deficiency, asthma or reactive airway Dz **Disp:** Prefilled, single-use, intranasal sprayer **SE:** Runny nose, nasal congestion, HA, cough **Notes:** 0.25 mL into each nostril; do not administer concurrently w/ other vaccines; avoid contact w/ immunocompromised individuals for 21 days

Insulin, Injectable **Uses:** *Type 1 or type 2 DM refractory to diet or PO hypoglycemic agents; acute life-threatening ↑ K^+* **Action:** Insulin supl **Dose:** Based on serum glucose; usually SQ; can give IV (only regular)/IM; type I typical start dose 0.5–1 units/kg/d; type 2 0.3–0.4 units/kg/d; renal failure may ↓ insulin needs **Caution:** [B, +] **Contra:** Hypoglycemia **Disp:** Table 6 **SE:** Highly purified insulins ↑ free insulin; monitor for several wks when changing doses/agents

Insulin Human Inhalation Powder (Exubera) Uses: * Type-1 DM in adults combo w/long-acting insulin; Type-2 DM monotherapy or w/other agents **Action:** Regulates glucose metabolism **Dose:** Premeal (mg) = BW(kg) × 0.05 mg/kg; round down to nearest whole mg; give w/in 10 min prior to meal; titrate based on glucose; 1 mg blister = 3 IU of SC regular human insulin; 3 mg blister = 8 IU of SC regular human insulin. **Caution:** [C, M] **Contra:** Smoker or if D/C smoking <6 months before start; D/C if smoking resumes; unstable or poorly controlled lung disease **Disp:** Unit dose blisters: 1, 3 mg; Exubera Inhaler **SE:** Hypoglycemia, dry mouth, chest pain, otitis media, cough, dyspnea, pharyngitis, rhinitis, sinusitis, epistaxis, ↑ sputum **Notes:** Assess pulmonary fxn before Tx and 6–12 months; store blisters at room temperature

Interferon Alfa (Roferon-A, Intron A) WARNING: Can cause or aggravate fatal or life-threatening neuropsychiatric, autoimmune, ischemic, and infectious disorders. Monitor patients closely. **Uses:** *Hairy cell leukemia, Kaposi sarcoma, melanoma, CML, chronic hepatitis C, chronic hep B, follicular NHL, condylomata acuminata,* **Action:** Antiproliferative; modulates host immune response; inhibits viral replication in infected cells **Dose:** Per protocols. *Adults.* Hairy cell leukemia: Alfa-2a (Roferon-A): 3 M units/d for 16—24 wk SQ/IM then 3 M units 3×/wk for up to 6–24 mo. Alfa-2b (Intron A). 2 M units/m² IM/ SQ 3×/wk for 2–6 mo *Chronic hepatitis B:* Alfa-2b (Intron A): 3 M units/m² SQ 3×/wk × 1 wk, then 6 M units/m² 3×/wk (Max 10M units 3×/wk, total duration 16–24 wks). *Follicular NHL* (Intron A) 5 M units SQ 3×/wk for 18 mo; *Melanoma* (Intron A) 20 M units m² IV × 5 days/wk for 4 wks, then 10 M units/m² SQ 3×/wk for 48 wks; *Kaposi sarcoma* (Intron A) 30 M units/m IM/SQ 3×/wk for 10–12 wks, then 36 M units IM/SQ 3×/wk; *Chronic hep C* (Intron A) 3m units 3×/wk for 16 wks (continue 18–24 mo if response) Roferon A: 3 M units 3×/wk for 12 mo SQ/IM; Condyloma acuminata (Intron A) 1 M unit/lesion (max 5 lesions) 3×/wk for 3 wks. *Peds.* CML: Alfa-2a (Roferon-A): 2.5–5 M units/m² IM qd **Contra:** Benzyl alcohol sensitivity, decompensated liver Dz, autoimmune Dz, immunosuppressed transplant recipients, neonates, infants **Disp:** Injectable forms (see also peg interferon) **SE:** Flulike Sxs; fatigue; anorexia in 20–30%; neurotox at high doses; neutralizing Ab (up to 40%) if on prolonged systemic therapy

Interferon Alfa-2b & Ribavirin Combo (Rebetron) WARNING: Can cause or aggravate fatal or life-threatening neuropsychiatric, autoimmune, ischemic, and infectious disorders. Monitor patients closely. Contraindicated in pregnant females & their male partners **Uses:** *Chronic hepatitis C in pts w/compensated liver Dz who relapse after α-interferon therapy **Action:** Combo antiviral agents (see individual agents) **Dose:** 3 M units Intron A SQ 3 × wk w/ 1,000–1,200 mg of Rebetron PO ÷ bid dose for 24 wk. *Pts <75 kg:* 1000 mg of Rebetron/d **Caution:** [X, ?] **Contra:** PRG, males w/ PRG female partner, autoimmune hepatitis, CrCl <50 mL/min **Disp:** *Pts <75 kg:* Combo packs: 6 vials Intron A (3 M Units/0.5 mL) w/ 6 syringes & EtOH swabs, 70 Rebetron caps; one 18-M unit multidose vial of Intron A inj (22.8 M units/3.8 mL; 3 M units/0.5 mL) & 6 syringes & swabs, 70 Rebetron caps; one 18 M units Intron A inj multidose pen (22.5 M units/1.5 mL; 3 M units/0.2 mL) w/ 6 needles & swabs, 70 Rebetron caps. *Pts >75 kg:* Identical except 84 Rebetron caps/pack **SE:** See warning, flulike syndrome, HA, anemia **Notes:** Monthly PRG test; instruct in self-administration of SQ Intron A

Interferon Alfacon-1 (Infergen) **WARNING:** Can cause or aggravate fatal or life-threatening neuropsychiatric, autoimmune, ischemic, and infectious disorders. Monitor patients closely. **Uses:** *Chronic hepatitis C* **Action:** Biologic response modifier **Dose:** 9 mcg SQ 3×/wk X 24 wk **Caution:** [C, M] **Contra:** *E. coli* product allergy **Disp:** Inj 9, 15 mcg **SE:** Flulike syndrome, depression, blood dyscrasias **Notes:** Allow >48 h between inj

Interferon beta 1a (Rebif) **Uses:** *MS, relapsing* **Action:** Biologic response modifier **Dose:** 44 mcg SC 3×/wk; start 8.8 mcg SC 3×/wk ×2wk, then 22 mcg SC 3×/wk × 2 wk **Caution:** [C, ?] W/ hepatic impair, depression, Sz disorder, thyroid Dz **Contra:** Human albumin allergy **Disp:** Inj SE: inj site rxn, HA, flu like Sx, malaise, fatigue, rigors, myalgia, depression w/suicidal ideation, hepatotoxicity, myelosuppression **Notes:** Dose >48 h apart; CBC 1, 3, and 6mo; TFTs q6mo w/hx thyroid dz

Interferon Beta-1b (Betaseron) **Uses:** *MS, relapsing-remitting & secondary progressive* **Action:** Biologic response modifier **Dose:** 0.25 mg SQ qod **Caution:** [C, ?] **Contra:** Human albumin allergy **Disp:** Powder for inj 0.3 mg **SE:** Flulike syndrome, depression, blood dyscrasias **Notes:** Monitor LFTs

Interferon γ-1b (Actimmune) **Uses:** *↓ Incidence of serious Infxns in chronic granulomatous Dz (CGD), osteopetrosis* **Action:** Biologic response modifier **Dose:** *Adults.* CGD: 50 mcg/m² SQ (1.5 million units/m²) BSA >0.5 m²; if BSA <0.5 m², give 1.5 mcg/kg/dose; given 3 × wk. *Peds.* BSA ≤0.5 m²: 1.5 mcg/kg/ SQ tid; BSA <0.5 m²: 50 mcg/m² SQ tid **Caution:** [C, ?] **Contra:** Allergy to *E. coli*-derived products **Disp:** Inj 100 mcg (2 million units) **SE:** Flulike syndrome, depression, blood dyscrasias

Ipecac Syrup [OTC] **Uses:** *Drug OD, certain cases of poisoning* **NOTE:** Usage is falling out of favor & is no longer recommended by some groups **Action:** Irritation of the GI mucosa; stimulation of the chemoreceptor trigger zone **Dose:** *Adults.* 15–30 mL PO, followed by 200–300 mL of H₂O; if no emesis in 20 min, repeat once. *Peds.* 6–12 y: 5–10 mL PO, followed by 10–20 mL/kg of H₂O; if no emesis in 20 min, repeat once. *1–12 y:* 15 mL PO followed by 10–20 mL/kg of H₂O; if no emesis in 20 min, repeat once **Caution:** [C, ?] **Contra:** Ingestion of petroleum distillates, strong acid, base, or other caustic agents; comatose/unconscious **Disp:** Syrup 15, 30 mL (OTC) **SE:** Lethargy, D, cardiotox, protracted vomiting **Notes:** Caution in CNS depressant OD; activated charcoal more effective (www.clintox.org/PosStatements/Ipecac.html)

Ipratropium (Atrovent) **Uses:** *Bronchospasm w/ COPD, rhinitis, rhinorrhea* **Action:** Synthetic anticholinergic similar to atropine **Dose:** *Adults & Peds*

>*12 y.* 2–4 puffs qid. *Nasal:* 2 sprays/nostril bid–tid **Caution:** [B, +/–] **Contra:** Allergy to soya lecithin/related foods **Disp:** Met-dose inhaler 18 mcg/dose; inhal soln 0.02%; nasal spray 0.03, 0.06%; nasal inhaler 20 mcg/dose **SE:** Nervousness, dizziness, HA, cough, bitter taste, nasal dryness **Notes:** Not for acute bronchospasm

Irbesartan (Avapro) Uses: *HTN, DN*, CHF **Action:** Angiotensin II receptor antagonist **Dose:** 150 mg/d PO, may to 300 mg/d **Caution:** [C (1st tri; D 2nd/3rd), ?/–] **Disp:** Tabs 75, 150, 300 mg **SE:** Fatigue, ↓ BP ↑ K

Irinotecan (Camptosar) Uses: *Colorectal* & lung CA **Action:** Topoisomerase I inhibitor; ↓DNA synthesis **Dose:** Per protocol; 125–350 mg/m² qwk–q3wk (↓ hepatic dysfunction, as tolerated per tox) **Caution:** [D, –] **Contra:** Allergy to component **Disp:** Inj 20 mg/mL **SE:** Myelosuppression, N/V/D, abdominal cramping, alopecia; D is dose limiting; Rx acute D w/ atropine; Rx subacute D w/ loperamide **Notes:** SN correlated to levels of metabolite SN-38

Iron Dextran (Dexferrum, INFeD) Uses: *Fe deficiency when cannot supplement PO* **Action:** Fe supl **Dose:** Estimate Fe deficiency, give IM/IV. Do 0.5-mL test dose; total replacement dose (mL) = 0.0476 × weight (kg) × [desired Hgb (g/dL) – measured Hgb (g/dL)] + 1 mL/5 kg weight (max 14 mL). *Adults.* Max daily dose. 100 mg Fe. *Peds.* Max daily dose: *<5 kg:* 25 mg Fe. *5–10 kg:* 50 mg Fe. *10–50 kg:* 100 mg Fe **Caution:** [C, M] **Contra:** Anemia w/o Fe deficiency. **Disp:** Inj 50 mg (Fe)/mL **SE:** Anaphylaxis, flushing, dizziness, inj site & inf Rxns, metallic taste **Notes:** Give deep IM using "Z-track" technique; IV preferred

Iron Sucrose (Venofer) Uses: *Fe deficiency anemia w/ chronic HD in those receiving erythropoietin* **Actions:** Fe replacement. **Dose:** 5 mL (100 mg) IV on dialysis, 1 mL (20 mg)/min max **Caution:** [C, M] **Contra:** Anemia w/o Fe deficiency **Disp:** 20 mg elemental Fe/mL, 5-mL vials. **SE:** Anaphylaxis, ↓ BP, cramps, N/V/D, HA **Notes:** Most pts require cumulative doses of 1000 mg; give at slow rate

Isoniazid (INH) Uses: *Rx & prophylaxis of TB* **Action:** Bactericidal; interferes w/ mycolic acid synthesis, disrupts cell wall **Dose:** *Adults.* Active TB: 5 mg/kg/24 h PO or IM (usually 300 mg/d) or DOT: 15mg/kg (max 900mg) 3×/wk. *Prophylaxis:* 300 mg/d PO for 6–12 mo or 900 mg 2×/wk. *Peds.* Active TB: 10–15 mg/kg/24 h PO or IM 300 mg/d max. *Prophylaxis:* 10 mg/kg/24 h PO; ↓ in hepatic/renal dysfunction **Caution:** [C, +] Liver Dz, dialysis; avoid EtOH **Contra:** Acute liver Dz, Hx INH hepatitis **Disp:** Tabs 100, 300 mg; syrup 50 mg/5 mL; inj 100 mg/mL **SE:** Hepatitis, peripheral neuropathy, GI upset, anorexia, dizziness, skin Rxn **Notes:** Use w/2–3 other drugs for active TB, based on INH resistance patterns when TB acquired & sensitivity results; prophylaxis usually w/ INH alone. IM rarely used. ↓ peripheral neuropathy w/ pyridoxine 50–100 mg/d. Check CDC guidelines (MMWR) for most current recommendations

Isoproterenol (Isuprel) Uses: *Shock, cardiac arrest, AV nodal block* **Action:** β₁- & β₂-receptor stimulant **Dose:** *Adults.* 2–10 mcg/min IV inf; titrate.

Peds. 0.2–2 mcg/kg/min IV inf; titrate. **Caution:** [C, ?] **Contra:** Angina, tachyarrhythmias (digitalis-induced or others) **Disp:** 0.02 mg/mL, 0.2 mg/mL **SE:** Insomnia, arrhythmias, HA, trembling, dizziness **Notes:** Pulse >130 bpm may induce arrhythmia

Isosorbide Dinitrate (Isordil, Sorbitrate, Dilatrate-SR) **Uses:** *Rx & prevent angina,* CHF (w/ hydralazine) **Action:** Relaxes vascular smooth muscle **Dose:** *Acute angina:* 5–10 mg PO (chew tabs) q2–3h or 2.5–10 mg SL PRN q5–10min; do not give >3 doses in a 15–30-min period. *Angina prophylaxis:* 5–40 mg PO q6h; do not give nitrates on a chronic q6h or qid basis >7–10 d; tolerance may develop; provide 10–12-h drug-free intervals **Caution:** [C, ?] **Contra:** Severe anemia, closed-angle glaucoma, postural ↓ BP, cerebral hemorrhage, head trauma (can ↑ ICP), w/ sildenafil, tadalafil, vardenafil **Disp:** Tabs 5, 10, 20, 30; SR tabs 40 mg; SL tabs 2.5, 5, 10 mg; SR caps 40 mg **SE:** HA, ↓ BP, flushing, tachycardia, dizziness **Notes:** Higher PO dose needed for same results as SL forms

Isosorbide Mononitrate (Ismo, Imdur) **Uses:** *Prevention/Rx of angina pectoris* **Action:** Relaxes vascular smooth muscle **Dose:** 5–10 mg PO bid, w/ the 2 doses 7 h apart or XR (Imdur) 30–60 mg/d PO, max 240 mg **Caution:** [C, ?] **Contra:** Head trauma/cerebral hemorrhage (can ↑ ICP), w/ sildenafil, tadalafil, vardenafil **Disp:** Tabs 10, 20 mg; XR 30, 60, 120 mg **SE:** HA, dizziness, ↓(BP

Isotretinoin [13-*cis* Retinoic Acid] (Accutane, Amnesteem, Claravis, Sotret) **WARNING:** Must not be used by PRG females; can induce severe birth defects; pt must be capable of complying w/ mandatory contraceptive measures; prescribed according to product-specific risk management system. Because of teratogenicity, Accutane is approved for marketing only under a special restricted distribution FDA program called iPLEDGE **Uses:** *Refractory severe acne* **Action:** Retinoic acid derivative **Dose:** 0.5–2 mg/kg/d PO ÷ bid (↓ in hepatic Dz, take w/ food) **Caution:** [X, –] Avoid tetracyclines **Contra:** Retinoid sensitivity, PRG **Disp:** Caps 10, 20, 30, 40 mg **SE:** Rare: Depression, psychosis, suicidal thoughts; dermatologic sensitivity, xerostomia, photosensitivity, LFTs, triglycerides **Notes:** Risk management program requires 2 (–) PRG tests before Rx & use of 2 forms of contraception 1 mo before, during, & 1 mo after therapy; to prescribe isotretinoin, the Prescriber must access the iPLEDGE system via the Internet (www.ipledgeprogram.com); monitor LFTs & lipids

Isradipine (DynaCirc) **Uses:** *HTN* **Action:** CCB **Dose:** *Adults.* 2.5–5 mg PO bid. **Caution:** [C, ?] **Contra:** Severe heart block, sinus bradycardia, CHF, dosing w/in several hours of IV β-blockers **Disp:** Caps 2.5, 5 mg; tabs CR 5, 10 mg **SE:** HA, edema, flushing, fatigue, dizziness, palpitations

Itraconazole (Sporanox) **WARNING:** Potential for negative inotropic effects on the heart; if signs or Sxs of CHF occur during administration, continued use should be assessed **Uses:** *Fungal Infxns (aspergillosis, blastomycosis, histoplasmosis, candidiasis)* **Action:** ↓ ergosterol synthesis **Dose:** 200 mg PO or IV qd–bid (capsule w/ meals or cola/grapefruit juice); PO soln on empty stomach; avoid antacids

Caution: [C, ?] Numerous interactions **Contra:** Inj. if CrCl <30 mL/min, Hx of CHF or ventricular dysfunction, w/H₂-antagonist, omeprazole **Disp:** Caps 100 mg; soln 10 mg/mL; inj 10 mg/mL **SE:** N, rash, hepatitis, ↓ K⁺, CHF (mostly w/ IV use) **Notes:** PO soln & caps not interchangeable; useful in pts who cannot take amphotericin B

Kaolin-Pectin (Kaodene, Kao-Spen, Kapectolin) [OTC] Uses: *Diarrhea* **Action:** Absorbent demulcent **Dose:** *Adults.* 60–120 mL PO after each loose stool or q3–4h PRN. *Peds.* 3–6 y: 15–30 mL/dose PO PRN. *6–12 y:* 30–60 mL/dose PO PRN **Caution:** [C, +] **Contra:** D secondary to pseudomembranous colitis **Disp:** Multiple OTC forms; also available w/ opium (Parepectolin CIII) **SE:** Constipation, dehydration

Ketoconazole (Nizoral, Nizoral AD Shampoo) [Shampoo–OTC] Uses: *Systemic fungal Infxns; topical for local fungal Infxns due to dermatophytes & yeast; shampoo for dandruff,* CAP when rapid ↓ testosterone needed (ie, cord compression) **Action:** ↓ fungal cell wall synthesis **Dose:** *Adults.* PO: 200 mg PO qd, ↑ to 400 mg PO qd for serious Infxn; CAP 400 mg PO tid (short-term). *Topical:* Apply qd (cream/shampoo) *Peds >2 y.* 5–10 mg/kg/24 h PO ÷ q12–24h (↓ in hepatic Dz) **Caution:** [C, +/–] Any agent that ↑ gastric pH prevents absorption; may enhance anticoagulants; w/ EtOH (disulfiram-like Rxn) numerous interactions **Contra:** CNS fungal Infxns (poor CNS penetration), w/astemizole, cisapride, triazolam **Disp:** Tabs 200 mg; topical cream 2%; shampoo 10% **SE:** N Notes: Monitor LFTs w/ systemic use

Ketoprofen (Orudis, Oruvail) WARNING: May ↑risk of cardiovascular events & GI bleeding Uses: *Arthritis, pain* **Action:** NSAID; ↓ prostaglandins **Dose:** 25–75 mg PO tid–qid, 300 mg/d/max; w/ food **Caution:** [B (D 3td tri), ?] **Contra:** NSAID/ASA sensitivity **Disp:** Tabs 12.5 mg; caps 25, 50, 75 mg; caps, SR 100, 150, 200 mg **SE:** GI upset, peptic ulcers, dizziness, edema, rash

Ketorolac (Toradol) WARNING: Indicated for short term (= 5 d) Rx of moderate–severe acute pain that requires opioid analgesia levels Uses: *Pain* **Action:** NSAID; ↓ prostaglandins **Dose:** 15–30 mg IV/IM q6h or 10 mg PO qid; max IV/IM 120 mg/d, max PO 40 mg/d; do not use for >5 d; ↓ for age & renal dysfunction **Caution:** [B (D 3rd tri), –] **Contra:** Peptic ulcer Dz, NSAID sensitivity, advanced renal Dz, CNS bleeding, anticipated major surgery, labor & delivery, nursing mothers **Disp:** Tabs 10 mg; inj 15 mg/mL, 30 mg/mL **SE:** Bleeding, peptic ulcer Dz, renal failure, edema, dizziness, allergy Notes: PO only as continuation of IM/IV therapy

Ketorolac Ophthalmic (Acular, Acular LS, Acular PF) Uses: *Ocular itching w/ seasonal allergies*; inflammation w/ cataract extraction; pain/photophobia w/ incisional refractive surgery (Acular PF); Pain w/ corneal refractive surgery (Acular LS) **Action:** NSAID **Dose:** 1 gt qid **Caution:** [C, +] **Disp:** Acular LS: 0.4%; Acular, Acular PF soln 0.5% **SE:** Local irritation

Ketotifen (Zaditor) Uses: *Allergic conjunctivitis* **Action:** H₁-receptor antagonist, mast cell stabilizer **Dose:** *Adults & Peds.* 1 gt in eye(s) q8–12h **Caution:** [C,?/–] **Disp:** Soln 0.025%/5 mL **SE:** Local irritation, HA, rhinitis

Labetalol (Trandate) Uses: *HTN* & hypertensive emergencies (IV) **Action:** α- & β-adrenergic blocking agent **Dose:** *Adults.* HTN: Initial, 100 mg PO bid, then 200–400 mg PO bid. *Hypertensive emergency:* 20–80 mg IV bolus, then 2 mg/min IV inf, titrate up to 300 mg. *Peds.* PO: 3–20 mg/kg/d in ÷ doses. *Hypertensive emergency:* 0.4–1.5 mg/kg/h IV cont inf **Caution:** [C (D in 2nd or 3rd tri), +] **Contra:** Asthma/COPD, cardiogenic shock, uncompensated CHF, heart block **Disp:** Tabs 100, 200, 300 mg; inj 5 mg/mL **SE:** Dizziness, nausea, ↓ BP, fatigue, CV effects

Lactic Acid & Ammonium Hydroxide [Ammonium Lactate] (Lac-Hydrin) Uses: *Severe xerosis & ichthyosis* **Action:** Emollient moisturizer **Dose:** Apply bid **Caution:** [B, ?] **Disp:** Cream, lotion, lactic acid 12% w/ ammonium hydroxide **SE:** Local irritation

Lactobacillus (Lactinex Granules) [OTC] Uses: * Control of D*, especially after antibiotic therapy **Action:** Replaces nl intestinal flora **Dose:** *Adults & Peds >3 y.* 1 packet, 1–2 caps, or 4 tabs QD–QID **Caution:** [A, +] **Contra:** Milk/lactose allergy **Disp:** Tabs; caps; EC caps; powder in packets (all OTC) **SE:** Flatulence

Lactulose (Constulose, Generlac, Enulose, others) Uses: *Hepatic encephalopathy; constipation* **Action:** Acidifies the colon, allows ammonia to diffuse into colon **Dose:** *Acute hepatic encephalopathy:* 30–45 mL PO q1h until soft stools, then tid–qid. *Chronic laxative therapy:* 30–45 mL PO tid–qid; adjust q1–2d to produce 2–3 soft stools/d. *Rectally:* 200 g in 700 mL of H₂O PR. *Peds.* Infants: 2.5–10 mL/24 h ÷ tid–qid. *Peds.* 40–90 mL/24 h ÷ tid–qid **Caution:** [B, ?] **Contra:** Galactosemia **Disp:** Syrup 10 g/15 mL, soln 10 g/15 mL, 10, 20 g/packet **SE:** Severe D, flatulence; life-threatening electrolyte disturbances

Lamivudine (Epivir, Epivir-HBV) **WARNING:** Lactic acidosis & severe hepatomegaly w/ steatosis reported w/ nucleoside analogus Uses: *HIV Infxn, chronic hepatitis B* **Action:** ↓ HIV RT & hepatitis B viral polymerase, resulting in viral DNA chain termination **Dose:** *HIV: Adults & Peds >16 y.* 150 mg PO bid or 300 mg PO qd. *Peds <16 y.* 4 mg/kg PO bid. *HBV: Adults.* 100 mg/d PO. *Peds 2–17 y.* 3 mg/kg/d PO, 100 mg max; ↓ in renal impair **Caution:** [C, -]: **Disp:** Tabs 100 mg (HBV) 150 mg, 300 mg; soln 5 mg/mL (HBV), 10 mg/mL (HBV) **SE:** HA, pancreatitis, GI upset, lactic acidosis, peripheral neuropathy

Lamotrigine (Lamictal) **WARNING:** Serious rashes requiring hospitalization & D/C of Rx reported; rash less frequent in adults Uses: *Partial Szs, bipolar disorder, Lennox–Gastaut syndrome* **Action:** Phenyltriazine antiepileptic, ↓ glutamate, stabilize neuronal membrane **Dose:** *Adults.* Szs: Initial 50 mg/d PO, then 50 mg PO bid for 2 wk, maint 300–500 mg/d in 2 ÷ doses. *Bipolar:* Initial 25 mg/d PO, 50 mg PO qd for 2 wk, 100 mg PO qd for 1 wk, maint 200 mg/d. *Peds.* 0.6 mg/kg in 2 ÷ doses for wk 1 & 2, then 1.2 mg/kg for wk 3 & 4, maint 15 mg/kg/d (max 400 mg/d)1–2 ÷ doses; ↓ in hepatic Dz or if w/ enzyme inducers or valproic acid **Caution:** [C, –] Interactions w/ other antiepileptics **Disp:** Tabs 25, 100, 150, 200 mg; chew tabs 2, 5, 25 mg **SE:** Photosensitivity, HA, GI upset, dizziness, ataxia, rash (potentially life-threatening in children >adults) **Notes:** ? value of therapeutic monitoring

Lansoprazole (Prevacid, Prevacid IV) **Uses:** *Duodenal ulcers, prevent & Rx NSAID gastric ulcers, IV alternative for ≤7 d /w erosive esophagitis.* *H. pylori* Infxn, erosive esophagitis, & hypersecretory conditions, GERD **Action:** Proton pump inhibitor **Dose:** 15–30 mg/d PO; NSAID ulcer prevention 15 mg/d PO ≤12 wk, NSAID ulcers 30 mg/d PO, ×8 wk; 30 mg IV qd ≤7 d change to PO for 6–8 wk; ↓ in severe hepatic impair **Caution:** [B, ?/–] **Disp:** Caps 15, 30 mg; granules for suspension 15, 30 mg, IV 30 mg; OD tabs 15, 30 mg **SE:** HA, fatigue **Notes:** For IV provided in-line filter must be used

Lanthanum Carbonate (Fosrenol) **Uses:** Hyperphosphatemia in renal disease * **Action:** Phosphate binder **Dose:** 750–1500 mg PO qd ÷ doses, w/ or immed after meal; titrate every 2–3 wk based on PO_4^{-2} levels **Caution:** [C, ?/–] No data in GI disease **Disp:** Chew tabs 250, 500, 750, 1000 mg **SE:** N/V, graft occlusion, HA ↓ BP **Notes:** Chew tabs before swallowing; separate from meds that interact with antacids by 2 h

Latanoprost (Xalatan) **Uses:** *Open angle glaucoma, ocular HTN* **Action:** Prostaglandin, ↑ outflow of aqueous humor **Dose:** 1 gt eye(s) hs **Caution:** [C, ?] Disp: 0.005% soln **SE:** May darken light irides; blurred vision, ocular stinging, & itching

Leflunomide (Arava) **WARNING:** PRG must be excluded prior to start of Rx **Uses:** *Active RA* **Action:** ↓ Pyrimidine synthesis Dose: Initial 100 mg/d PO for 3 d, then 10–20 mg/d **Caution:** [X, –] **Contra:** PRG Disp: Tabs 10, 20, 100 mg **SE:** D, Infxn, HTN, alopecia, rash, nausea, joint pain, hepatitis **Notes:** Monitor LFTs during initial therapy

Lenalidomide (Revlimid) **WARNING:** Significant teratogen; patient must be enrolled in RevAssist risk reduction program **Uses:** *MDS* multiple myeloma **Action:** Thalidomide analog, immune modulator **Dose:** *Adults.* 10 mg PO daily; swallow whole w/water **Caution:** [X,–] w/ renal impair **Disp:** Caps 5, 10 mg **SE:** D, pruritus, rash, fatigue, myelosuppression, thromboembolism, ↑ LFT **Notes:** Monitor for myelosuppression, thromboembolism, hepatotoxicity; routine PRG tests required; Rx only in 1-mo increments; limited distribution network; males must use condom and not donate sperm; use contraception at least 4 wks beyond D/C

Lepirudin (Refludan) **Uses:** *HIT* **Action:** Direct thrombin inhibitor **Dose:** Bolus 0.4 mg/kg IV, then 0.15 mg/kg/h inf (↓ dose & inf rate if CrCl <60 mL/min) **Caution:** [B, ?/–] Hemorrhagic event or severe HTN **Contra:** Active bleeding **Disp:** Inj 50 mg **SE:** Bleeding, anemia, hematoma **Notes:** Adjust based on aPTT ratio, maintain aPTT 1.5–2.0

Letrozole (Femara) **Uses:** *Advanced breast CA in postmenopausal* **Action:** Nonsteroidal aromatase inhibitor **Dose:** 2.5 mg/d PO **Caution:** [D, ?] **Contra:** PRG Disp: Tabs 2.5 mg **SE:** Anemia, nausea, hot flashes, arthralgia **Notes:** Monitor CBC, thyroid Fxn, electrolytes, LFT, & renal monitoring

Leucovorin (Wellcovorin) Uses: *OD of folic acid antagonist; megaloblastic anemia, augment 5-FU impaired MTX elimination* Action: Reduced folate source; circumvents action of folate reductase inhibitors (eg, MTX) Dose: *Adults & Peds.* Per protocol. Caution: [C, ?/–] Contra: Pernicious anemia Disp: Tabs 5, 10, 15, 25 mg; inj 50, 100, 200, 350, 500 SE: Allergic Rxn, N/V/D, fatigue Notes: Many dosing schedules for leucovorin rescue following MTX therapy; do not use intrathecally/intraventrically

Leuprolide (Lupron, Lupron DEPOT, Lupron DEPOT-Ped, Viadur, Eligard) Uses: *Advanced CAP (all products except Depot-Ped), endometriosis (Lupron), uterine fibroids (Lupron), & CPP (Lupron-Ped)* Action: LHRH agonist; paradoxically ↓ release of gonadotropin, resulting in ↓ pituitary gonadotropins (↓ LH); in men ↓ testosterone Dose: *Adults.* CAP: Lupron Depot: 7.5 mg IM q28d or 22.5 mg IM q3mo or 30 mg IM q4mo; Eligard: 7.5 mg IM/SQ q28d or 22.5 mg IM q3mo or 30 mg IM/SQ q4mo; Eligard 45 mg SQ 6 mo; Viadur implant (CAP only); insert in inner upper arm w/ local anesthesia, replace q12mo. *Endometriosis (Lupron DEPOT):* 3.75 mg IM qmo X6. *Fibroids:* 3.75 mg IM qmo X3. *Peds.* CPP (Lupron-Ped): 50 mcg/kg/d SQ inj; ↑ by 10 mcg/kg/d until total down-regulation achieved. *DEPOT: <25 kg:* 7.5 mg IM q4wk. *>25–37.5 kg:* 11.25 mg IM q4wk. *>37.5 kg:* 15 mg IM q4wk Caution: [X, ?] w/ impending cord compression in CAP Contra: Undiagnosed vaginal bleeding, implant dosage form in women & peds; PRG Disp: Inj 5 mg/mL; Lupron DEPOT 3.75 (1 mo for fibroids, endometriosis); Lupron DEPOT for CAP: 7.5 mg (1 mo), 11.25 mg (3 mo), 22.5 (3 mo), 30 mg (4 mo); Eligard depot for CAP: 7.5 mg (1 mo); 22.5 mg (3 mo), 30 mg (4 mo), 45 mg (6 mo); Viadur 65 mg 12-mo SQ implant, Lupron-Ped 7.5, 11.25, 15 mg SE: Hot flashes, gynecomastia, N/V, alopecia, anorexia, dizziness, HA, insomnia, paresthesias, depression exacerbation, peripheral edema, & bone pain (transient "flare Rxn" at 7–14 d after the 1st dose [LH/testosterone surge before suppression]) Notes: Nonsteroidal antiandrogen (eg, bicalutamide) may block flare

Levalbuterol (Xopenex) Uses: *Asthma (Rx & prevention of bronchospasm)* Action: Sympathomimetic bronchodilator Dose: *Adult > 12 yrs:* 0.63-1.25 mg neb q6–8h; *Peds.* > 4 yrs: 1–2 puffs q4-6h Caution: [C, ?] Disp: Multidose inhaler 45 mcg/puff (15 gm); Soln for inhal 0.31, 0.63, 1.25 mg/3 mL 1.25 mg/0.5 mL SE: Tachycardia, nervousness, trembling, flu syndrome Notes: *R* - isomer of albuterol, may ↓ CV side effects compared with albuterol

Levetiracetam (Keppra) Uses: *Partial onset Szs* Action: Unknown Dose: *Adults.* 500 mg PO bid, may ↑ 3000 mg/d max; *Peds.* 4–16 y: 10–20 mg/kg/d ÷ in 2 doses, 60 mg/kg/d max (↓ in renal insuff) Caution: [C, ?/–] Contra: Component allergy Disp: Tabs 250, 500, 750, 1000 mg, Sol 100 mg/mL SE: Dizziness & somnolence; impaired coordination

Levobunolol (A-K Beta, Betagan) Uses: *Glaucoma* Action: β-Adrenergic blocker Dose: 1 gt qd–bid Caution: [C, ?] Disp: Soln 0.25, 0.5% SE: Ocular stinging or burning Notes: Possible systemic effects if absorbed

Levocabastine (Livostin) Uses: *Allergic seasonal conjunctivitis* **Action:** Antihistamine **Dose:** 1 gt in eye(s) qid ≤ 2 wk **Caution:** [C, +/–] **Disp:** 0.05% gtt **SE:** Ocular discomfort

Levofloxacin (Levaquin, Quixin & Iquix Ophthalmic) Uses: * Lower resp tract Infxns, sinusitis, UTI; topical for bacterial conjunctivitis, skin Infxns* **Action:** Quinolone antibiotic, ↓ DNA gyrase. *Spectrum:* Excellent gram(+) except MRSA & *E. faecium;* excellent gram(–) except *S. maltophilia* & *Acinetobacter* sp; poor anaerobic **Dose:** 250–500 mg/d PO or IV; community acquired pneumonia 750 mg/day for 5 d; ophth 1–2 gtt in eye(s) q2h while awake for 2 d, then q4h while awake for 5 d, ↓ in renal impair, avoid antacids if PO **Caution:** [C, –] Interactions w/ cation-containing products (eg, antacids) **Contra:** Quinolone sensitivity **Disp:** Tabs 250, 500, 750 mg; premixed IV 250, 500, 750 mg, inj 25 mg/mL; Leva-Pak 750 mg × 5 d; Sol: 25 mg/mL ophth soln 0.5% (Quixin), 1.5% (Iquix) **SE:** N/D, dizziness, rash, GI upset, photosensitivity

Levonorgestrel (Plan B) Uses: *Emergency contraceptive ("morning-after pill")*; prevents PRG if taken <72 h after unprotected sex/contraceptive fails **Action:** Progestin **Dose:** 0.75 mg q12h × 2 **Caution:** [X, M] **Contra:** Known/suspected PRG, abnormal uterine bleeding **Disp:** Tab, 0.75 mg, 2 blister pack **SE:** N/V, abdominal pain, fatigue, HA, menstrual changes. **Notes:** Will not induce abortion; ↑ risk of ectopic PRG

Levonorgestrel Implant (Norplant II, Jadelle) Uses: *Contraceptive* **Action:** Progestin **Dose:** Implant 150 mg in midforearm **Caution:** [X, +/–] **Contra:** Undiagnosed abnormal uterine bleeding, Hepatic Dz, thromboembolism, Hx of intracranial HTN, breast CA, renal impair **Disp:** 75 mg implant × 2 **SE:** Uterine bleeding HA, acne, nausea **Notes:** Prevents PRG for up to 5 y; remove if PRG desired

Levorphanol (Levo-Dromoran) [C-II] Uses: *Moderate–severe pain; chronic pain* **Action:** Narcotic analgesic **Dose:** 2–4 mg PO PRN q6–8h; 1–2 mg IM/SQ PRN q6–8h; ↓ in hepatic impair **Caution:** [B/D (prolonged use/high doses at term), ?] **Contra:** Component allergy **Disp:** Tabs 2 mg; inj 2 mg/mL **SE:** Tachycardia, ↓ BP, drowsiness, GI upset, constipation, resp depression, pruritus

Levothyroxine (Synthroid, Levoxyl, others) Uses: * Hypothyroidism, myxedema coma* **Action:** Supplement L-thyroxine **Dose:** *Adults.* Hypothyroid Initial, 12.5–50 mcg/d PO; ↑ by 25–50 mcg/d every mo; usual 100–200 mcg/d. Myxedema: 200–500 mcg IV, then 100–300 mcg/d *Peds.* Hypothyroid: 0–3 mo: 10–15 mcg/kg/24 h PO. *3–6 mo:* 8–10 mcg/kg/d PO; 6–12 mo: 6–8 mcg/kg/d PO; 1–5 yr: 5–6 mcg/kg/d PO; 6–12 yr: 4–5 mcg/kd/d PO; > 12 yr: 2–3 mcg/kd/d PO. Reduce dose by 50% if IV; titrate based on response & thyroid tests; dose can ↑ rapidly in young/middle-aged **Caution:** [A, +] **Contra:** Recent MI, uncorrected adrenal insuff **Disp:** Tabs 25, 50, 75, 88, 100, 112, 125, 137, 150, 175, 200, 300 mcg; inj 200, 500 mcg **SE:** Insomnia, weight loss, alopecia, arrhythmia **Notes:** Take w/ full glass of water (prevents choking)

Lidocaine (Anestacon Topical, Xylocaine, others) Uses: *
Local anesthetic; Rx cardiac arrhythmias* **Action:** Anesthetic; class IB antiarrhythmic **Dose:** *Adults.* Antiarrhythmic, ET: 5 mg/kg; follow w/ 0.5 mg/kg in 10
min if effective. *IV load:* 1 mg/kg bolus over 2–3 min; repeat in 5–10 min;
200–300 mg/h max; cont inf 20–50 mcg/kg/min or 1–4 mg/min. *Peds.* Antiarrhythmic, ET, load: 1 mg/kg; repeat in 10–15 min 5 mg/kg max total, then IV inf 20–50
mcg/kg/min. *Topical:* Apply max 3 mg/kg/dose. *Local inj anesthetic:* Max 4.5
mg/kg (Table 3, page 215) **Caution:** [C, +] **Contra:** Do not use lidocaine w/ epi on
digits, ears, or nose (risk of vasoconstriction & necrosis); heart block **Disp:** *Inj
local:* 0.5, 1, 1.5, 2, 4, 10, 20%. *Inj IV:* 1% (10 mg/mL), 2% (20 mg/mL); admix-
ture 4, 10, 20%. *IV inf:* 0.2%, 0.4%; cream 2%; gel 2, 2.5%; oint 2.5, 5%; liq 2.5%;
soln 2, 4%; viscous 2% **SE:** Dizziness, paresthesias, & convulsions associated w/
tox **Notes:** 2nd line to amiodarone in ECC; dilute ET dose 1–2 mL w/ NS; epi may
be added for local anesthesia to ↑ effect & ↓ bleeding; for IV forms, ↓ w/ liver Dz
or CHF; see Table 2 for levels

Lidocaine/Prilocaine (EMLA, LMX) Uses: *Topical anesthetic*; adjunct to phlebotomy or dermal procedures **Action:** Topical anesthetic **Dose:**
Adults. EMLA cream, anesthetic disc (1 g/10 cm²): Thick layer 2–2.5 g to intact
skin, cover w/ occlusive dressing (eg, Tegaderm) for at least 1 h. *Anesthetic disc:*
1 g/10 cm² for at least 1 h. *Peds.* Max dose: <3 mo or <5 kg: 1 g/10 cm² for 1 h.
3–12 mo & >5 kg: 2 g/20 cm² for 4 h. *1–6 y & >10 kg:* 10 g/100 cm² for 4 h. *7–12
y & >20 kg:* 20 g/200 cm² for 4 h **Caution:** [B, +] Methemoglobinemia **Contra:**
Use on mucous membranes, broken skin, eyes; allergy to amide-type anesthetics
Disp: Cream 2.5% lidocaine/2.5% prilocaine; anesthetic disc (1 g) **SE:** Burning,
stinging, methemoglobinemia **Notes:** Longer contact time ↑ effect

Lindane (Kwell) [OTC] Uses: *Head lice, crab lice, scabies* **Action:** Ec-
toparasiticide & ovicide **Dose:** *Adults & Peds.* Cream or lotion: Thin layer after
bathing, leave for 8–12 h, pour on laundry. *Shampoo:* Apply 30 mL, develop a lather
w/ warm water for 4 min, comb out nits **Caution:** [C, +/–] **Contra:** Open wounds,
Sz disorder **Disp:** Lotion 1%; shampoo 1% **SE:** Arrhythmias, Szs, local irritation, GI
upset **Notes:** Caution w/ overuse (may be absorbed); may repeat Rx in 7 d

Linezolid (Zyvox) Uses: *Infxns caused by gram(+) bacteria (including
vancomycin-resistant enterococcus, VRE), pneumonia, skin Infxns* **Action:**
Unique, binds ribosomal bacterial RNA; bactericidal for strep, bacteriostatic for
enterococci & staph. *Spectrum:* Excellent gram(+) including VRE & MRSA **Dose:**
Adults. 400–600 mg IV or PO q12h. *Peds.* 10 mg/kg IV or PO q8h (q12h in
preterm neonates) **Caution:** [C, ?/–] w/ reversible MAOI, avoid foods w/ tyramine
& cough/cold products w/ pseudoephedrine; w/ myelosuppression **Disp:** Inj 2
mg/mL; tabs 400, 600 mg; susp 100 mg/5 mL **SE:** HTN, N/D, HA, insomnia, GI
upset, myelosuppression, tongue discoloration **Notes:** Follow weekly CBC

Liothyronine (Cytomel) Uses: *Hypothyroidism, goiter, myxedema
coma, thyroid suppression therapy* **Action:** T₃ replacement **Dose:** *Adults.* Initial

25 mcg/24 h, titrate q1–2wk to response & TFT; maint of 25–100 mcg/d PO. *Myxedema coma:* 25–50 mcg IV. **Peds.** Initial 5 mcg/24 h, titrate by 5-mcg/24-h increments at 1–2-wk intervals; maint 20–75 mcg/24 h PO qd; ↓ in elderly **Caution:** [A, +] **Contra:** Recent MI, uncorrected adrenal insuff, uncontrolled HTN **Disp:** Tabs 5, 25, 50 mcg; inj 10 mcg/mL **SE:** Alopecia, arrhythmias, CP, HA, sweating **Notes:** Monitor TFT

Lisinopril (Prinivil, Zestril) Uses: *HTN, CHF, prevent DN & AMI* **Action:** ACE inhibitor **Dose:** 5–40 mg/24 h PO qd–bid. *AMI:* 5 mg w/in 24 h of MI, then 5 mg after 24 h, 10 mg after 48 h, then 10 mg/d; ↓ in renal insuff **Caution:** [D, –] **Contra:** ACE inhibitor sensitivity **Disp:** Tabs 2.5, 5, 10, 20, 30, 40 mg **SE:** Dizziness, HA, cough, ↓ BP, angioedema, ↑ K⁺ **Notes:** To prevent DN, start when urinary microalbuminemia begins

Lithium Carbonate (Eskalith, Lithobid, others) Uses: *Manic episodes of bipolar Dz* **Action:** Effects shift toward intraneuronal metabolism of catecholamines **Dose:** *Adults.* Acute mania: 600–1200 mg/d PO ÷tid–qid (max 2.4 g/d) or 900 mg SR bid **Peds 2–12 y.** 15–60 mg/kg/d in 3–4 ÷ doses; must titrate; ↓ in renal insuff, elderly **Caution:** [D, –] Many drug interactions **Contra:** Severe renal impair or CV Dz, lactation **Disp:** Caps 150, 300, 600 mg; tabs 300 mg; SR tabs 300, CR tabs 450 mg; syrup 300 mg/5 mL **SE:** Polyuria, polydipsia, nephrogenic DI, tremor; Na retention or diuretic use may ↑tox; arrhythmias, dizziness **Notes:** See Table 2 for levels.

Lodoxamide (Alomide) Uses: *Vernal conjunctivitis/keratitis* **Action:** Stabilizes mast cells **Dose:** *Adults & Peds >2 y.* 1–2 gtt in eye(s) qid ≤3 mo **Caution:** [B, ?] **Disp:** Soln 0.1% **SE:** Ocular burning, stinging, HA

Lomefloxacin (Maxaquin) Uses: *UTI, acute exacerbation of chronic bronchitis, prophylaxis in transurethral procedures* **Action:** Quinolone antibiotic; ↓ DNA gyrase. *Spectrum:* Good gram(–) including *H. influenzae* except *Stenotrophomonas maltophilia, Acinetobacter* sp, & some *P. aeruginosa* **Dose:** 400 mg/d PO, ↓ in renal insuff, avoid antacids **Caution:** [C, –] Interactions w/ cation-containing products **Contra:** Allergy to other quinolones, children <18 y **Disp:** Tabs 400 mg **SE:** Photosensitivity, Szs, HA, dizziness

Loperamide (Imodium) [OTC] Uses: *Diarrhea* **Action:** Slows intestinal motility **Dose:** *Adults.* Initial 4 mg PO, then 2 mg after each loose stool, up to 16 mg/d. **Peds.** *2–5 y, 13–20 kg:* 1 mg PO tid. *6–8 y, 20–30 kg:* 2 mg PO bid. *8–12 y, >30 kg:* 2 mg PO tid **Caution:** [B, +] Not for acute diarrhea caused by *Salmonella, Shigella,* or *C. difficile* **Contra:** Pseudomembranous colitis, bloody diarrhea **Disp:** Caps 2 mg; tabs 2 mg; liq 1 mg/5 mL (OTC) **SE:** Constipation, sedation, dizziness

Lopinavir/Ritonavir (Kaletra) Uses: *HIV Infxn* **Action:** Protease inhibitor **Dose:** *Adults.* TX naïve: 2 tab PO qd or 1 tab PO bid; TX experienced pt: 1 tab PO bid (↑ dose if taken w/ amprenavir, efavirenz, fosamprenavir, nelfinavir, nevirapine). **Peds.** 7–15 kg: 12/3 mg/kg PO bid. *15–40 kg:* 10/2.5 mg/kg PO bid.

>40 kg: Adult dose (w/ food) **Caution:** [C, ?/–] Numerous interactions **Contra:** w/drugs dependent on CYP3A or CYP2D6 **Disp:** Tab 200 mg/50 mg, soln 400 mg/100 mg/5 mL **SE:** Soln has EtOH, avoid disulfiram, metronidazole; GI upset, asthenia, ↑ cholesterol/triglycerides, pancreatitis; protease metabolic syndrome

Loracarbef (Lorabid) Uses: *Upper & lower resp tract, skin, urinary tract* **Action:** 2nd-gen cephalosporin; ↓ cell wall synthesis. *Spectrum:* Weaker than 1st-gen against gram(+), enhanced gram(–)**Dose: Adults.** 200–400 mg PO qd-bid. **Peds.** 7.5–15 mg/kg/d PO ÷ bid; on empty stomach; ↓ in severe renal insuff **Caution:** [B, +] **Disp:** Caps 200, 400 mg; susp 100, 200 mg/5 mL **SE:** D

Loratadine (Claritin, Alavert) Uses: *Allergic rhinitis, chronic idiopathic urticaria* **Action:** Nonsedating antihistamine **Dose: Adults.** 10 mg/d PO **Peds.** 2–5 y: 5 mg PO qd. >6 y: Adult dose; on empty stomach↓ ↓ in hepatic insuff **Caution:** [B, +/–] **Contra:** Component allergy **Disp:** Tabs 10 mg (OTC); rapidly disintegrating Reditabs 10 mg; syrup 1 mg/mL **SE:** HA, somnolence, xerostomia

Lorazepam (Ativan, others) [C-IV] Uses: *Anxiety & anxiety w/ depression; preop sedation; control status epilepticus*; EtOH withdrawal; antiemetic **Action:** Benzodiazepine; antianxiety agent **Dose: Adults.** Anxiety: 1–10 mg/d PO in 2–3 ÷ doses. *Preop:* 0.05 mg/kg to 4 mg max IM 2 h before surgery. *Insomnia:* 2–4 mg PO hs. *Status epilepticus:* 4 mg/dose IV PRN q10–15 min; usual total dose 8 mg. *Antiemetic:* 0.5–2 mg IV or PO q4–6h PRN. *EtOH withdrawal:* 2–5 mg IV or 1–2 mg PO initial depending on severity; titrate **Peds.** Status epilepticus: 0.05 mg/kg/dose IV, repeat at 1–20 min intervals × 2 PRN. *Antiemetic, 2–15 y:* 0.05 mg/kg (to 2 mg/dose) pre chemo; ↓ in elderly; do not administer IV >2 mg/min or 0.05 mg/kg/min **Caution:** [D, ?/–] **Contra:** Severe pain, severe ↓ BP, sleep apnea, NA glaucoma, allergy to propylene glycol or benzyl alcohol **Disp:** Tabs 0.5, 1, 2 mg; soln, PO conc 2 mg/mL; inj 2, 4 mg/mL **SE:** Sedation, ataxia, tachycardia, constipation, resp depression **Notes:** ≤10 min for effect if IV

Losartan (Cozaar) Uses: *HTN,* CHF, DN **Action:** Angiotensin II antagonist **Dose:** 25–50 mg PO qd-bid, max 100 mg; ↓ in elderly/hepatic impair **Caution:** [C (1st tri), D 2nd & 3rd tri), ?/–] **Disp:** Tabs 25, 50, 100 mg **SE:** ↓ BP in pts on diuretics; GI upset, angioedema

Lovastatin (Mevacor, Altocor) Uses: *Hypercholesterolemia* **Action:** HMG-CoA reductase inhibitor **Dose:** 20 mg/d PO w/ PM meal; may ↑ at 4-wk intervals to 80 mg/d max or 60 mg ER tab; take w/ meals **Caution:** [X, –] Avoid w/ grapefruit juice, gemfibrozil. **Contra:** Active liver Dz **Disp:** Tabs 10, 20, 40 mg; ER tabs 10, 20, 40, 60 mg **SE:** HA & GI intolerance common; promptly report any unexplained muscle pain, tenderness, or weakness (myopathy) **Notes:** Maintain cholesterol-lowering diet; monitor LFT q12wk × 1 y, then q6mo

Lubiprostone (Amitiza) Uses: *Chronic idiopathic constipation in adults* **Action:** Selective Cl channel activator **Dose: Adults.** 24 mcg PO bid w/ food **Contra:** Mechanical GI obstruction **Caution:** [C,?/-] Severe D, severe renal or moderate-severe hepatic impair **Disp:** Gelcaps 24 mcg **SE:** N, HA, D, GI distention, abd pain **Notes:** Requires (-) pregnancy test before Tx; utilize contraception; periodically reassess drug need; not for chronic use

Lutropin Alfa (Luveris) **Uses:** *Infertility* **Action:** Recombinant LH **Dose:** 75 units SC w/ 75–150 units FSH, 2 separate inj max 14 d **Caution:** [X, ?/M] **Contra:** Primary ovarian failure, uncontrolled thyroid/adrenal dysfunction, intracranial lesion, abnormal uterine bleeding, hormone-dependent GU tumor, ovarian cyst, PRG **Disp:** Inj 75 units **SE:** HA, N, ovarian hyperstimulation syndrome, breast pain, ovarian cysts; ↑ risk of multiple births **Notes:** Rotate inj sites; do not exceed 14 d duration unless signs of imminent follicular development

Lymphocyte Immune Globulin [Antithymocyte Globulin, ATG] (Atgam) **Uses:** *Allograft rejection in transplant pts, aplastic anemia if not candidates for BMT* **Action:** ↓ circulating T lymphocytes **Dose:** *Adults.* Prevent rejection: 15 mg/kg/day IV ×14 d, then qod ×7; initial w/in 24 h before/after transplant. *Rx rejection:* Same except use 10–15 mg/kg/d; max 28 doses in 21 d. *Peds.* 5–25 mg/kg/d IV. **Caution:** [C, ?] **Contra:** Hx Rxn to other equine γ-globulin preparation, leukopenia, thrombocytopenia **Disp:** Inj 50 mg/mL **SE:** D/C w/ severe thrombocytopenia/leukopenia; rash, fever, chills, ↓ BP, HA, ↑ K⁺ **Notes:** Test dose: 0.1 mL 1:1000 dilution in NS

Magaldrate (Riopan, Lowsium) [OTC] **Uses:** *Hyperacidity associated w/ peptic ulcer, gastritis, & hiatal hernia* **Action:** Low-Na antacid **Dose:** 5–10 mL PO between meals & hs **Caution:** [B, ?] **Contra:** Ulcerative colitis, diverticulitis, ileostomy/colostomy, renal insuff (Mg content) **Disp:** Susp (OTC) **SE:** GI upset **Notes:** <0.3 mg Na/tab or tsp

Magnesium Citrate (various) [OTC] **Uses:** *Vigorous bowel preparation*; constipation **Action:** Cathartic laxative **Dose:** *Adults.* 120–300 mL PO PRN. *Peds.* 0.5 mL/kg/dose to 200 mL PO max; w/ a beverage **Caution:** [B, +] **Contra:** Severe renal Dz, heart block, N/V, rectal bleeding **Disp:** Effervescent soln (OTC) **SE:** Abdominal cramps, gas

Magnesium Hydroxide (Milk of Magnesia) [OTC] **Uses:** *Constipation*, hyperacidity, Mg replacement **Action:** NS laxative **Dose:** *Adults.* Antacid 5–15 mL PO PRN qid, 2–4 tab PO PRN QID; laxative 30–60 mL PO qd or in ÷ doses *Peds.* <2 yrs 0.5 mL/kg/dose PO PRN (follow dose w/ 8 oz of H₂O) **Caution:** [B, +] **Contra:** Renal insuff, intestinal obstruction, ileostomy/colostomy **Disp:** Chew tabs 311 mg; liq 400, 800 mg/5 mL (OTC) **SE:** D, abdominal cramps

Magnesium Oxide (Mag-Ox 400, others) [OTC] **Uses:** *Replace low Mg levels* **Action:** Mg supl **Dose:** 400–800 mg/d ÷ qd–qid w/ full glass of H₂O **Caution:** [B, +] **Contra:** Ulcerative colitis, diverticulitis, ileostomy/colostomy, heart block, renal insuff **Disp:** Caps 140 mg; tabs 400 mg (OTC) **SE:** D, N

Magnesium Sulfate (various) **Uses:** * Replacement for low Mg levels; preeclampsia & premature labor; refractory ↓ K⁺ & ↓ Ca²⁺* **Action:** Mg supl **Dose:** *Adults.* 3 gm PO q6h × 4 *PRN; Supl:* 1–2 g IM or IV; repeat PRN. *Preeclampsia/premature labor:* 4 g load then 1–4 g/h IV inf. *Peds.* 25–50 mg/kg/dose IM or IV q4–6h for 3–4 doses; repeat PRN; ↓ dose w/ low urine output or renal insuff **Caution:** [B, +] **Contra:** Heart block, renal failure **Disp:** Inj 10, 20, 40, 80, 125, 500 mg/mL; bulk powder **SE:** CNS depression, D, flushing, heart block

Mannitol (various) **Uses:** *Cerebral edema, ↑intraocular pressure, renal impair, poisonings* **Action:** Osmotic diuretic **Dose:** *Adults. Test dose:* 0.2 g/kg/dose IV over 3–5 min; if no diuresis w/in 2 h, D/C. *Oliguria:* 50 g–100 g IV over 90 min; ↑ IOP: 0.5–2 gm/kg IV over 30 min. *Cerebral edema:* 0.25–1.5 g/kg/dose IV >30 min. **Caution:** [C, ?] w/ CHF or volume overload **Contra:** Anuria, dehydration, heart failure, PE **Disp:** Inj 5, 10, 15, 20, 25% **SE:** May exacerbate CHF, N/V/D **Notes:** monitor for volume depletion

Measles, Mumps, Rubella and Varicella Virus Vaccine Live (Proquad) **Uses:** *Simultaneous vaccination against measles, mumps, rubella, & varicella in peds 12 mo–12 y or for second dose of MMR* **Action:** Active immunization, live attenuated virus **Dose:** 1 vial SQ inj **Caution:** [N/A] Hx of cerebral injury or Szs (febrile reaction) **Contra:** Hx anaphylaxis to neomycin, blood dyscrasia, lymphoma, leukemia, immunosuppressive steroids, febrile illness, untreated TB **Disp:** SE: Fever, inj site Rxn, rash **Notes:** Allow 1 mo between inj & any other measles vaccine

Mecasermin (Increlex) **Uses:** *Growth failure in IGF-1 deficiency or HGH antibodies* **Action:** Human IGF-1 **Dose:** *Peds.* 0.04–0.09 mg/kg SQ BID; may ↑ by 0.04 mg/kg to 0.12 mg/kg; take w/in 20 min of meal **Caution:** [C,+/–] **Disp:** Vial 40 mg **SE:** HA, inj site rxn, V, hypoglycemia **Notes:** Rapid dose ↑ may cause hypoglycemia; limited distribution network

Mechlorethamine (Mustargen) WARNING: Highly toxic, handle w/ care **Uses:** *Hodgkin Dz & NHL, cutaneous T-cell lymphoma (mycosis fungoides), lung CA, CML, malignant pleural effusions,* & CLL **Action:** Alkylating agent (bifunctional) **Dose:** Per protocol; 0.4 mg/kg single dose or 0.1 mg/kg/d for 4 d; 6 mg/m² 1–2 × mo **Caution:** [D, ?] **Contra:** Known infectious Dz **Disp: Inj 10 mg** SE: Myelosuppression, thrombosis, thrombophlebitis at site; tissue damage w/ extravasation (Na thiosulfate used topically to treat); N/V, skin rash, amenorrhea, sterility (especially in men), secondary leukemia if treated for Hodgkin Dz **Notes:** Highly volatile; administer w/in 30–60 min of prep

Meclizine (Antivert) **Uses:** *Motion sickness; vertigo* **Action:** Antiemetic, anticholinergic, & antihistaminic properties **Dose:** *Adults & Peds >12 y.* 12.5–100 mg PO tid–qid PRN **Caution:** [B, ?] **Disp:** Tabs 12.5, 25, 50 mg; chew tabs 25 mg; caps 25, 30 mg (OTC) **SE:** Drowsiness, xerostomia, & blurred vision

Medroxyprogesterone (Provera, Depo-Provera) WARNING: May cause loss of bone density; associated w/ duration of use **Uses:** *Contraception; secondary amenorrhea, abnormal uterine bleeding (AUB) caused by hormonal imbalance; endometrial CA* **Action:** Progestin supl **Dose:** *Contraception:* 150 mg IM q3mo depo or 104 mg SQ q3 mo (depo SQ). *Secondary amenorrhea:* 5–10 mg/d

PO for 5–10 d. *AUB:* 5–10 mg/d PO for 5–10 d beginning on the 16th or 21st d of menstrual cycle. *Endometrial CA:* 400–1000 mg/wk IM; ↓ in hepatic insuff **Caution:** [X, +] **Contra:** Hx of thromboembolic disorders, hepatic Dz, PRG **Disp:** Tabs 2.5, 5, 10 mg; depot inj 150, 400 mg/mL; depo SQ inj 104 mg/10.65 mL **SE:** Breakthrough bleeding, spotting, altered menstrual flow, anorexia, edema, thromboembolic complications, depression, weight gain **Notes:** Perform breast exam & Pap smear before contraceptive therapy; obtain PRG test if last inj >3 mo

Megestrol Acetate (Megace) Uses: * Breast/endometrial CAs; appetite stimulant in cachexia (CA & HIV)* **Action:** Hormone; progesterone analog **Dose:** *CA:* 40–320 mg/d PO in ÷ doses. *Appetite:* 800 mg/d PO ÷ dose **Caution:** [X, –] Thromboembolism **Contra:** PRG **Disp:** Tabs 20, 40 mg; soln 40 mg/mL **SE:** DVT; edema, menstrual bleeding; photosensitivity, insomnia, rash, myelosuppression **Notes:** Do not D/C abruptly

Meloxicam (Mobic) WARNING: May ↑ risk of cardiovascular events & GI bleeding Uses: *Osteoarthritis, RA, JRA* **Action:** NSAID w/ ↑ COX-2 activity **Dose:** *Adult:* 7.5–15 mg/d PO; *Peds* (>2 yr): 0.125 mg/kg/d, max 7.5 mg; ↓ in renal insuff; take w/food **Caution:** [C, D (3rd trimester) ?/–] Peptic ulcer, NSAID, or ASA sensitivity **Disp:** Tabs 7.5 mg; susp. 7.5 mg/5 mL **SE:** HA, dizziness, GI upset, GI bleeding, edema

Melphalan [L-PAM] (Alkeran) WARNING: Severe BM depression, leukemogenic, & mutagenic Uses: *Multiple myeloma, ovarian CAs,* breast & testicular CA, melanoma; allogenic & ABMT (high dose) **Action:** Alkylating agent (bifunctional) **Dose:** (Per protocol) 6 mg/d or 0.15 - 0.25 mg/kg/d for 4–7 d, repeat 4–6 wk intervals, or 1 mg/kg X1 q4–6wk; 0.15 mg/kg/d for 5 d q6wk. *High-dose high-risk multiple myeloma:* Single dose 140 mg/m². *ABMT:* 140–240 mg/m² IV; ↓ in renal insuff **Caution:** [D, ?] **Contra:** Allergy or resistance **Disp:** Tabs 2 mg; inj 50 mg **SE:** ↓ BM, secondary leukemia, alopecia, dermatitis, stomatitis, & pulmonary fibrosis; rare allergic Rxns **Notes:** Take PO on empty stomach

Memantine (Namenda) Uses: *Moderate/severe Alzheimer Dz* **Action:** N-methyl-D-aspartate receptor antagonist **Dose:** Target 20 mg/d, start 5 mg/d, ↑ 5 mg/d to 20 mg/d, wait >1 wk before ↑ dose; use ÷ doses >5 mg/d **Caution:** [B, ?/–] Hepatic/mild–moderate renal impair **Disp:** Tabs 5, 10 mg, combo pak: 5 mg × 28 + 10 mg × 21; sol 2 mg/mL **SE:** Dizziness **Notes:** Renal clearance ↓ by alkaline urine (↓ 80% @pH 8)

Meningococcal Polysaccharide Vaccine (Menomune) Uses: *Immunize against N. meningitidis (meningococcus)*; OK in some complement deficiency, asplenia, lab workers w/ exposure; college students by some professional groups **Action:** Active immunization **Dose:** *Adults & Peds >2 y.* 0.5 mL SQ (not IM, intradermally or IV) **Caution:** [C, ?/–] **Contra:** Thimerosal sensitivity **Disp:** Inj **SE:** Local inj site Rxns, HA **Notes:** Active against meningococcal serotypes A, C, Y, & W-135; not group B; keep epi (1:1000) available for anaphylactic/allergic Rxns

Meperidine (Demerol) [C–II] Uses: *Moderate–severe pain* Action: Narcotic analgesic Dose: *Adults.* 50–150 mg PO or IM/SQ q3–4h PRN. *Peds.* 1–1.5 mg/kg/dose PO or IM/SQ q3–4h PRN, up to 100 mg/dose; ↓ in elderly/renal impair Caution: [C/D (prolonged use or high dose at term), +] ↓ Sz threshold Contra: w/ MAOIs, renal failure Disp: Tabs 50, 100 mg; syrup 50 mg/5 mL; inj 10, 25, 50, 75, 100 mg/mL SE: Resp depression, Szs, sedation, constipation Notes: Analgesic effects potentiated w/ hydroxyzine; 75 mg IM = 10 mg morphine IM

Meprobamate (Equinil, Miltown) [C-IV] Uses: *Short-term relief of anxiety* Action: Mild tranquilizer; antianxiety Dose: *Adults.* 400 mg PO tid-qid, max 2400 mg/d–. *Peds 6–12 y.* 100–200 mg bid–tid; ↓ in renal/liver impair Caution: [D, +/–] Contra: NA glaucoma, porphyria, PRG Disp: Tabs 200, 400 mg SE: May cause drowsiness, syncope, tachycardia, edema

Mercaptopurine [6-MP] (Purinethol) Uses: *Acute leukemias,* 2nd-line Rx of CML & NHL, maint ALL in children, immunosuppressant w/ autoimmune Dzs (Crohn Dz) Action: Antimetabolite, mimics hypoxanthine Dose: 80–100 mg/m^2/d or 2.5–5 mg/kg/d; maint 1.5–2.5 mg/kg/d; w/ allopurinol requires a 67–75% ↓ dose of 6-MP (interference w/ xanthine oxidase metabolism); ↓ in renal/hepatic insuff; take on empty stomach Caution: [D, ?] Contra: Severe hepatic Dz, BM suppression, PRG Disp: Tabs 50 mg SE: Mild hematotox, mucositis, stomatitis, D rash, fever, eosinophilia, jaundice, hepatitis Notes: Handle properly; ensure adequate hydration

Meropenem (Merrem) Uses: * Intraabdominal Infxns, bacterial meningitis* Action: Carbapenem; ↓ cell wall synthesis, a β-lactam. *Spectrum:* Excellent gram(+) (except MRSA & *E. faecium*); excellent gram(−) including extended-spectrum β-lactamase producers; good anaerobic Dose: *Adults.* 1 to 2 g IV q8h. *Peds.* >3 mo, <50 kg 10–40 mg/kg IV q 8h; ↓ in renal insuff Caution: [B, ?] Contra: β-Lactam sensitivity Disp: Inj 1 g, 500 mg SE: Less Sz potential than imipenem; D, thrombocytopenia Notes: Overuse ↑ bacterial resistance

Mesalamine (Rowasa, Asacol, Pentasa) Uses: * Mild–moderate distal ulcerative colitis, proctosigmoiditis, proctitis* Action: Unknown; may inhibit prostaglandins Dose: *Rectal:* 60 mL QHS, retain 8 h (enema), 500 mg bid–tid or 1000 mg qhs (supp) *PO:* Cap: 1 gm PO qid, Tab: 1.6–2.4 g/d ÷ doses (tid–qid); ↓ initial dose in elderly Caution: [B, M] Contra: Salicylate sensitivity Disp: Tabs 400 mg; caps 250, 500 mg supp 500, 1000 mg; rectal susp 4 g/60 mL SE: Yellow-brown urine, HA, malaise, abdominal pain, flatulence, rash, pancreatitis, pericarditis

Mesna (Mesnex) Uses: * Prevent hemorrhagic cystitis due to ifosfamide or cyclophosphamide* Action: Antidote, reacts with acrolein and other metabolites to form stable compounds Dose: Per protocol; dose as % of ifosfamide or cyclophosphamide dose *IV bolus:* 20% (eg, 10–12 mg/kg) IV at 0, 4 and 8 h, then 40% at 0, 1, 4 and 7 h; *IV inf:* 20% prechemo, 50–100% w/chemo, then 25–50% for 12 h following chemo; *Oral:* 20% IV dose at hour 0, 4, and 8 h (mix with juice)

Caution: [B; ?/–] **Contra:** Thiol sensitivity **Disp:** Inj 100 mg/mL; tablets 400 mg **SE:** ↓ BP, allergic Rxns, HA, GI upset, taste perversion **Notes:** Hydration helps ↓ hemorrhagic cystitis; higher dose for BMT

Mesoridazine (Serentil)   WARNING: Can prolong QT interval in dose-related fashion; torsades de pointes reported **Uses:** *Schizophrenia,* acute & chronic alcoholism, chronic brain syndrome **Action:** Phenothiazine antipsychotic **Dose:** Initial, 25–50 mg PO or IV tid; ↑ to 300–400 mg/d max **Caution:** [C, ?/–] **Contra:** Phenothiazine sensitivity; concomitant administration w/ drugs that cause QT$_c$ prolongation, CNS depression **Disp:** Tabs 10, 25, 50, 100 mg; PO conc 25 mg/mL; inj 25 mg/mL **SE:** Low incidence of EPS; ↓ BP, xerostomia, constipation, skin discoloration, tachycardia, lowered Sz threshold, blood dyscrasias, pigmentary retinopathy at high doses

Metaproterenol (Alupent, Metaprel)   **Uses:** * Asthma & reversible bronchospasm* **Action:** Sympathomimetic bronchodilator **Dose:** *Adults.* Inhal: 1–3 inhal q3–4h, 12 inhal max/24 h; wait 2 min between inhal. *PO:* 20 mg q6–8h. *Peds.* Inhal: 0.5 mg/kg/dose, 15 mg/dose max inhaled q4–6h by neb or 1–2 puffs q4–6h. *PO:* 0.3–0.5 mg/kg/dose q6–8h **Caution:** [C, ?/–] **Contra:** Tachycardia, other arrhythmias **Disp:** Aerosol 0.65 mg/inhal; soln for inhal 0.4, 0.6; tabs 10, 20 mg; syrup 10 mg/5 mL **SE:** Nervousness, tremor, tachycardia, HTN **Notes:** Fewer β₁ effects than isoproterenol & longer acting

Metaxalone (Skelaxin)   **Uses:** * Painful musculoskeletal conditions* **Action:** Centrally acting skeletal muscle relaxant **Dose:** 800 mg PO tid–qid **Caution:** [C, ?/] anemia **Contra:** Severe hepatic/renal impair **Disp:** Tabs 400, 800 mg **SE:** N/V, HA, drowsiness, hepatitis

Metformin (Glucophage, Glucophage XR)   WARNING: Associated w/ lactic acidosis **Uses:** *Type 2 DM* **Action:** ↓ Hepatic glucose production & intestinal absorption of glucose; ↑ insulin sensitivity **Dose:** *Adults.* Initial: 500 mg PO bid; or 850 mg qd, may ↑ to 2,550 mg/d max; take w/ AM & PM meals; can convert total daily dose to qd dose of XR *Peds 10–16 y.* 500 mg PO bid, ↑ 500 mg/wk to 2,000 mg/d max in ÷ doses; do not use XR formulation in peds **Caution:** [B, +/–] avoid EtOH; hold dose before & 48 h after ionic contrast **Contra:** SCr >1.4 in females or >1.5 in males; hypoxemic conditions (eg acute CHF/sepsis) **Disp:** Tabs 500, 850, 1000 mg; XR tabs 500, 750, 1,000 mg **SE:** Anorexia, N/V, rash, lactic acidosis (rare, but serious)

Methadone (Dolophine) [C-II]   **Uses:** * Severe pain; detox, maint of narcotic addiction* **Action:** Narcotic analgesic **Dose:** *Adults.* 2.5–10 mg IM q3–8h or 5–15 mg PO q8h; titrate as needed *Peds.* 0.7 mg/kg/24 h PO or IM ÷ q8h; ↑ slowly to avoid resp depression; ↓ in renal impair **Caution:** [B/D (prolonged use/high doses at term), + (w/ doses =/> 20 mg/24 h)], severe liver Dz **Disp:** Tabs 5, 10, 40 mg; PO soln 5, 10 mg/5 mL; PO conc 10 mg/mL; inj 10 mg/mL **SE:** Resp depression, sedation, constipation, urinary retention, ventricular arrhythmias **Notes:** Equianalgesic w/ parenteral morphine; longer half-life; prolongs QT interval

Methenamine (Hiprex, Urex, others) Uses: *Suppress/eliminate bacteriuria associated w/ chronic/ recurrent UTI* Action: Converted to formaldehyde & ammonia in acidic urine; nonspecific bactericidal action Dose: *Adults.* Hippurate: 0.5–1 gm bid. *Mandelate:* 1 g qid PO pc & hs *Peds 6–12 y.* Hippurate: 25–50 mg/kg/d PO ÷ bid. *Mandelate:* 50–75 mg/kg/d PO ÷ qid (take w/ food, ascorbic acid w/ adequate hydration) Caution: [C, +] Contra: Renal insuff, severe hepatic Dz, & severe dehydration; sulfonamide allergy Disp: *Methenamine hippurate* (Hiprex, Urex): Tabs 1 g. *Methenamine mandelate:* 500 mg, 1g EC tabs SE: Rash, GI upset, dysuria, ↑ LFTs

Methimazole (Tapazole) Uses: *Hyperthyroidism, thyrotoxicosis,* prep for thyroid surgery or radiation Action: Blocks T_3 & T_4 formation Dose: *Adults.* Initial: 15–60 mg/d PO ÷ tid. *Maint:* 5–15 mg PO qd. *Peds.* Initial: 0.4–0.7 mg/kg/24 h PO ÷ tid. *Maint:* ⅓–⅔ of initial dose PO qd; w/ food Caution: [D, +/–] Contra: Breast-feeding Disp: Tabs 5, 10, 20 mg SE: GI upset, dizziness, blood dyscrasias Notes: Follow clinically & w/ TFT

Methocarbamol (Robaxin) Uses: *Relief of discomfort associated w/ painful musculoskeletal conditions* Action: Centrally acting skeletal muscle relaxant Dose: *Adults.* 1.5 g PO qid for 2–3 d, then 1-g PO qid maint therapy; IV form rarely indicated. *Peds.* 15 mg/kg/dose IV, may repeat PRN (OK for tetanus only), max 1.8 g/m²/d for 3 d Caution: Sz disorders [C, +] Contra: MyG, renal impair Disp: Tabs 500, 750 mg; inj 100 mg/mL SE: Can discolor urine; drowsiness, GI upset

Methotrexate (Folex, Rheumatrex) Uses: *ALL, AML, leukemic meningitis, trophoblastic tumors (chorioepithelioma, choriocarcinoma, hydatidiform mole), breast, lung, head & neck CAs, Burkitt's lymphoma, mycosis fungoides, osteosarcoma, Hodgkin Dz & NHL, psoriasis; RA* Action: ↓ Dihydrofolate reductase-mediated production of tetrahydrofolate Dose: *CA:* Per protocol. *RA:* 7.5 mg/wk PO 1/wk 1 or 2.5 mg q12h PO for 3 doses/wk; ↓ in renal/hepatic impair Caution: [D, –] Contra: Severe renal/hepatic impair, PRG/lactation Disp: Tabs 2.5, 5, 7.5, 10, 15 mg; inj 2.5, 10, 25 mg/mL, powder 20 mg SE: Myelosuppression, N/V/D, anorexia, mucositis, hepatotox (transient & reversible; may progress to atrophy, necrosis, cirrhosis), rashes, dizziness, malaise, blurred vision, alopecia, photosensitivity, renal failure, pneumonitis; rarely, pulmonary fibrosis; chemical arachnoiditis & HA w/ IT delivery Notes: Monitor CBC, LFTs, Cr, MTX levels & CXR; "high dose" > 500 mg/m² requires leucovorin rescue to ↓ tox; w/intrathecal, use preservative-free/alcohol-free solution

Methyldopa (Aldomet) Uses: *HTN* Action: Centrally acting antihypertensive Dose: *Adults.* 250–500 mg PO bid–tid (max 2–3 g/d) or 250 mg–1 g IV q6–8h. *Peds.* 10 mg/kg/24 h PO in 2–3 ÷ doses (max 40 mg/kg/24 h ÷ q6–12h) or 5–10 mg/kg/dose IV q6–8h to total dose of 20–40 mg/kg/24 h; ↓ in renal insuff/elderly Caution: [B (PO), C (IV), +] Contra: Liver Dz; MAOIs Disp: Tabs 125, 250, 500 mg; inj 50 mg/mL SE: Discolors urine; initial transient sedation/drowsiness frequent, edema, hemolytic anemia, hepatic disorders

Methylergonovine (Methergine) Uses: *Postpartum bleeding (uterine subinvolution)* Action: Ergotamine derivative Dose: 0.2 mg IM after placental delivery, may repeat 2–4-h intervals or 0.2–0.4 mg PO q6–12h for 2–7 d Caution: [C, ?] Contra: HTN, PRG Disp: Injectable 0.2 mg/mL; tabs 0.2 mg SE: HTN, N/V Notes: Give IV over >1 min w/BP monitoring

Methylphenidate, Oral (Concerta, Ritalin, Ritalin SR, others) [CII] Uses: *ADHD, narcolepsy* depression Action: CNS stimulant Dose: *Adults.* Narcolepsy: 10 mg PO 2–3 times/day, 60 mg/day max. Depression: 2.5 mg QAM; ↑ slowly, 20 mg/day max; use regular release only *Peds.* Based on product; Initial total daily dose of 15–20 mg, 90 mg/day max; administer once (ER/SR) to BID (regular) Caution: [C,+/–] Hx alcoholism or drug abuse; separate from MAOIs by 14 days Disp: Tabs 5, 10, 20 mg; Tabs SR (Ritalin SR) 20 mg; ER tabs (Concerta) 18, 27, 36, 54 mg SE: CV or CNS stimulation Notes: Titrate dose; take 30–45 min before meals; do not chew or crush; Concerta "ghost tablet" may appear in stool; see insert to convert to ER dose; see also transdermal methylphenidate; abuse and diversion concerns

Methylphenidate, transdermal (Daytrana)[CII] Uses: *ADHD in children 6–12 yrs* Action: CNS stimulant Dose: *Peds.* Apply to hip in AM (2 h before desired effect), remove 9 h later Caution: [C,+/–] sensitization may preclude subsequent use of oral forms; abuse and diversion concerns Disp: Patches 10, 15, 20, 30 mg SE: Local reactions, stimulation Notes: Titrate dose in weekly increments; effects last several hours following removal

Methylprednisolone (Solu-Medrol) [See Steroids page 175 and Table 4]

Metoclopramide (Reglan, Clopra, Octamide) Uses: *Diabetic gastroparesis, symptomatic GERD, chemo N/V, facilitate small-bowel intubation & UGI radiologic evaluation* stimulate gut in prolonged postop ileus Action: ↑ UGI motility; blocks dopamine in chemoreceptor trigger zone Dose: *Adults.* Gastroparesis: 10 mg PO 30 min ac & hs for 2–8 wk PRN, or same dose IV for 10 d, then PO. Reflux: 10–15 mg PO 30 min ac & hs. Antiemetic: 1–3 mg/kg/dose IV 30 min before chemo, then q2h × 2 doses, then q3h X3 doses. *Peds.* Reflux: 0.1 mg/kg/dose PO qid. Antiemetic: 1–2 mg/kg/dose IV as adults Caution: [B, –] Drugs w/ extrapyramidal ADRs Contra: Sz disorders, GI obstruction Disp: Tabs 5, 10 mg; syrup 5 mg/5 mL; inj 5 mg/mL SE: Dystonic Rxns common w/ high doses, (Rx w/IV diphenhydramine); restlessness, D, drowsiness

Metolazone (Mykrox, Zaroxolyn) Uses: *Mild–moderate essential HTN & edema of renal Dz or cardiac failure* Action: Thiazide-like diuretic; ↓ distal tubule Na reabsorption Dose: *HTN:* 2.5–5 mg/d PO (Zaroxolyn), 0.5–1 mg/day PO (Mykrox) *Edema:* 2.5–20 mg/d PO. *Peds.* 0.2–0.4 mg/kg/d PO ÷ q12h–qd Caution: [D, +] Contra: Thiazide/sulfonamide sensitivity, anuria Disp: *Tabs:* Mykrox (rapid acting) 0.5 mg, Zaroxolyn 2.5, 5, 10 mg SE: Monitor fluid/electrolytes; dizziness, ↓ BP, tachycardia, CP, photosensitivity Notes: Mykrox & Zaroxolyn not bioequivalent

Metoprolol (Lopressor, Toprol XL) **WARNING:** Do not acutely stop therapy as marked worsening of angina can result **Uses:** *HTN, angina, AMI, CHF* **Action:** β-adrenergic receptor blocker **Dose:** *Angina:* 50–200 mg PO bid max 400mg/d *HTN:* 50–200 mg PO BID max 450 mg/d. *AMI:* 5 mg IV q2 min × 3 doses, then 50 mg PO q6h × 48 h, then 100 mg PO bid. *CHF:* 12–25 mg/d PO X2 wk, ↑ at 2-wk intervals to 200 mg/max, use low dose in pts w/ greatest severity; ↓ in hepatic failure; take w/meals **Caution:** [C, +] Uncompensated CHF, bradycardia, heart block **Contra:** Arrhythmia w/ tachycardia **Disp:** Tabs 25, 50, 100 mg; ER tabs 25, 50, 100, 200 mg; inj 1 mg/mL **SE:** Drowsiness, insomnia, ED, bradycardia, bronchospasm

Metronidazole (Flagyl, MetroGel) **Uses:** *Bone/joint, endocarditis, intraabdominal, meningitis, & skin Infxns; amebiasis; trichomoniasis; bacterial vaginosis* **Action:** Interferes w/ DNA synthesis. *Spectrum:* Excellent anaerobic *C. difficile*, also *H. pylori* in combo therapy **Dose:** *Adults.* Anaerobic Infxns: 500 mg IV q6–8h. *Amebic dysentery:* 750 mg/d PO for 5–10 d. *Trichomoniasis:* 250 mg PO tid for 7 d or 2 g PO × 1. *C. difficile Infxn:* 500 mg PO or IV q8h for 7–10 d (PO preferred; IV only if pt NPO). *Vaginosis:* 1 applicatorful intravag bid or 500 mg PO bid for 7 d. *Acne rosacea/skin:* Apply bid. **Peds.** Anaerobic Infxns: 15 mg/kg/24 h PO or IV ÷ q6h. *Amebic dysentery:* 35–50 mg/kg/24 h PO in 3 ÷ doses for 5–10 d; ↓ in hepatic impair **Caution:** [B, M] Avoid EtOH **Contra:** First tri of PRG **Disp:** Tabs 250, 500 mg; XR tabs 750 mg; caps 375 mg; topical lotion & gel 0.75%; intravag gel 0.75% (5 g/applicator 37.5 mg in 70-g tube), cream 1% **SE:** Disulfiram-like Rxn; dizziness, HA, GI upset, anorexia, urine discoloration **Notes:** For Trichomoniasis, Rx pt's partner; no aerobic bacteria activity; use in combo w/ serious mixed Infxns

Mexiletine (Mexitil) **Uses:** *Suppression of symptomatic ventricular arrhythmias*; diabetic neuropathy **Action:** Class IB antiarrhythmic **Dose:** *Adults.* 200–300 mg PO q8h; 1200 mg/d max. **Peds.** 2.5–5 mg/kg PO q 8h; w/ food or antacids **Caution:** [C, +] May worsen severe arrhythmias; interactions w/ hepatic inducers & suppressors requires dosage changes **Contra:** Cardiogenic shock or 2nd-/3rd-degree AV block w/o pacemaker **Disp:** Caps 150, 200, 250 mg **SE:** Lightheadedness, dizziness, anxiety, incoordination, GI upset, ataxia, hepatic damage, blood dyscrasias; monitor LFTs

Mezlocillin (Mezlin) **Uses:** *Infxns caused by susceptible gram(−) bacteria (skin, bone, resp tract, urinary tract, abdomen, septicemia)* **Action:** Bactericidal; ↓ cell wall synthesis. *Spectrum:* Gram(−) *Klebsiella, Proteus, E. coli, Enterobacter, P. aeruginosa, & Serratia* **Dose:** *Adults.* 3 g IV q4–6h. **Peds.** 300 mg/kg/d ÷ q4–6h; ↓ in renal/hepatic impair **Caution:** [B, M] **Contra:** PCN sensitivity **Disp:** Inj **SE:** GI upset, thrombocytopenia **Notes:** Often used w/ aminoglycoside

Miconazole (Monistat, others) **Uses:** *Candidal Infxns, dermatomycoses (various tinea forms)* **Action:** Fungicide; alters fungal membrane permeability **Dose:** Apply to area bid for 2–4 wk. *Intravag:* 1 applicatorful or supp hs for 3 (4% or 200 mg) or 7 d (2% or 100 mg) **Caution:** [C, ?] Azole sensitivity **Disp:** Topical cream 2%; lotion 2%; powder 2%; spray 2%; vag supp 100, 200 mg; vag cream 2%, 4% [OTC] **SE:** Vag burning, may ↑ warfarin **Notes:** Antagonistic to amphotericin B in vivo

Midazolam (Versed) [C-IV]   **Uses:** *Preop sedation, conscious sedation for short procedures & mechanically ventilated pts, induction of general anesthesia* **Action:** Short-acting benzodiazepine **Dose:** *Adults.* 1–5 mg IV or IM; titrate to effect. *Peds.* Preop: > 6 mo 0.25–1 mg/kg PO, 20 mg max, *Conscious sedation:* 0.08 mg/kg × 1. > 6 mo 0.1–0.2 mg/kg IM x1 max 10 mg. *General anesthesia:* 0.025–0.1 mg/kg IV q2min for 1–3 doses PRN to induce anesthesia (↓ in elderly, w/ narcotics or CNS depressants) **Caution:** [D, +/–] w/CYP3A4 substrate (Table 13), multiple drug interactions **Contra:** NA glaucoma; w/amprenavir, nelfinavir, ritonavir **Disp:** Inj 1, 5 mg/mL; syrup 2 mg/mL **SE:** Resp depression; ↓ BP w/ conscious sedation, N **Notes:** Reversal w/ flumazenil; monitor for resp depression

Mifepristone [RU 486] (Mifeprex)   **WARNING:** Pt counseling & information required; associated w/ fatal infections & bleeding **Uses:** *Terminate intrauterine pregnancies of <49 d* **Action:** Antiprogestin; ↑ prostaglandins, results in uterine contraction **Dose:** Administered w/ 3 office visits: day 1, three 200-mg tabs PO; day 3 if no abortion, two 200-mg tabs PO; on or about day 14, verify termination of PRG **Caution:** [X, –] **Contra:** Anticoagulation therapy, bleeding disorders **Disp:** Tabs 200 mg **SE:** Abdominal pain & 1–2 wk of uterine bleeding **Notes:** Under physician's supervision only

Miglitol (Glyset)   **Uses:** *Type 2 DM* **Action:** α-Glucosidase inhibitor; delays digestion of carbohydrates **Dose:** Initial 25 mg PO tid; maint 50–100 mg tid (w/ 1st bite of each meal) **Caution:** [B, –] **Contra:** DKA, obstructive/inflammatory GI disorders; SCr >2 **Disp:** Tabs 25, 50, 100 mg **SE:** Flatulence, D, abdominal pain **Notes:** Use alone or w/ sulfonylureas

Milrinone (Primacor)   **Uses:** *CHF* **Action:** Positive inotrope & vasodilator; little chronotropic activity **Dose:** 50 mcg/kg, then 0.375–0.75 mcg/kg/min IV inf; ↓ in renal impair **Caution:** [C, ?] **Contra:** Allergy to drug or amrinone **Disp:** Inj 200 mcg/mL, 1 mg/ml **SE:** Arrhythmias, ↓ BP, HA **Notes:** Monitor fluid/electrolyte,BP, HR

Mineral Oil [OTC]   **Uses:** *Constipation* **Action:** Emollient laxative **Dose:** *Adults.* 15–45 mL PO PRN. *Peds >6 y.* 5–20 mL PO q day **Caution:** [C, ?] N/V, difficulty swallowing, bedridden pts **Contra:** Colostomy/ileostomy, appendicitis, diverticulitis, UC **Disp:** Liq [OTC] **SE:** Lipid pneumonia, anal incontinence, ↓ vitamin absorption

Minoxidil (Loniten, Rogaine)   **Uses:** *Severe HTN; male & female pattern baldness* **Action:** Peripheral vasodilator; stimulates vertex hair growth **Dose:** *Adults.* PO: (HTN) 2.5–80 mg PO ÷ qd –bid max 100mg/day. *Topical:* (Baldness) Apply bid to area. *Peds.* 0.2–1 mg/kg/24 h ÷ PO q12–24h, max 50 mg/day); ↓ PO in elderly **Caution:** [C, +] **Contra:** Pheochromocytoma, component allergy **Disp:** Tabs 2.5, 5, 10 mg; topical soln (Rogaine) 2%, 5% **SE:** Pericardial effusion & volume overload w/ PO use; hypertrichosis w/chronic use, edema, ECG changes, weight gain

Mirtazapine (Remeron, Remeron SolTab) **WARNING:** Closely monitor for worsening depression or emergence of suicidality, particularly in ped pts **Uses:** *Depression* **Action:** Tetracyclic antidepressant **Dose:** 15 mg PO hs, up to 45 mg/d hs **Caution:** [C, ?] **Contra:** MAOIs w/in 14 d **Disp:** Tabs 15, 30, 45 mg; rapid dissolving tabs 15 mg, 30 mg **SE:** Somnolence, ↑ cholesterol, constipation, xerostomia, weight gain, agranulocytosis **Notes:** Do not ↑ dose at intervals of less than 1–2 wk; handle rapid tabs with dry hands, do not cut or chew

Misoprostol (Cytotec) **Uses:** * Prevent NSAID-induced gastric ulcers*; induce labor, incomplete & therapeutic abortion **Action:** Prostaglandin w/ antisecretory & mucosal protective properties **Dose:** *Ulcer prevention:* 200 mcg PO qid w/ meals; in females, start 2nd or 3rd day of next nl menstrual period; 25–50 mcg for induction of labor (term); 400 mcg on day 3 of mifepristone for PRG termination (take w/ food) **Caution:** [X, –] **Contra:** PRG, component allergy **Disp:** Tabs 100, 200 mcg **SE:** Can cause miscarriage w/ potentially dangerous bleeding; HA, GI Sxs common (D, abdominal pain, constipation)

Mitomycin (Mutamycin) **Uses:** *Stomach, pancreas,* breast, colon CA; squamous cell carcinoma of the anus; non-small-cell lung, head & neck, cervical; bladder CA (intravesically) **Action:** Alkylating agent; may generate oxygen free radicals w/ DNA strand breaks **Dose:** Per protocol; 20 mg/m² q6–8wk or 10 mg/m² in combo w/ other myelosuppressive drugs; bladder CA 20–40 mg in 40 mL NS via a urethral catheter once/wk × 8 wk, followed by monthly × 12 mo for 1 y; ↓ in renal/hepatic impair **Caution:** [D, –] **Contra:** Thrombocytopenia, leukopenia, coagulation disorders, SCr >1.7 mg/dL **Disp:** Inj 5, 20, 40 mg **SE:** Myelosuppression (may persist 3–8 wk after, may be cumulative; minimize by lifetime dose <50–60 mg/m²), N/V, anorexia, stomatitis, & renal tox; microangiopathic hemolytic anemia w/ progressive renal failure (similar to hemolytic–uremic syndrome); venoocclusive liver Dz, interstitial pneumonia, alopecia; extravasation Rxns; contact dermatitis

Mitoxantrone (Novantrone) **Uses:** *AML (w/ cytarabine), ALL, CML, CAP, MS,* breast CA, & NHL **Action:** DNA-intercalating agent; ↓ DNA topoisomerase II **Dose:** Per protocol; ↓ in hepatic impair, leukopenia, thrombocytopenia **Caution:** [D, –] reports of secondary AML (monitor CBC) **Contra:** PRG **Disp:** Inj 2 mg/mL **SE:** Myelosuppression, N/V, stomatitis, alopecia (infrequent), cardiotox, urine discoloration **Notes:** Maintain hydration; cardiac monitoring prior to each dose

Modafinil (Provigil) **Uses:** * Improve wakefulness in pts w/ narcolepsy & excess daytime sleepiness* **Action:** Alters dopamine & norepinephrine release, ↓ GABA-mediated neurotransmission **Dose:** 200 mg PO q AM; ↓ dose 50% w/el-

Moxifloxacin **135**

derly/hepatic impair **Caution:** [C,?/–] CV Dz; ↑ effects of warfarin, diazepam, phenytoin; ↓ OCP, cyclosporine & theophylline effects **Contra:** Component allergy **Disp:** Tablets 100 mg, 200 mg **SE:** HA, N, D, paresthesias, rhinitis, agitation

Moexipril (Univasc) Uses: *HTN, post-MI,* DN **Action:** ACE inhibitor **Dose:** 7.5–30 mg in 1–2 ÷ doses 1 h ac **Caution:** [C (1st tri, D 2nd & 3rd tri), ?] **Contra:** ACE inhibitor sensitivity **Disp:** Tabs 7.5, 15 mg; ↓ in renal impair **SE:** ↓ BP, edema, angioedema, HA, dizziness, cough

Molindone (Moban) Uses: *Psychotic disorders* **Action:** Piperazine phenothiazine **Dose:** *Adults.* 50–75 mg/d PO, ↑ to 225 mg/d if necessary. *Peds.* 3–5 y: 1–2.5 mg/d PO in 4 ÷ doses, 5–12 y: 0.5–1.0 mg/kg/d in 4 ÷ doses **Caution:** [C, ?] NA glaucoma **Contra:** Drug/EtOH CNS depression **Disp:** Tabs 5, 10, 25, 50 mg; **SE:** ↓ BP, tachycardia, arrhythmias, EPS, Szs, constipation, xerostomia, blurred vision

Montelukast (Singulair) Uses: *Prophylaxis & Rx of chronic asthma, seasonal allergic rhinitis* **Action:** Leukotriene receptor antagonist **Dose:** *Asthma: Adults & Peds > 15 y:* 10 mg/d PO taken in PM. *Peds.* 2–5 y: 4 mg/d PO taken in PM. *6–14 y:* 5 mg/d PO in PM. **Caution:** [B, M] **Contra:** Component allergy **Disp:** Tabs 10 mg; chew tabs 4, 5 mg; granules 4 mg/packet **SE:** HA, dizziness, fatigue, rash, GI upset, Churg–Strauss syndrome **Notes:** Not for acute asthma

Morphine (Avinza XR, Duramorph, Infumorph, MS Contin, Kadian SR, Oramorph SR, Palladone, Roxanol) [C-II] Uses: *Relief of severe pain* **Action:** Narcotic analgesic **Dose:** Adults. PO: 5–30 mg q4h PRN; SR tabs 15–60 mg q8–12h (do not chew/crush). *IV/IM:* 2.5–15 mg q2–6h; supp 10–30 mg q4h. *IT.* (Duramorph, Infumorph): Per protocol *Peds.* > 6 mo 0.1–0.2 mg/kg/dose IM/IV q2–4h PRN to 15 mg/dose max; 0.2–0.5 mg/kg PO q 4–6h prn, 0.3–0.6 mg/kg SR tabs PO q12h **Caution:** [B (D w/prolonged use or high doses at term), +/–] **Contra:** Severe asthma, resp depression, GI obstruction **Disp:** Immediate-release tabs 15, 30 mg; MS Contin CR tabs 15, 30, 60, 100, 200 mg; Oramorph SR CR tabs 15, 30, 60, 100 mg; Kadian SR caps 20, 30, 50, 60, 100 mg; Avinza XR caps 30, 60, 90, 120 mg; soln 10, 20, 100 mg/5 mL; supp 5, 10, 20 mg; inj 2, 4, 5, 8, 10, 15, 25, 50 mg/mL; Duramorph/Infumorph inj 0.5, 1 mg/mL; supp 5, 10, 20, 30 mg **SE:** Narcotic SE (resp depression, sedation, constipation, N/V, pruritus); granulomas w/ IT **Notes:** May require scheduled dosing to relieve severe chronic pain; do not crush/chew SR/CR forms

Morphine liposomal (DepoDur) Uses: *Long-lasting epidural analgesia* **Action:** ER morphine analgesia **Dose:** 10–20 mg lumbar epidural inj (c-section 10 mg after cord clamped) **Caution:** [C,+/–] elderly, biliary Dz (sphincter of Oddi spasm) **Contra:** Ileus, resp depression, asthma, obstructed airway, suspected/known head injury ↑ ICP, allergy to morphine. **Disp:** Inj 10 mg/mL **SE:** Hypoxia, resp depression, ↓ BP, retention, N/V, constipation, flatulence, pruritus, pyrexia, anemia, HA, dizziness, tachycardia, insomnia, ileus **Notes:** Effect ≤48 h; not for IT/IV/IM

Moxifloxacin (Avelox, Vigamox ophthalmic) Uses: *Acute sinusitis & bronchitis, skin/soft tissue Infxns, conjunctivitis, & community-acquired*

pneumonia* **Action:** 4th-gen quinolone; ↓ DNA gyrase. *Spectrum:* Excellent gram(+) except MRSA & *E. faecium;* good gram(–) except *P. aeruginosa, S. maltophilia,* & *Acinetobacter* sp; good anaerobic coverage **Dose:** 400 mg/d PO/IV; avoid cation products, antacids. *Ophth:* 1 gt tid X7d; take PO 4 h before or 8 h after antacids **Caution:** [C, ?/–] Quinolone sensitivity; interactions w/ Mg, Ca, Al,Fe-containing products & class IA & III antiarrhythmic agents **Contra:** Quinolone/component sensitivity **Disp:** Tabs 400 mg, inj, ophth 0.5% **SE:** Dizziness, N, QT prolongation, Szs, photosensitivity, tendon rupture

Multivitamins (Table 15)

Mupirocin (Bactroban) **Uses:** *Impetigo; eradicate MRSA in nasal carriers* **Action:** ↓ bacterial protein synthesis **Dose:** *Topical:* Apply small amount to area 2–5 x/day X 5–14 d. *Nasal:* Apply bid in nostrils × 5d **Caution:** [B, ?] **Contra:** Do not use w/ other nasal products **Disp:** Oint 2%; cream 2% **SE:** Local irritation, rash

Muromonab-CD3 (Orthoclone OKT3) **WARNING:** Can cause anaphylaxis; monitor fluid status **Uses:** *Acute rejection following organ transplantation* **Action:** Murine Ab, blocks T-cell Fxn **Dose:** Per protocol *Adults.* 5 mg/d IV for 10–14 d. *Peds.* 0.1 mg/kg/d IV for 10–14 d **Caution:** [C, ?/–] Murine sensitivity, fluid overload **Contra:** Heart failure/fluid overload, Hx of Szs, PRG, uncontrolled HTN **Disp:** Inj 5 mg/5 mL **SE:** Anaphylaxis, pulm edema, fever/chills w/1st dose (premedicate w/ steroid/APAP/antihistamine) **Notes:** Monitor during inf; use 0.22-micron filter

Mycophenolic Acid (CellCept, Myfortic) **WARNING:** ↑Risk of Infxns, possible development of lymphoma **Uses:** *Prevent rejection after renal transplant* **Action:** Cytostatic to lymphocytes **Dose:** *Adults.* 720 mg PO bid; *Peds.* BSA 400–720 mg/m²: 750 mg PO bid; ↓ in renal insuff/neutropenia; take on empty stomach **Caution:** [C, ?/–] **Contra:** Component allergy **Disp:** DR tabs 180, 360 mg **SE:** N/V/D, pain, fever, HA, Infxn, HTN, anemia, leukopenia, edema

Mycophenolate Mofetil (CellCept) **WARNING:** ↑ Risk of Infxns, possible development of lymphoma **Uses:** *Prevent organ rejection after transplant* **Action:** ↓ immunologically mediated inflammatory responses **Dose:** *Adults.* 1 g PO bid; *Peds.* BSA 1.2–1.5 m²: 750 mg PO bid; *BSA >1.5 m²:* 1 g PO bid; may taper up to 600 mg/m² PO bid; used w/ steroids & cyclosporine; ↓ in renal insuff or neutropenia. *IV:* Infuse over >2 h. *PO:* Take on empty stomach, do not open capsules **Caution:** [C, ?/–] **Contra:** Component allergy; IV use in polysorbate 80 allergy **Disp:** Caps 250, 500 mg; susp 200mg/mL, inj 500 mg **SE:** N/V/D, pain, fever, HA, Infxn, HTN, anemia, leukopenia, edema

Nabilone (Cesamet)[CII] **WARNING:** Psychotomimetic rxns, may persist for 72 h following d/c; caregivers should be present during initial use or dosage modification; patients should not operate heavy machinery; avoid alcohol, sedatives, hypnotics, other psychoactive substances **Uses:** *Refractory chemo-induced emesis* **Action:** Synthetic cannabinoid **Dose:** *Adults.* 1 – 2 mg PO bid 1-3 h be-

fore chemo, 6 mg/d max; may continue for 48 h beyond final chemo dose **Caution:** [C,?/-] elderly, HTN, heart failure, underlying psychiatric illness, substance abuse; high protein binding and first-pass metabolism may lead to drug interactions **Disp:** Caps 1 mg **SE:** Drowsiness, vertigo, xerostomia, euphoria, ataxia, HA, difficulty concentrating, tachycardia, ↓ BP **Notes:** May require initial dose evening before chemo; Rx only quantity for single cycle

Nabumetone (Relafen) **WARNING:** May ↑risk of cardiovascular events & GI bleeding **Uses:** *Arthritis & pain* **Action:** NSAID; ↓ prostaglandins **Dose:** 1000–2000 mg/d ÷ qd–bid w/ food **Caution:** [C (D 3rd tri), +] **Contra:** Peptic ulcer, NSAID sensitivity, severe hepatic Dz **Disp:** Tabs 500, 750 mg **SE:** Dizziness, rash, GI upset, edema, peptic ulcer

Nadolol (Corgard) **Uses:** *HTN & angina* **Action:** Competitively blocks β-adrenergic receptors (β_1,β_2) **Dose:** 40–80 mg/d; ↑ to 240 mg/d (angina) or 320 mg/d (HTN) PRN; ↓ in renal insuff & elderly **Caution:** [C (1st tri; D if 2nd or 3rd tri), +] **Contra:** Uncompensated CHF, shock, heart block, asthma **Disp:** Tabs 20, 40, 80, 120, 160 mg **SE:** Nightmares, paresthesias, ↓ BP, bradycardia, fatigue

Nafcillin (Nallpen) **Uses:** *Infxns due to susceptible strains of Staphylococcus & Streptococcus* **Action:** Bactericidal β-lactamase-resistant penicillin; ↓ cell wall synthesis. *Spectrum:* Good gram(+) except MRSA and entrococcus, no gram (-), poor anaerobe **Dose:** *Adults.* 1–2 g IV q4–6h. *Peds.* 50–200 mg/kg/d ÷ q4–6h **Caution:** [B, ?] PCN allergy **Disp:** Inj powder 1, 2 gm **SE:** Interstitial nephritis, D, fever, N **Notes:** No adjustments for renal Fxn

Naftifine (Naftin) **Uses:** *Tinea pedis, cruris, & corporis* **Action:** Allylamine antifungal, ↓ cell membrane ergosterol synthesis **Dose:** Apply bid **Caution:** [B, ?] **Contra:** Component sensitivity **Disp:** 1% cream; gel **SE:** Local irritation

Nalbuphine (Nubain) **Uses:** *Moderate–severe pain; preop & obstetric analgesia* **Action:** Narcotic agonist–antagonist; ↓ ascending pain pathways **Dose:** *Adults.* 10–20 mg IM or IV q4–6h PRN; max of 160 mg/d; max single dose, 20 mg. *Peds.* 0.2 mg/kg IV or IM, 20 mg max; ↓ in hepatic insuff **Caution:** [B (D if prolonged/high doses at term), ?] **Contra:** Sulfite sensitivity **Disp:** Inj 10, 20 mg/mL **SE:** CNS depression, drowsiness; caution w/ opiate use

Naloxone (Narcan) **Uses:** *Opioid addiction (diagnosis) & OD* **Action:** Competitive narcotic antagonist **Dose:** *Adults.* 0.4–2.0 mg IV, IM, or SQ q5min; max total dose, 10 mg. *Peds.* 0.01–1 mg/kg/dose IV, IM, or SQ; repeat IV q3min × 3 doses PRN **Caution:** [B, ?] May precipitate acute withdrawal in addicts **Disp:** Inj 0.4, 1.0 mg/mL; neonatal inj 0.02 mg/mL **SE:** ↓ BP, tachycardia, irritability, GI upset, pulmonary edema **Notes:** If no response after 10 mg, suspect nonnarcotic cause

Naltrexone (ReVia) **Uses:** *EtOH & narcotic addiction* **Action:** Competitively binds to opioid receptors **Dose:** 50 mg/d PO; do not give until opioid-free for 7–10 d **Caution:** [C, M] **Contra:** Acute hepatitis, liver failure, opioid use **Disp:** Tabs 50 mg **SE:** May cause hepatotox; insomnia, GI upset, joint pain, HA, fatigue

Naphazoline & Antazoline (Albalon-A Ophthalmic, others), Naphazoline & Pheniramine Acetate (Naphcon A) Uses: *Relieve ocular redness & itching caused by allergy* **Action:** Vasoconstrictor & antihistamine **Dose:** 1–2 gtt up to qid **Caution:** [C, +] **Contra:** Glaucoma, children <6 y, & w/ contact lenses **Disp:** Soln 15 mL **SE:** CV stimulation, dizziness, local irritation

Naproxen (Aleve [OTC], Naprosyn, Anaprox) WARNING: May ↑ risk of cardiovascular events & GI bleeding Uses: *Arthritis & pain* **Action:** NSAID; ↓ prostaglandins **Dose:** *Adults & Peds >12 y.* 200–500 mg bid–tid to 1500 mg/d max; ↓ in hepatic impair **Caution:** [B (D 3rd tri), +] **Contra:** NSAID sensitivity, peptic ulcer **Disp:** Tabs: 200, 250, 375, 500 mg; delayed release: 375 mg, 500 mg; controlled release: 375 mg, 500 mg; susp 125 mL/5 mL. **SE:** Dizziness, pruritus, GI upset, peptic ulcer, edema

Naratriptan (Amerge) Uses: *Acute migraine attacks* **Action:** Serotonin 5-HT$_1$ receptor antagonist **Dose:** 1–2.5 mg PO once; repeat PRN in 4 h; ↓ in mild renal/hepatic insuff, take w/ fluids **Caution:** [C, M] **Contra:** Severe renal/hepatic impair, avoid w/ angina, ischemic heart Dz, uncontrolled HTN, cerebrovascular syndromes, & ergot use **Disp:** Tabs 1, 2.5 mg **SE:** Dizziness, sedation, GI upset, paresthesias, ECG changes, coronary vasospasm, arrhythmias

Natalizumab (Tysabri) WARNING: Cases of progressive multifocal leukoencephalopathy (PML) reported Uses: *Relapsing MS to delay disability and ↓ recurrences* **Action:** Adhesion molecule inhibitor **Dose:** *Adults.* 300 mg IV q4 wk; second-line Tx only **Contra:** PML; immune compromise or w/immunosuppressant **Caution:** [C,?/-] baseline MRI to rule out PML **Disp:** Vial 300 mg **SE:** Infxn, immunosuppression; infusion rxn precluding subsequent use; HA, fatigue, arthralgia **Notes:** Give slowly to ↓ rxns; limited distribution (TOUCH risk mgmt program); d/c immediately w/signs of PML (weakness, paralysis, vision loss, impaired speech, cognitive ↓); evaluate at 3 and 6 mos, then q 6 mos thereafter

Nateglinide (Starlix) Uses: *Type 2 DM* **Action:** ↑ Pancreatic insulin release **Dose:** 120 mg PO tid 1–30 min pc; ↓ to 60 mg tid if near target HbA$_{1c}$, (take 1–30 min ac) **Caution:** [C, –]. w/CYP2C9/3A4 metabolized drug (Table 13) **Contra:** DKA, type 1 DM **Disp:** Tabs 60, 120 mg **SE:** Hypoglycemia, URI; salicylates, nonselective β-blockers may enhance hypoglycemia

Nedocromil (Tilade) Uses: *Mild–moderate asthma* **Action:** Anti-inflammatory agent **Dose:** *Inhal:* 2 inhal qid **Caution:** [B, ?/–] **Contra:** Component allergy **Disp:** Met-dose inhaler **SE:** Chest pain, dizziness, dysphonia, rash, GI upset, Infxn **Notes:** Not for acute asthma

Nefazodone WARNING: Fatal hepatitis & liver failure possible, D/C if LFT >3× ULN, do not retreat; closely monitor for worsening depression or emergence of suicidality, particularly in ped pts Uses: *Depression* **Action:** ↓ Neuronal uptake of serotonin & norepinephrine **Dose:** Initial 100 mg PO bid; usual 300–600 mg/d in 2 ÷ doses **Caution:** [C, ?] **Contra:** MAOIs, pimozide, cisapride, carbamazepine **Disp:** Tabs 50, 100, 150, 200, 250, 500 mg **SE:** Postural ↓ BP & allergic Rxns; HA, drowsiness, xerostomia, constipation, GI upset, liver failure **Notes:** Monitor LFTs, HR, BP

Nelarabine (Arranon) **WARNING:** Neurotoxicity possible, which may be fatal **Uses:** *T-cell ALL or T-cell LBL unresponsive >2 other regimens* **Action:** Nucleoside analog **Dose:** *Adults.* 1500 mg/m² IV over 2 hr days 1, 3, 5 of 21-day cycle *Peds.* 650 mg/m² IV over 1 hr days 1–5 of 21-day cycle **Caution:** [D,?/-] **Disp:** Vial 250 mg **SE:** Neuropathy, ataxia, seizures, coma, hematologic toxicity, GI upset, HA, blurred vision **Notes:** Prehydration, urinary alkalinization, and allopurinol before dose; monitor CBC

Nelfinavir (Viracept) **Uses:** *HIV Infxn* **Action:** Protease inhibitor causes immature, noninfectious virion production **Dose:** *Adults.* 750 mg PO tid or 1250 mg PO bid, *Peds.* 20–30 mg/kg PO tid; take w/ food **Caution:** [B, ?] Many drug interactions **Contra:** Phenylketonuria, triazolam/midazolam use or drug dependent on CYP3A4 (Table 13) **Disp:** Tabs 250, 625 mg; powder 50 mg/g; **SE:** Food ↑ absorption; interacts w/ St. John's wort; dyslipidemia, lipodystrophy, D, rash

Neomycin, Bacitracin, & Polymyxin B (Neosporin Ointment) (See Bacitracin, Neomycin, & Polymyxin B Topical, page 43)

Neomycin, Colistin, & Hydrocortisone (Cortisporin-TC Otic Drops); Neomycin, Colistin, Hydrocortisone, & Thonzonium (Cortisporin-TC Otic Suspension) **Uses:** *External otitis,* *Infxns of mastoid/fenestration cavities* **Action:** Antibiotic w/antiinflammatory **Dose:** *Adults.* 4–5 gtt in ear(s) tid–qid. *Peds.* 3–4 gtt in ear(s) tid–qid **Caution:** [C, ?] **Disp:** Otic gtt & susp **SE:** Local irritation

Neomycin & Dexamethasone (AK-Neo-Dex Ophthalmic, NeoDecadron Ophthalmic) **Uses:** *Steroid-responsive inflammatory conditions of the cornea, conjunctiva, lid, & anterior segment* **Action:** Antibiotic w/ anti-inflammatory corticosteroid **Dose:** 1–2 gtt in eye(s) q3–4h or thin coat tid–qid until response, then ↓ to qd **Caution:** [C, ?] **Disp:** Cream neomycin 0.5%/dexamethasone 0.1%; oint neomycin 0.35%/dexamethasone 0.05%; soln neomycin 0.35%/dexamethasone 0.1% **SE:** Local irritation **Notes:** Use under ophthalmologist's supervision

Neomycin & Polymyxin B (Neosporin Cream) [OTC] **Uses:** *Infxn in minor cuts, scrapes, & burns* **Action:** Bactericidal **Dose:** Apply bid–qid **Caution:** [C, ?] **Contra:** Component allergy **Disp:** Cream neomycin 3.5 mg/polymyxin B 10,000 units/g **SE:** Local irritation **Notes:** Different from Neosporin oint

Neomycin, Polymyxin B, & Dexamethasone (Maxitrol) **Uses:** *Steroid-responsive ocular conditions w/ bacterial Infxn* **Action:** Antibiotic w/ anti-inflammatory corticosteroid **Dose:** 1–2 gtt in eye(s) q4–6h; apply oint in eye(s) tid–qid **Caution:** [C, ?] **Disp:** Oint neomycin sulfate 3.5 mg/polymyxin B sulfate 10,000 units/dexamethasone 0.1%/g; susp identical/5 mL **SE:** Local irritation **Notes:** Use under supervision of ophthalmologist

Neomycin-Polymyxin Bladder Irrigant [Neosporin GU Irrigant]
Uses: *Continuous irrigant for prophylaxis against bacteriuria & gram(−) bacteremia associated w/ indwelling catheter use* **Action:** Bactericidal; not for *Serratia* and streptococci **Dose:** 1 mL irrigant in 1 L of 0.9% NaCl; cont bladder irrigation w/ 1 L of soln/24 h **Caution:** [D] **Contra:** Component allergy **Disp:** Soln neomycin sulfate 40 mg & polymyxin B 200,000 units/mL; amp 1, 20 mL **SE:** Neomycin ototox or nephrotox (rare) **Notes:** Potential for bacterial/fungal super Infxn; not for inj

Neomycin, Polymyxin, & Hydrocortisone (Cortisporin Ophthalmic & Otic)
Uses: *Ocular & otic bacterial Infxns* **Action:** Antibiotic & antiinflammatory **Dose:** *Otic:* 3–4 gtt in the ear(s) tid–qid. *Ophth:* Apply a thin layer to the eye(s) or 1 gt qd–qid **Caution:** [C, ?] **Disp:** Otic susp; ophth soln; ophth oint **SE:** Local irritation

Neomycin, Polymyxin B, & Prednisolone (Poly-Pred Ophthalmic)
Uses: *Steroid-responsive ocular conditions w/ bacterial Infxn* **Action:** Antibiotic & anti-inflammatory **Dose:** 1–2 gtt in eye(s) q4–6h; apply oint in eye(s) tid–qid **Caution:** [C, ?] **Disp:** Susp neomycin 0.35%/polymyxin B 10,000 units/prednisolone 0.5%/mL **SE:** Irritation **Notes:** Use under supervision of ophthalmologist

Neomycin Sulfate (Mycinguent) [OTC]
Uses: *Hepatic coma, bowel prep* **Action:** Aminoglycoside, poorly absorbed PO; ↓ GI bacterial flora **Dose:** *Adults.* 3–12 g/24 h PO in 3–4 ÷ doses. *Peds.* 50–100 mg/kg/24 h PO in 3–4 ÷ doses **Caution:** [C, ?/−] renal failure, neuromuscular disorders, hearing impair **Contra:** Intestinal obstruction **Disp:** Tabs 500 mg; PO soln 125 mg/5 mL **SE:** Hearing loss w/ long-term use; rash, N/V **Notes:** Do not use parenterally (↑ tox); part of the Condon bowel prep

Nepafenac (Nevanac)
Uses: *Inflammation post-cataract surgery* **Action:** NSAID **Dose:** *Adults.* 1 gtt in eye(s) TID 1 day before, and 14 days after surgery **Contra:** NSAID or aspirin sensitivity **Caution:** [C,?/-] may ↑ bleeding time, delay healing, cause keratitis **Disp:** Susp 3 mL **SE:** Capsular opacity, visual changes, foreign body sensation, inc. IOP **Notes:** Prolonged use ↑ corneal risk; shake well before use, separate from other drops by >5 min.

Nesiritide (Natrecor)
Uses: *Acutely decompensated CHF* **Action:** Human B-type natriuretic peptide **Dose:** 2 mcg/kg IV bolus, then 0.01 mcg/kg/min IV **Caution:** [C, ?/−] When vasodilators are not appropriate **Contra:** SBP <90, cardiogenic shock **Disp:** Vials 1.5 mg **SE:** ↓ BP, HA, GI upset, arrhythmias, ↑ Cr **Notes:** Requires continuous BP monitoring; some studies indicate ↑in mortality

Nevirapine (Viramune)
WARNING: Reports of fatal hepatotox even after short-term use; severe life-threatening skin reactions (Stevens–Johnson, toxic epidermal necrolysis, & allergic Rxns); monitor closely during 1st 8 wk of Rx

Uses: *HIV Infxn* **Action:** Nonnucleoside RT inhibitor **Dose:** *Adults.* Initial 200 mg/d PO × 14 d, then 200 mg bid. *Peds.* <8 y: 4 mg/kg/d × 14 d, then 7 mg/kg bid. >8 y: 4 mg/kg/d × 14 d, then 4 mg/kg bid (w/o regard to food) **Caution:** [C, +/−] OCP **Disp:** Tabs 200 mg; susp 50 mg/5 mL **SE:** Life-threatening rash; HA, fever, D, neutropenia, hepatitis. **Notes:** HIV resistance when given as monotherapy; always use in combo w/at least 1 additional antiretroviral agent. Not recommended in women if CD_4 > 250 or men >400 unless benefit >> risk of hepatotoxicity

Niacin (Niaspan, Slo-Niacin) **Uses:** * Adjunct in significant hyperlipidemia* **Action:** Nicotinic acid, Vit B_3; ↓ Lipolysis; ↓ esterification of triglycerides; ↑ lipoprotein lipase **Dose:** 1–6 g ÷ doses PO tid; 9 g/d max (w/ food) **Caution:** [A (C if doses >RDA), +] **Contra:** Liver Dz, peptic ulcer, arterial hemorrhage **Disp:** SR caps 125, 250, 300, 400, 500 mg; tabs 25, 50, 100, 250, 500 mg; SR tabs 150, 250, 500, 750 mg; elixir 50 mg/5 mL **SE:** Upper body/facial flushing & warmth; GI upset, flatulence, exacerbate peptic ulcer; HA, paresthesias, liver damage, gout, or altered glucose control in DM. **Notes:** Flushing ↓ by taking aspirin or NSAID 30–60 min prior to dose

Nicardipine (Cardene) **Uses:** *Chronic stable angina & HTN*; prophylaxis of migraine **Action:** CCB **Dose:** *Adults.* PO. 20–40 mg PO tid. *SR:* 30–60 mg PO bid. *IV:* 5 mg/h IV cont inf; ↑ by 2.5 mg/h q15min to max 15 mg/h. *Peds.* PO: 20–30 mg PO q 8h. *IV:* 0.5–5 mcg/kg/min; ↓ in renal/hepatic impair **Caution:** [C, ?/−] Heart block, CAD **Contra:** Cardiogenic shock **Disp:** Caps 20, 30 mg; SR caps 30, 45, 60 mg; inj 2.5 mg/mL **SE:** Flushing, tachycardia, ↓ BP, edema, HA **Notes:** *PO-to-IV conversion.* 20 mg tid = 0.5 mg/h, 30 mg tid = 1.2 mg/h, 40 mg tid = 2.2 mg/h; take w/ food (not high fat)

Nicotine Gum (Nicorette) [OTC] **Uses:** *Aid to smoking cessation, relieve nicotine withdrawal* **Action:** Systemic delivery of nicotine **Dose:** Chew 9–12 pieces/d PRN; max 30 pieces/d **Caution:** [C, ?] **Contra:** Life-threatening arrhythmias, unstable angina **Disp:** 2 mg, 4 mg/piece; mint, orange, original flavors **SE:** Tachycardia, HA, GI upset, hiccups **Notes:** Must stop smoking & perform behavior modification for max effect

Nicotine Nasal Spray (Nicotrol NS) **Uses:** *Aid to smoking cessation, relieve nicotine withdrawal* **Action:** Systemic delivery of nicotine **Dose:** 0.5 mg/actuation; 1–2 sprays/h, 10 sprays/h max **Caution:** [D, M] **Contra:** Life-threatening arrhythmias, unstable angina **Disp:** Nasal inhaler 10 mg/mL **SE:** Local irritation, tachycardia, HA, taste perversion **Notes:** Must stop smoking & perform behavior modification for max effect

Nicotine Transdermal (Habitrol, Nicoderm CQ [OTC], Nicotrol [OTC]) **Uses:** *Aid to smoking cessation; relief of nicotine withdrawal* **Action:** Systemic delivery of nicotine **Dose:** Individualized; 1 patch (14–22 mg/d) & taper over 6 wk **Caution:** [D, M] **Contra:** Life-threatening arrhythmias, unstable angina **Disp:** Habitrol & Nicoderm CQ 7, 14, 21 mg of nicotine/24 h; Nicotrol 5, 10, 15 mg/24 h **SE:** Insomnia, pruritus, erythema, local site

Rxn, tachycardia **Notes:** Nicotrol worn for 16 h to mimic smoking patterns; others worn for 24 h; must stop smoking & perform behavior modification for max effect

Nifedipine (Procardia, Procardia XL, Adalat, Adalat CC)
Uses: *Vasospastic or chronic stable angina & HTN*; tocolytic **Action:** CCB **Dose:** *Adults.* SR tabs 30–90 mg/d. *Tocolysis:* 10–20 mg PO q4–6h. *Peds.* 0.6–0.9 mg/kg/24 h ÷ tid–qid **Caution:** [C, +] Heart block, aortic stenosis **Contra:** Immediate-release preparation for urgent or emergent HTN; acute MI **Disp:** Caps 10, 20 mg; SR tabs 30, 60, 90 mg **SE:** HA common on initial Rx; reflex tachycardia may occur w/ regular release dosage forms; peripheral edema, ↓ BP, flushing, dizziness **Notes:** Adalat CC & Procardia XL not interchangeable; SL administration not OK

Nilutamide (Nilandron) **WARNING:** Interstitial pneumonitis possible; most cases in 1st 3 mo; follow CXR before Rx **Uses:** *Combo w/ surgical castration for metastatic CAP* **Action:** Nonsteroidal antiandrogen **Dose:** 300 mg/d PO in ÷ doses × 30 d, then 150 mg/d **Caution:** [no used in females] **Contra:** Severe hepatic impair, resp insuff **Disp:** Tabs 150 mg **SE:** See warning, Interstitial pneumonitis, hot flashes, ↓ libido, impotence, N/V/D, gynecomastia, hepatic dysfunction **Notes:** May cause Rxn when taken w/ EtOH, follow LFT

Nimodipine (Nimotop) **Uses:** *Prevent vasospasm following subarachnoid hemorrhage* **Action:** CCB **Dose:** 60 mg PO q4h for 21 d; ↓ in hepatic failure **Caution:** [C, ?] **Contra:** Component allergy **Disp:** Caps 30 mg **SE:** ↓ BP, HA, constipation **Notes:** Give via NG tube if caps cannot be swallowed whole

Nisoldipine (Sular) **Uses:** *HTN* **Action:** CCB **Dose:** 10–60 mg/d PO; do not take w/ grapefruit juice or high-fat meal; ↓ start doses w/ elderly or hepatic impair **Caution:** [C, ?] **Disp:** ER tabs 10, 20, 30, 40 mg **SE:** Edema, HA, flushing

Nitazoxanide (Alinia) **Uses:** *Cryptosporidium or Giardia*–induced diarrhea in pts 1–11 y* **Action:** Antiprotozoal interferes w/ pyruvate ferredoxin oxidoreductase *Spectrum: Cryptosporidium or Giardia* **Dose:** *Peds 12–47 mo.* 5 mL (100 mg) PO q 12h × 3 d. *4–11 y:* 10 mL (200 mg) PO q 12h × 3 d; take w/ food **Caution:** [B, ?] **Disp:** 100 mg/5 mL PO susp **SE:** Abdominal pain **Notes:** Susp contains sucrose, interacts w/ highly protein-bound drugs

Nitrofurantoin (Macrodantin, Furadantin, Macrobid) **WARNING:** Pulmonary reactions possible **Uses:** *Prevention & Rx UTI* **Action:** Bacteriostatic; interferes w/ carbohydrate metabolism. *Spectrum:* some gram(+), susceptible gram(–) & bacteria; *Pseudomonas, Serratia,* & most sp. *Proteus*-resistant **Dose:** *Adults.* Suppression: 50–100 mg/d PO. *Rx:* 50–100 mg PO qid. *Peds.* 4–7 mg/kg/24 h in 4 ÷ doses (w/ food/milk/antacid) **Caution:** [B, +] Avoid w/CrCl <50 mL/min, pregnant at term **Contra:** Renal failure, infants <1 mo **Disp:** Caps 25, 50, 100 mg; susp 25 mg/5 mL **SE:** GI effects, dyspnea, various acute/chronic pulmonary reactions, peripheral neuropathy **Notes:** Macrocrystals (Macrodantin) cause < N than other forms

Nitroglycerin (Nitrostat, Nitrolingual, Nitro-Bid Ointment, Nitro-Bid IV, Nitrodisc, Transderm-Nitro, others) **Uses:** *Angina pectoris, acute & prophylactic therapy, CHF, BP control* **Action:** Relaxes vascular smooth muscle, dilates coronary arteries **Dose: *Adults.*** SL: 1 tab q5 min SL PRN for 3 doses. *Translingual:* 1–2 met-doses sprayed onto PO mucosa q3–5min, max 3 doses. *PO:* 2.5–9 mg tid. *IV:* 5–20 mcg/min, titrated to effect. *Topical:* Apply ½ in. of oint to chest wall tid, wipe off at night. *TD:* 0.2–0.4 mg/h/patch qd. ***Peds.*** 1 mcg/kg/min IV, titrate. **Caution:** [B, ?] Restrictive cardiomyopathy **Contra:** *IV:* Pericardial tamponade, constrictive pericarditis. *PO:* w/ sildenafil, tadalafil, vardenafil, head trauma, closed-angle glaucoma **Disp:** SL tabs 0.3, 0.4, 0.6 mg; translingual spray 0.4 mg/dose; SR caps 2.5, 6.5, 9, 13 mg; SR tabs 2.6, 6.5, 9.0 mg; inj 0.5, 5, 10 mg/mL; oint 2%; TD patches 0.1, 0.2, 0.4, 0.6 mg/h; buccal CR 2, 3 mg **SE:** HA, ↓ BP, lightheadedness, GI upset **Notes:** Nitrate tolerance w/ chronic use after 1–2 wk; minimize by providing nitrate-free period qd, using shorter-acting nitrates tid, & removing long-acting patches & oint before sleep to ↓ tolerance

Nitroprusside (Nipride, Nitropress) **Uses:** *Hypertensive crisis, CHF, controlled ↓ BP periop (↓ bleeding),* aortic dissection, pulmonary edema **Action:** ↓ Systemic vascular resistance **Dose: *Adult & Peds.*** 0.5–10 mcg/kg/min IV inf, titrate; usual dose 3 mcg/kg/min **Caution:** [C, ?] ↓ cerebral perfusion **Contra:** High output failure, compensatory HTN **Disp:** Inj 25 mg/mL **SE:** Excessive hypotensive effects, palpitations, HA **Notes:** Thiocyanate (metabolite w/renal excretion) w/ tox at 5–10 mg/dL, more likely if used for >2–3 d; w/aortic dissection use w/ β-blocker

Nizatidine (Axid, Axid AR [OTC]) **Uses:** *Duodenal ulcers, GERD, heartburn* **Action:** H_2 receptor antagonist **Dose: *Adults.*** Active ulcer: 150 mg PO bid or 300 mg PO hs; maint 150 mg PO hs. *GERD:* 300 mg PO bid; maint 150 mg PO bid. *Heartburn:* 75 mg PO bid. ***Peds.*** GERD: 10 mg/kg PO bid in ÷ doses, 150 mg bid max/↓ in renal impair **Caution:** [B, +] **Contra:** H_2-receptor antagonist sensitivity **Disp:** Caps 75 [OTC], 150, 300 mg; sol 15 mg/mL **SE:** Dizziness, HA, constipation, D

Norepinephrine (Levophed) **Uses:** *Acute ↓ BP, cardiac arrest (adjunct)* **Action:** Peripheral vasoconstrictor of arterial/venous beds **Dose: *Adults.*** 8–12 mcg/min IV, titrate. ***Peds.*** 0.05–0.1 mg/kg/min, titrate **Caution:** [C, ?] **Contra:** ↓ BP due to hypovolemia **Disp:** Inj 1 mg/mL **SE:** Bradycardia, arrhythmia **Notes:** Correct volume depletion as much as possible before vasopressors; interaction w/ TCAs leads to severe HTN; use large vein to avoid extravasation; phentolamine 5–10 mg/10 mL NS injected locally for extravasation

Norethindrone Acetate/Ethinyl Estradiol (FemHRT) **WARNING:** Estrogens & progestins should not be used for the prevention of CV Dz; the WHI study reported ↑ risks of MI, breast CA, & DVT in postmenopausal women during 5 y of treatment with estrogens combined with medroxyprogesterone acetate relative to placebo **Uses:** *Tx moderate–severe vasomotor Sxs associated w/ menopause; prevent osteoporosis* **Action:** Hormone replacement **Dose:** 1 tablet qd **Caution:** [X, –] **Contra:** PRG; Hx breast CA; estrogen-dependent tumor; abnormal genital bleeding; Hx DVT, PE, or related disorders; recent (w/in past year) arterial thromboembolic Dz (CVA, MI) **Disp:** 1 mg norethindrone/5 mcg ethinyl estradiol tablets **SE:** Thrombosis, dizziness, HA, libido changes **Notes:** Use in women w/ intact uterus

Norfloxacin (Noroxin, Chibroxin ophthal) Uses: *Complicated & uncomplicated UTI due to gram(–) bacteria, prostatitis, gonorrhea,* infectious D, conjunctivitis **Action:** Quinolone, ↓ DNA gyrase, bactericidal. *Spectrum:* Broad gram (+) and (-) *E. faecalis, E. coli, K. pneumoniae, P. mirabilis, P. aeruginosa, S. epidermidis, S. saprophyticus* **Dose:** 400 mg PO bid (↓ in renal impair). *Gonorrhea:* 800 mg single dose. *Prostatitis:* 400 mg PO bid. *Gastroenteritis, travelers D* 400 mg PO × 3–5 d *Adults, Peds > 1 y:* 1 gtt each eye qid for 7 d **Caution:** [C, –] Tendinitis/tendon rupture, quinolone sensitivity **Contra:** Hx allergy or tendinitis w/ fluoroquinolones **Disp:** Tabs 400 mg; ophth 3 mg/mL **SE:** Photosensitivity, HA, GI; ocular burning w/ ophth **Notes:** Interactions w/ antacids, theophylline, caffeine; good conc in the kidney & urine, poor blood levels; not for urosepsis

Norgestrel (Ovrette) Uses: *PO contraceptive* **Action:** Prevent follicular maturation & ovulation **Dose:** 1 tab/d; begin day 1 of menses **Caution:** [X, ?] **Contra:** Thromboembolic disorders, breast CA, PRG, severe hepatic Dz **Disp:** Tabs 0.075 mg **SE:** Edema, breakthrough bleeding, thromboembolism **Notes:** Progestin-only products have ↑ risk of failure in prevention of PRG

Nortriptyline (Aventyl, Pamelor) Uses: *Endogenous depression* **Action:** TCA; ↑ synaptic CNS levels of serotonin &/or norepinephrine **Dose:** *Adults.* 25 mg PO tid–qid; >150 mg/d not OK. *Elderly.* 10–25 mg hs. *Peds.* 6–7 y: 10 mg/d. *8–11 y:* 10–20 mg/d. *>11 y:* 25–35 mg/d, ↓ w/ hepatic insuff **Caution:** [D, +/–] NA glaucoma, CV Dz **Contra:** TCA allergy, use w/ MAOI **Disp:** Caps 10, 25, 50, 75 mg; soln 10 mg/5 mL **SE:** Anticholinergic (blurred vision, retention, xerostomia) **Notes:** Max effect seen after 2 wk

Nystatin (Mycostatin) Uses: *Mucocutaneous *Candida* Infxns (oral, skin, vaginal)* **Action:** Alters membrane permeability. *Spectrum:* Susceptible *Candida* sp **Dose:** *Adults & children.* PO: 400,000–600,000 U PO "swish & swallow" qid. *Vaginal:* 1 tab vaginally hs × 2 wk. *Topical:* Apply bid–tid to area. *Peds.* Infants: 200,000 Units PO q6h. **Caution:** [B (C PO), +] **Disp:** PO susp 100,000 units/mL; PO tabs 500,000 units; troches 200,000 units; vaginal tabs 100,000 U; topical cream/oint 100,000 units/g, powder 100,000 units/gram **SE:** GI upset, Stevens–Johnson syndrome **Notes:** Not absorbed PO; not for systemic Infxns

Octreotide (Sandostatin, Sandostatin LAR) Uses: *↓ severe diarrhea associated w/ carcinoid & neuroendocrine GI tumors (eg, VIPoma, ZE syndrome)*; bleeding esophageal varices **Action:** Long-acting peptide; mimics natural hormone somatostatin **Dose:** *Adults.* 100–600 mcg/d SQ/IV in 2–4 ÷ doses; start 50 mcg qd–bid. *Sandostatin LAR (depot):* 10–30 mg IM q4wk. *Peds.* 1–10 mcg/kg/24 h SQ in 2–4 ÷ doses. **Caution:** [B, +] Hepatic/renal impair **Disp:** Inj 0.05, 0.1, 0.2, 0.5, 1 mg/mL; 10, 20, 30 mg/5 mL depot **SE:** N/V, abdominal discomfort, flushing, edema, fatigue, cholelithiasis, hyper/hypoglycemia, hepatitis

Ofloxacin (Floxin, Ocuflox Ophthalmic) Uses: *Lower resp tract, skin & skin structure, & UTI, prostatitis, uncomplicated gonorrhea, & *Chlamydia* Infxns; topical (bacterial conjunctivitis; otitis externa; if perforated ear drum >12 y)* Action: Bactericidal; ↓ DNA gyrase. Broad spectrum gram (+) and (-): *S. pneumoniae, S. aureus, S. pyogenes, H. influenzae, P. mirabilis, N. gonorrhoeae, C. trachomatis, E. coli* Dose: *PO: Adults.* 200–400 mg PO bid or IV q12h. *Ophth: Adults & Peds >1 y.* 1–2 gtt in eye(s) q2–4h for 2 d, then qid × 5 more d. *Otic: Adults & Peds >12 y.* 10 gtt in ear(s) bid for 10 d. *Peds 1–12 y.* 5 gtt in ear(s) bid for 10 d. ↓ in renal impair, take on empty stomach Caution: [C, ↓] ↓ absorption w/ antacids, sucralfate, Al-, Ca-, Mg-, Fe-, or Zn-containing drugs Contra: Quinolone allergy Disp: Tabs 200, 300, 400 mg; inj 20, 40 mg/mL; ophth & otic 0.3% SE: N/V/D, photosensitivity, insomnia, HA Notes: Use ophth form in ears

Olanzapine (Zyprexa, Zyprexa Zydis) WARNING: Mortality in elderly w/ dementia-related psychosis Uses: *Bipolar mania, schizophrenia,* psychotic disorders, acute agitation in schizophrenia Action: Dopamine & serotonin antagonist; p inj 10 mg Dose: *Bipolar/schizophrenia:* 5–10 mg/d, ↑ weekly PRN, 20 mg/d max *Agitation:* 10–20 mg IMq2–4h PRN, 40 mg day/max Caution: [C, –] Disp: Tabs 2.5, 5, 7.5, 10, 15, 20 mg; PO disint. tabs 5, 10, 15, 20 mg Inj 10 mg SE: HA, somnolence, orthostatic ↓ BP, tachycardia, dystonia, xerostomia, constipation Notes: Takes weeks to titrate dose; smoking ↓ levels; may be confused w/ Zyrtec

Olopatadine (Patanol) Uses: *Allergic conjunctivitis* Action: H₁-receptor antagonist Dose: 1–2 gtt in eye(s) bid q6–8h Caution: [C, ?] Disp: Soln 0.1% 5 mL SE: Local irritation, HA, rhinitis Notes: Do not instill w/ contacts in

Olsalazine (Dipentum) Uses: *Maint remission in UC* Action: Topical anti-inflammatory Dose: 500 mg PO bid (w/ food) Caution: [C, M] Salicylate sensitivity Disp: Caps 250 mg SE: D, HA, blood dyscrasias, hepatitis

Omalizumab (Xolair) Uses: *Moderate–severe asthma in >/=12 y w/ reactivity to an allergen & when Sxs inadequately controlled w/ inhaled steroids* Action: Anti-IgE Ab Dose: 150–375 mg SQ q2–4wk (dose/frequency based on serum IgE level & BW, see package insert) Caution: [B,?/–] Contra: Component allergy Disp: 75, 150 mg single-use 5-mL vial SE: Site Rxn, sinusitis, HA, anaphylaxis reported in 3 pts Notes: Continue other asthma medications as indicated

Omega-3 fatty acid [fish oil](Omacor) Uses: *Prevent secondary MI, hypertriglyceridemia when diet fails* Action: Omega-3 fatty acid ethyl esters, ↓ thrombus, ↓ inflammation, ↓ triglycerides Dose: *Post MI:* 1 cap/day; *Hypertriglyceridemia:* 2 caps/d, ↑ to 4/d PRN Caution: [?,-] w/ anticoagulant use, w/bleed risk Contra: Hypersensitivity to components Disp: 1000-mg gelcap SE: Dyspepsia, N, GI pain, rash Notes: Only FDA approved fish oil supplement; not for exogenous hypertriglyceridemia (type 1 hyperchylomicronaemia); many OTC products (see page 202)

Omeprazole (Prilosec, Zegerid) Uses: *Duodenal/gastric ulcers, ZE syndrome, GERD,* *H. pylori* Infxns Action: Proton-pump inhibitor Dose: 20–40 mg PO qd–bid Zegerid powder/hac; in small cup w/ 2 Tbsp H_2O (not food or other liquids) refill and drink Caution: [C, –] Disp: DR tabs 20 mg; DR caps 10, 20, 40 mg; Zegerid powder for oral suspension: 20, 40 mg SE: HA, D Notes: Combo (ie, antibiotic) Rx for *H. pylori*

Ondansetron (Zofran, Zofran ODT) Uses: *Prevent chemo-associated & postop N/V* Action: Serotonin receptor antagonist Dose: *Chemo: Adults & Peds.* 0.15 mg/kg/dose IV prior to chemo, then 4 & 8 h after 1st dose or 4–8 mg PO tid; 1st dose 30 min prior to chemo & give on a schedule, not PRN. *Postop: Adults.* 4 mg IV immediately before anesthesia or postop. *Peds.* <40 kg: 0.1 mg/kg. *>40 kg:* 4 mg IV ↓ dose w/ hepatic impair Caution: [B, +/–] Disp: Tabs 4, 8, 24 mg, soln 4 mg/5 mL, inj 2 mg/ml, 32 mg/50 mL; Zofran ODT tab, 4, 8 mg. SE: D, HA, constipation, dizziness

Oprelvekin (Neumega) Uses: *Prevent severe thrombocytopenia w/ chemo* Action: ↑Proliferation & maturation of megakaryocytes (interleukin-11) Dose: *Adults.* 50 mcg/kg/d SQ for 10–21 d. *Peds* >12 y: 75–100 mcg/kg/d SQ for 10–21 d. *<12 y:* Use only in clinical trials. Caution: [C, ?/–] Disp: 5 mg powder for inj SE: Tachycardia, palpitations, arrhythmias, edema, HA, dizziness, insomnia, fatigue, fever, N, anemia, dyspnea, allergic reactions including anaphylaxis

Oral Contraceptives, Biphasic, Monophasic, Triphasic, Progestin Only (Table 7) Uses: *Birth control & regulation of anovulatory bleeding* Action: *Birth control:* Suppresses LH surge, prevents ovulation; progestins thicken cervical mucus; ↓ fallopian tubule cilia, ↓ endometrial thickness to ↓ chances of fertilization. *Anovulatory bleeding:* Cyclic hormones mimic body's natural cycle & regulate endometrial lining, results in regular bleeding q28d; may also ↓ uterine bleeding & dysmenorrhea Dose: 28-d cycle pills take qd; 21-d cycle pills take qd, no pills during last 7 d of cycle (during menses); some available as transdermal patch Caution: [X, +] Migraine, HTN, DM, sickle cell Dz, gallbladder Dz Contra: Undiagnosed vaginal bleeding, PRG, estrogen-dependent malignancy, hypercoagulation disorders, liver Dz, hemiplegic migraine, smokers >35 y Disp: 28-d cycle pills (21 active pills + 7 placebo/Fe supl); 21-d cycle pills (21 active pills) SE: Intramenstrual bleeding, oligomenorrhea, amenorrhea, ↑ appetite/weight gain, ↓ libido, fatigue, depression, mood swings, mastalgia, HA, melasma, ↑ vaginal discharge, acne/greasy skin, corneal edema, nausea Notes: Taken correctly, 99.9% effective for preventing PRG; no STDs prevention, use additional barrier contraceptive; long term, can ↓ risk of ectopic PRG, benign breast Dz, ovarian & uterine CA. *Rx for menstrual cycle control:* Start w/ monophasic; take for 3 mo before switching to another brand; if bleeding continues, change to pill w/ higher estrogen dose. *Rx for birth control:* Choose pill w/ lowest SE profile for particular pt; SEs numerous, due to Sxs of estrogen excess or progesterone deficiency; each pill's side effect profile is unique (see insert)

Orlistat (Xenical) Uses: *Manage obesity w/ BMI = 30 kg/m^2 or = 27 kg/m^2 w/ other risk factors; type 2 DM, dyslipidemia* **Action:** Reversible inhibitor of gastric & pancreatic lipases. **Dose:** 120 mg PO tid w/ a fat-containing meal **Caution:** [B, ?] May ↓ cyclosporine & warfarin dose requirements **Contra:** Cholestasis, malabsorption **Disp:** Capsules 120 mg **SE:** Abdominal pain/discomfort, fatty/oily stools, fecal urgency **Notes:** Do not use if meal contains no fat; GI effects ↑ w/ higher-fat meals; supplement w/ fat-soluble vitamins

Orphenadrine (Norflex) Uses: *Muscle spasms* **Action:** Central atropine-like effects cause indirect skeletal muscle relaxation, euphoria, analgesia **Dose:** 100 mg PO bid, 60 mg IM/IV q12h **Caution:** [C, +] **Contra:** Glaucoma, GI obstruction, cardiospasm, MyG **Disp:** Tabs 100 mg; SR tabs 100 mg; inj 30 mg/mL **SE:** Drowsiness, dizziness, blurred vision, flushing, tachycardia, constipation

Oseltamivir (Tamiflu) Uses: *Prevention & Rx influenza A & B* **Action:** ↓ viral neuraminidase **Dose:** *Adults.* 75 mg PO bid for 5 d. *Peds.* PO bid dosing: <14 kg: 30 mg. *16–23 kg:* 45 mg. *24–40 kg:* 60 mg; *>40 kg:* As adults; ↓ in renal impair **Caution:** [C, ?/–] Contra: Component allergy **Disp:** Caps 75 mg, powder 12 mg/mL **SE:** N/V, insomnia **Notes:** Initiate w/in 48 h of Sx onset or exposure

Oxacillin (Prostaphlin) Uses: *Infxns due to susceptible *S. aureus* & *Streptococcus** **Action:** Bactericidal; ↓ cell wall synthesis. *Spectrum:* Excellent gram(+), poor gram(–)**Dose:** *Adults.* 250–500 mg (1 g severe) IM/IV q4–6h. *Peds.* 150–200 mg/kg/d IV ÷ q4 6h; ↓ in significant renal Dz **Caution:** [B, M] **Contra:** PCN sensitivity **Disp:** Powder for inj 500 mg, 1, 2, 10 g, soln 250 mg/5 mL **SE:** GI upset, interstitial nephritis, blood dyscrasias

Oxaliplatin (Eloxatin) WARNING: Administer w/ supervision of physician experienced in chemo. Appropriate management is possible only w/ adequate diagnostic & Rx facilities. Anaphylactic-like Rxns reported Uses: *Adjuvant Rx stage-III colon CA (primary resected) & metastatic colon CA w/ 5-FU* **Action:** Metabolized to platinum derivatives, crosslinks DNA **Dose:** Per protocol; see insert. *Premedicate:* Antiemetics w/ or w/o dexamethasone **Caution:** [D, –] see Warning **Contra:** Allergy to components or platinum **Disp:** injection 50, 100 mg **SE:** Anaphylaxis, granulocytopenia, paresthesia, N/V/D, stomatitis, fatigue, neuropathy, hepatotox **Notes:** 5-FU & Leucovorin are given in combo; epi, corticosteroids, & antihistamines alleviate severe Rxns

Oxaprozin (Daypro, Daypro ALTA) WARNING: May ↑risk of cardiovascular events & GI bleeding Uses: *Arthritis & pain* **Action:** NSAID; ↓ prostaglandins synthesis **Dose:** 600–1200 mg/QD (÷ dose may help GI tolerance); ↓ in renal/hepatic impair **Caution:** [C (D in 3rd tri or near term), ?], peptic ulcer, bleeding disorders **Contra:** ASA/NSAID sensitivity peri-operative pain w/CABG **Disp:** Daypro ALTA tab 600 mg; caplets 600 mg **SE:** CNS inhibition, sleep disturbance, rash, GI upset, peptic ulcer, edema, renal failure, anaphylactoid reaction with aspirin triad (asthmatic w/rhinitis, nasal polyps and bronchospasm w/NSAID use)

Oxazepam (Serax) [C-IV] Uses: *Anxiety, acute EtOH withdrawal,* anxiety w/ depressive Sxs **Action: Benzodiazepine** Dose: *Adults.* 10–15 mg PO tid–qid; severe anxiety & EtOH withdrawal may require up to 30 mg qid. *Peds.* 1 mg/kg/d ÷ doses **Caution:** [D, ?] **Disp:** Caps 10, 15, 30 mg; tabs 15 mg **SE:** Sedation, ataxia, dizziness, rash, blood dyscrasias, dependence **Notes:** Avoid abrupt D/C; metabolite of diazepam (Valium)

Oxcarbazepine (Trileptal) Uses: *Partial Szs,* bipolar disorders **Action:** Blocks voltage-sensitive Na⁺ channels, stabilization of hyperexcited neural membranes **Dose:** *Adults.* 300 mg PO bid, ↑ weekly to target maint 1200–2400 mg/d. *Peds.* 8–10 mg/kg bid, 500 mg/d max, ↑ weekly to target maint dose; ↓in renal insuff **Caution:** [C, –] Cross-sensitivity to carbamazepine; reports of fatal skin and multiorgan hypersensitivity Rxns **Contra:** Components sensitivity **Disp:** Tabs 150, 300, 600 mg; Susp 300 mg/5 mL **SE:** ↓ Na⁺, HA, dizziness, fatigue, somnolence, GI upset, diplopia, mental concentration difficulties **Notes:** Do not abruptly D/C, check Na⁺ if fatigue reported; advise about symptoms of Stevens–Johnson syndrome and topic epidermal necrolysis

Oxiconazole (Oxistat) Uses: *Tinea pedis, cruris, & corporis* **Action:** Antifungal antibiotic. Spectrum: Most strains of *Epidermophyton floccosum, Trichophyton mentagrophytes, Trichophyton rubrum, Malassezia furfur* **Dose:** Apply bid **Caution:** [B, M] **Contra:** Component allergy **Disp:** Cream 1%; lotion **SE:** Local irritation

Oxybutynin (Ditropan, Ditropan XL) Uses: *Symptomatic relief of urgency, nocturia, & incontinence w/ neurogenic or reflex neurogenic bladder* **Action:** Direct smooth muscle antispasmodic; ↑ bladder capacity **Dose:** *Adults & Peds > 5 y.* 5 mg PO tid–qid; XL 5 mg PO qd; ↑ to 30 mg/d PO (5 & 10 mg/tab). *Peds 1–5 y.* 0.2 mg/kg/dose bid–qid (syrup 5 mg/5 mL); ↓ in elderly; periodic drug holidays OK **Caution:** [B, ? (use w/ caution)] **Contra:** Glaucoma, MyG, GI or GU obstruction, ulcerative colitis, megacolon **Disp:** Tabs 5 mg; XL tabs 5, 10, 15 mg; syrup 5 mg/5 mL **SE:** Anticholinergic (drowsiness, xerostomia, constipation, tachycardia)

Oxybutynin Transdermal System (Oxytrol) Uses: *Rx OAB* **Action:** Smooth muscle antispasmodic; ↑ bladder capacity **Dose:** One 3.9 mg/d system apply 2×/wk to abdomen, hip, or buttock **Caution:** [B, ?/–] **Contra:** Urinary or gastric retention, uncontrolled NA glaucoma **Disp:** 3.9 mg/d transdermal system **SE:** Anticholinergic effects, itching/redness at site **Notes:** Avoid reapplication to the same site w/in 7 d

Oxycodone [Dihydrohydroxycodeinone] (OxyContin, OxyIR, Roxicodone) [C-II] WARNING: Swallow whole, do not crush; high abuse potential **Uses:** *Moderate/severe pain, usually in combo w/ nonnarcotic analgesics* **Action:** Narcotic analgesic **Dose:** *Adults.* 5 mg PO q6h PRN.

Peds. 6–12 y: 1.25 mg PO q6h PRN. *>12 y:* 2.5 mg q6h PRN. ↓ w/ severe liver Dz **Caution:** [B (D if prolonged use or near term), M] **Contra:** Allergy, resp depression **Disp:** Immediate-release caps (OxyIR) 5 mg; tabs (Percolone) 5 mg; CR (OxyContin) 10, 20, 40, 80 mg, liq 5 mg/5 mL; soln conc 20 mg/mL **SE:** ↓BP, sedation, dizziness, GI upset, constipation, risk of abuse **Notes:** OxyContin for chronic CA pain; sought after as drug of abuse

Oxycodone & Acetaminophen (Percocet, Tylox) [C-II] Uses:
Moderate–severe pain **Action:** Narcotic analgesic **Dose:** *Adults.* 1–2 tabs/caps PO q4–6h PRN (acetaminophen max dose 4 g/d). *Peds.* Oxycodone 0.05–0.15 mg/kg/dose q 4–6h PRN, up to 5 mg/dose **Caution:** [B (D prolonged use or near term), M] **Contra:** Allergy, resp depression **Disp:** Percocet tabs, mg oxycodone/mg APAP: 2.5/325, 5/325, 7.5/325, 10/325, 7.5/500, 10/650; Tylox caps 5 mg oxycodone, 500 mg APAP; soln 5 mg oxycodone & 325 mg APAP/5 mL **SE:** ↓BP, sedation, dizziness, GI upset, constipation

Oxycodone & Aspirin (Percodan, Percodan-Demi) [C-II]
Uses: *Moderate–moderately severe pain* **Action:** Narcotic analgesic w/ NSAID **Dose:** *Adults.* 1–2 tabs/caps PO q4–6h PRN. *Peds.* Oxycodone 0.05–0.15 mg/kg/dose q 4–6h PRN, up to 5 mg/dose; ↓ in severe hepatic failure **Caution:** [B (D prolonged use or near term), M] Peptic ulcer **Contra:** Component allergy **Disp:** Percodan 4.5 mg oxycodone hydrochloride, 0.38 mg oxycodone terephthalate, 325 mg ASA; Percodan-Demi 2.25 mg oxycodone hydrochloride, 0.19 mg oxycodone terephthalate, 325 mg ASA **SE:** Sedation, dizziness, GI upset, constipation

Oxycodone/Ibuprofen (Combunox) [C-II] Uses: *Short term (not
≥7 d) management of acute moderate–severe pain* **Action:** Narcotic w/NSAID **Dose:** Initial **Caution:** [C, –] w/ impaired renal/hepatic Fxn; COPD, CNS depression **Contra:** Paralytic ileus, 3rd tri PRG, allergy to ASA or NSAIDs, where opioids are contraindicated **Disp:** Tabs 5 mg oxycodone/400 mg ibuprofen **SE:** N/V, somnolence, dizziness, sweating, flatulence, ↑ LFTs **Notes:** Monitor renal Fxn; abuse potential w/ oxycodone

Oxymorphone (Numorphan) [C-II] Uses: *Moderate/severe pain,
sedative* **Action:** Narcotic analgesic **Dose:** 0.5 mg IM, SQ, IV initial, 1–1.5 mg q4–6h PRN. *PR:* 5 mg q4–6h PRN **Caution:** [B, ?] **Contra:** ↑ ICP, severe resp depression **Disp:** Inj 1, 1.5 mg/mL; supp 5 mg **SE:** ↓ BP, sedation, GI upset, constipation, histamine release **Notes:** Chemically related to hydromorphone

Oxytocin (Pitocin) Uses: *Induce labor, control postpartum hemorrhage*;
promote milk letdown in lactating women **Action:** Stimulate muscular contractions of the uterus & milk flow during nursing **Dose:** 0.001–0.002 units/min IV inf; titrate 0.02 units/min max. *Breast-feeding:* 1 spray in both nostrils 2–3 min before feeding **Caution:** [Uncategorized, No anomalies expected, +/–] **Contra:** Where vaginal delivery not favorable, fetal distress **Disp:** Inj 10 units/mL; nasal soln 40 units/mL **SE:** Uterine rupture, fetal death; arrhythmias, anaphylaxis, H_2O intox **Notes:** Monitor vital signs; nasal form for breast-feeding only

Paclitaxel (Taxol, Abraxane)   Uses: *Ovarian & breast CA* CAP **Action:** Mitotic spindle poison promotes microtubule assembly & stabilization against depolymerization **Dose:** Per protocols; use glass or polyolefin containers (eg, nitroglycerin tubing set); PVC sets leach plasticizer; ↓ in hepatic failure; **Caution:** [D, –] **Contra:** Neutropenia <1500 WBC/mm^3; solid tumors **Disp:** Inj 6 mg/mL, 5 mg/mL albumin bound (Abraxane) **SE:** Myelosuppression, peripheral neuropathy, transient ileus, myalgia, bradycardia, ↓ BP, mucositis, N/V/D, fever, rash, HA, phlebitis; hematologic tox schedule-dependent; leukopenia dose-limiting by 24-h inf; neurotox limited w/ short (1–3 h) inf; allergic Rxns (dyspnea, ↓ BP, urticaria, rash) **Notes:** Maintain hydration; allergic Rxn usually w/in 10 min of inf; minimize w/ corticosteroid, antihistamine pretreatment

Palivizumab (Synagis)   Uses: *Prevent RSV Infxn* **Action:** MoAb **Dose:** *Peds.* 15 mg/kg IM monthly, typically Nov–Apr **Caution:** [C, ?] Renal/hepatic dysfunction **Contra:** Component allergy **Disp:** Vials 50, 100 mg **SE:** URI, rhinitis, cough, ↑ LFT, local irritation

Palifermin (Kepivance)   Uses: Oral mucositis w/ BMT * **Action:** Synthetic keratinocyte GF **Dose:** *Phase 1:* 60 mcg/kg IV qd ×3, 3rd dose 24–48 h before chemo *Phase 2:* 60 mcg/kg IV qd ×3, immediately after stem cell infusion **Caution:** [C, ?/–] **Contra:** N/A **Disp:** Inj 6.25 mg **SE:** Unusual mouth sensations, tongue thickening, rash, ↑ amylase & lipase **Notes:** *E coli*-derived; separate phases by 4 d; safety unknown w/ nonhematologic malignancies

Palonosetron (Aloxi)   WARNING: May ↑ QT$_c$ interval Uses: *Prevention acute & delayed N/V w/ emetogenic chemo* **Action:** 5HT3-receptor antagonist **Dose:** 0.25 mg IV 30 min prior to chemo; do not repeat w/in 7 d **Caution:** [B, ?] **Contra:** Component allergy **Disp:** 0.25 mg/5 mL vial **SE:** HA, constipation, dizziness, abdominal pain, anxiety

Pamidronate (Aredia)   Uses: *↑ Ca^{2+} of malignancy, Paget Dz, palliate symptomatic bone metastases* **Action:** ↓ Nl & abnormal bone resorption **Dose:** ↑ *Ca^{2+}:* 60 mg IV over 4 h or 90 mg IV over 24 h. *Paget Dz:* 30 mg/d IV slow inf for 3 d **Caution:** [C, ?/–] Avoid invasive dental procedures w/use **Contra:** PRG **Disp:** Powder for inj 30, 60, 90 mg **SE:** Fever, inj site Rxn, uveitis, fluid overload, HTN, abdominal pain, N/V, constipation, UTI, bone pain, ↓K$^+$, ↓Ca^{2+}, ↓Mg^{2+}, hypophosphatemia; jaw osteonecrosis, dental exam pretherapy

Pancrelipase (Pancrease, Cotazym, Creon, Ultrase)   Uses: *Exocrine pancreatic secretion deficiency (eg, CF, chronic pancreatitis, pancreatic insuff), steatorrhea of malabsorption* **Action:** Pancreatic enzyme supl **Dose:** 1–3 caps (tabs) w/ meals & snacks; ↑ to 8 caps (tabs); do not crush or chew EC products; dose-dependent on digestive requirements of pt; avoid antacids **Caution:** [C, ?/–] **Contra:** Pork product allergy **Disp:** Caps, tabs **SE:** N/V, abdominal cramps **Notes:** Individualize therapy

Pancuronium (Pavulon)   Uses: *Paralysis w/ mechanical ventilation* **Action:** Nondepolarizing neuromuscular blocker **Dose:** *Adults.* 2–4 mg IV q2–4h

PRN. **Peds.** 0.02–0.1 mg/kg/dose q2–4h PRN; ↓ in renal/hepatic impair; intubate pt & keep on controlled ventilation; use adequate sedation or analgesia **Caution:** [C, ?/–] **Contra:** Component or bromide sensitivity **Disp:** Inj 1, 2 mg/mL **SE:** Tachycardia, HTN, pruritus, other histamine reactions

Pantoprazole (Protonix)
Uses: *GERD, erosive gastritis,* ZE syndrome, PUD **Action:** Proton-pump inhibitor **Dose:** 40 mg/d PO; do not crush/chew tabs; 40 mg IV/d (not >3 mg/min, use Protonix filter) **Caution:** [B, ?/–] **Disp:** Tabs, delayed release 20, 40 mg; powder for inj 40 mg **SE:** Chest pain, anxiety, GI upset, ↑ LFTs

Paregoric [Camphorated Tincture of Opium] [C-III]
Uses: *Diarrhea,* pain, & neonatal opiate withdrawal syndrome **Action:** Narcotic **Dose:** **Adults.** 5–10 mL PO qd–qid PRN. **Peds.** 0.25–0.5 mL/kg qd–qid. **Neonatal withdrawal :** 3–6 gtt PO q3–6 h PRN to relieve Sxs for 3–5 d, then taper over 2–4 wk **Caution:** [B (D w/ prolonged use/high dose near term, +] **Contra:** Tincture in children; convulsive disorder **Disp:** Liq 2 mg morphine = 20 mg/20 mL opium/5 mL **SE:** ↓ BP, sedation, constipation **Notes:** Contains anhydrous morphine from opium; short-term use only

Paroxetine (Paxil, Paxil CR)
WARNING: Closely monitor for worsening depression or emergence of suicidality, particularly in ped pts **Uses:** *Depression, OCD, panic disorder, social anxiety disorder,* PMDD **Action:** SSRI **Dose:** 10–60 mg PO single daily dose in AM; CR 25 mg/d PO; ↑ 12.5 mg/wk (max range 26–62.5 mg/d) **Caution:** [B, ?/?] **Contra:** MAOI **Disp:** Tabs 10, 20, 30, 40 mg, susp 10 mg/5 mL; CR 12.5, 25, 37.5 mg **SE:** Sexual dysfunction, HA, somnolence, dizziness, GI upset, D, xerostomia, tachycardia

Pegfilgrastim (Neulasta)
Uses: *↓ Frequency of Infxn in pts w/ nonmyeloid malignancies receiving myelosuppressive anti-CA drugs that cause febrile neutropenia* **Action:** Granulocyte and macrophage stimulating factor **Dose:** **Adults.** 6 mg SQ × 1/chemo cycle. **Peds.** 100 mcg/kg SQ × 1/chemo cycle **Caution:** [C, M] in sickle cell **Contra:** Allergy to E. coli derived proteins or filgrastim **Disp:** Syringes: 6 mg/0.6 mL **SE:** Splenic rupture HA, fever, weakness, fatigue, dizziness, insomnia, edema, N/V/D, stomatitis, anorexia, constipation, taste perversion, dyspepsia, abdominal pain, granulocytopenia, neutropenic fever, ↑ LFT & uric acid, arthralgia, myalgia, bone pain, ARDS, alopecia, aggravation of sickle cell Dz **Notes:** Never give between 14 d before & 24 h after dose of cytotoxic chemo

Peg Interferon Alfa-2a (Pegasys)
Uses: *Chronic hepatitis C w/ compensated liver Dz* **Action:** Biologic response modifier **Dose:** 180 mcg (1 mL) SQ qwk × 48 wk; ↓ in renal impair **Caution:** [C, /?–] **Contra:** Autoimmune hepatitis, decompensated liver Dz **Disp:** 180 mcg/mL inj **SE:** Depression, insomnia, suicidal behavior, GI upset, neutro & thrombocytopenia, alopecia, pruritus **Notes:** May aggravate neuropsychiatric, autoimmune, ischemic, & infectious disorders; Copegus is ribavirin product

Peg Interferon Alfa-2b (PEG-Intron) **WARNING:** Can cause or aggravate fatal or life-threatening neuropsychiatric, autoimmune, ischemic, and infectious disorders. Monitor patients closely **Uses:** *Rx hepatitis C* **Action:** Immune modulation **Dose:** 1 mcg/kg/wk SQ; 1.5 mcg/kg/wk combined w/ribavirin **Caution:** [C, ?/–] w/psychiatric Hx **Contra:** Autoimmune hepatitis, decompensated liver Dz, hemoglobinopathy **Disp:** Vials 50, 80, 120, 150 mcg/0.5 mL; Redipen 50, 80,120,150 mcg/5 mL; reconstitute w/0.7 mL provided sterile water diluent **SE:** Depression, insomnia, suicidal behavior, GI upset, neutropenia, thrombocytopenia, alopecia, pruritus **Notes:** Give hs or w/APAP to ↓ flulike Sxs; monitor CBC/platelets; use immediately or store in refrigerator × 24 h; do not freeze

Pemetrexed (Alimta) **Uses:** *W/ cisplatin in nonresectable mesothelioma* NSCLC **Action:** Antifolate antineoplastic **Dose:** 500 mg/m^2 IV over 10 min every 3 wk; hold if CrCl <45 mL/min; give w/ vitamin B$_{12}$ (1000 mcg IM every 9 wk) & folic acid (350–1000 mcg PO qd); start 1 wk before; dexamethasone 4 mg PO bid × 3 start 1 d before each Rx **Caution:** [D, –] Renal/hepatic/BM impair **Contra:** Component sensitivity **Disp:** 500-mg vial **SE:** Neutropenia, thrombocytopenia, N/V/D, anorexia, stomatitis, renal failure, neuropathy, fever, fatigue, mood changes, dyspnea, anaphylactic reactions **Notes:** Avoid NSAIDs, follow CBC/platelets

Pemirolast (Alomast) **Uses:** *Allergic conjunctivitis* **Action:** Mast cell stabilizer **Dose:** 1–2 gtt in each eye qid **Caution:** [C, ?/–] **Disp:** 0.1% (1 mg/ml) in 10-mL bottles **SE:** HA, rhinitis, cold/flu symptoms, local irritation **Notes:** Wait 10 min before inserting contacts

Penbutolol (Levatol) **Uses:** *HTN* **Action:** β-adrenergic receptor blocker, β$_1$, β$_2$ **Dose:** 20–40 mg/d; ↓ in hepatic insuff **Caution:** [C (1st tri; D if 2nd/3rd tri), M] **Contra:** Asthma, cardiogenic shock, cardiac failure, heart block, bradycardia **Disp:** Tabs 20 mg **SE:** Flushing, ↓ BP, fatigue, hyperglycemia, GI upset, sexual dysfunction, bronchospasm

Penciclovir (Denavir) **Uses:** *Herpes simplex (herpes labialis/cold sores)* **Action:** Competitive inhibitor of DNA polymerase **Dose:** Apply at 1st sign of lesions, then q2h × 4 d **Caution:** [B, ?/–] **Contra:** Allergy **Disp:** Cream 1% [OTC] **SE:** Erythema, HA **Notes:** Do not apply to mucous membranes

Penicillin G, Aqueous (Potassium or Sodium) (Pfizerpen, Pentids) **Uses:** *Bacteremia, endocarditis, pericarditis, resp tract Infxns, meningitis, neurosyphilis, skin/skin structure Infxns* **Action:** Bactericide; ↓ cell wall synthesis. *Spectrum:* Most gram(+) (not staphylococci), streptococci, *N. meningitidis*, syphilis, clostridia, & anaerobes (not *Bacteroides*) **Dose:** *Adults.* 400,000–800,000 units PO qid; IV doses vary depending on indications; range 0.6–24 MU/d in ÷ doses q4h. *Peds.* Newborns <1 wk: 25,000–50,000 units/kg/dose IV q12h. *Infants 1 wk–<1 mo:* 25,000–50,000 units/kg/dose IV q8h. *Children:* 100,000–300,000 units/kg/24h IV ÷ q4h; ↓ in renal impair **Caution:** [B, M] **Contra:** Allergy **Disp:** Tabs 200,000, 250,000, 400,000, 800,000 units; susp 200,000,

400,000 units/5 mL; powder for inj **SE:** Allergic Rxns; interstitial nephritis, D, Szs **Notes:** Contains 1.7 mEq of K⁺/MU

Penicillin G Benzathine (Bicillin) Uses: *Single-dose regimen for streptococcal pharyngitis, rheumatic fever, glomerulonephritis prophylaxis, & syphilis* **Action:** Bactericidal; ↓ cell wall synthesis. *Spectrum:* See Penicillin G **Dose:** *Adults.* 1.2–2.4 million units deep IM inj q2–4wk. *Peds.* 50,000 units/kg/dose, 2.4 million units/dose max; deep IM inj q2–4 wk **Caution:** [B, M] **Contra:** Allergy **Disp:** Inj 300,000, 600,000 units/mL; Bicillin L-A benzathine salt only; Bicillin C-R combo of benzathine & procaine (300,000 units procaine w/ 300,000 units benzathine/mL or 900,000 units benzathine w/ 300,000 units procaine/2 mL) **SE:** Inj site pain, acute interstitial nephritis, anaphylaxis **Notes:** Sustained action, detectable levels up to 4 wk; drug of choice for noncongenital syphilis

Penicillin G Procaine (Wycillin, others) Uses: *Infxns of respir tract, skin/soft tissue, scarlet fever, syphilis* **Action:** Bactericidal; ↓ cell wall synthesis. *Spectrum:* PCN G-sensitive organisms that respond to low, persistent serum levels **Dose:** *Adults.* 0.6–4.8 million units/d in ÷ doses q12–24h; give probenecid at least 30 min prior to PCN to prolong action. *Peds.* 25,000–50,000 units/kg/24h IM ÷ qd–bid **Caution:** [B, M] **Contra:** Allergy **Disp:** Inj 300,000, 500,000, 600,000 units/mL **SE:** Pain at inj site, interstitial nephritis, anaphylaxis **Notes:** Long-acting parenteral PCN; levels up to 15 h

Penicillin V (Pen-Vee K, Veetids, others) Uses: Susceptible streptococci Infxns, otitis media, URIs, skin/soft tissue Infxns (PCN-sensitive staph) **Action:** Bactericidal; ↓ cell wall synthesis *Spectrum:* Most gram(+), including strep **Dose:** *Adults.* 250–500 mg PO q6h, q8h, q12h *Peds.* 25–50 mg/kg/25h PO in 4 doses; ↓ in renal impair; on empty stomach **Caution:** [B, M] **Contra:** Allergy **Disp:** Tabs 125, 250, 500 mg; susp 125, 250 mg/5 mL **SE:** GI upset, interstitial nephritis, anaphylaxis, convulsions **Notes:** Well-tolerated PO PCN; 250 mg = 400,000 units of PCN G

Pentamidine (Pentam 300, NebuPent) Uses: *Rx & prevention of PCP* **Action:** ↓ DNA, RNA, phospholipid, & protein synthesis **Dose:** *Rx: Adults & Peds.* 4 mg/kg/24 h IV qd for 14–21 d. *Prevention: Adults & Peds >5 y.* 300 mg once q4wk, give via Respirgard II neb; ↓ w/IV in renal impair **Caution:** [C, ?] **Contra:** Component allergy **Disp:** Inj 300 mg/vial; aerosol 300 mg **SE:** Associated w/ pancreatic cell necrosis w/ hyperglycemia; pancreatitis, CP, fatigue, dizziness, rash, GI upset, renal impair, blood dyscrasias (leukopenia & thrombocytopenia) **Notes:** Follow CBC, glucose, pancreatic Fxn monthly for 1st 3 mo; monitor for ↓ BP following IV dose

Pentazocine (Talwin, Talwin Compound, Talwin NX) [C-IV] Uses: *Moderate–severe pain* **Action:** Partial narcotic agonist–antagonist **Dose:** *Adults.* 30 mg IM or IV; 50–100 mg PO q3–4h PRN. *Peds.* 5–8 y: 15 mg IM q4h PRN. *8–14 y:* 30 mg IM q4h PRN; ↓ in renal/hepatic impair **Caution:** [C (1st tri, D w/ prolonged use/high dose near term), +/–] **Contra:** Allergy **Disp:** Talwin

Compound tab 12.5 mg + 325 mg ASA; Talwin NX 50 mg + 0.5 mg naloxone; inj 30 mg/mL **SE:** Considerable dysphoria; drowsiness, GI upset, xerostomia, Szs **Notes:** 30–60 mg IM = 10 mg of morphine IM; NX has naloxone to curb abuse by nonoral route

Pentobarbital (Nembutal, others) [C-II] Uses: *Insomnia, convulsions,* induce coma following severe head injury **Action:** Barbiturate **Dose:** *Adults.* Sedative: 20–40 mg PO or PR q6–12h. *Hypnotic:* 100–200 mg PO or PR hs PRN. *Induced coma:* Load 5–10 mg/kg IV, then maint 1–3 mg/kg/h IV inf (keep serum level 20–50 mg/mL). *Peds.* Hypnotic: 2–6 mg/kg/dose PO hs PRN. *Induced coma:* As adult **Caution:** [D, +/–] Severe hepatic impair **Contra:** Allergy **Disp:** Caps 50, 100 mg; elixir 18.2 mg/5 mL (= 20 mg pentobarbital); supp 30, 60, 120, 200 mg; inj 50 mg/mL **SE:** Resp depression, ↓ BP w/ aggressive IV use for cerebral edema; bradycardia, ↓ BP, sedation, lethargy, resp ↓, hangover, rash, Stevens–Johnson syndrome, blood dyscrasias **Notes:** Tolerance to sedative–hypnotic effect w/in 1–2 wk

Pentosan Polysulfate Sodium (Elmiron) Uses: * Relief of pain/discomfort associated w/ interstitial cystitis* **Action:** Bladder wall buffer **Dose:** 100 mg PO tid on empty stomach w/ H_2O 1 h ac or 2 h pc **Caution:** [B, ?/–] **Contra:** Allergy **Disp:** Caps 100 mg **SE:** Alopecia, N/D, HA, ↑ LFTs, anticoagulant effects, thrombocytopenia **Notes:** Reassess after 3 mo

Pentoxifylline (Trental) Uses: *Symptomatic management of peripheral vascular Dz* **Action:** ↓ Blood cell viscosity by restoring erythrocyte flexibility **Dose:** *Adults.* 400 mg PO tid pc; Rx for at least 8 wk for full effect; ↓ to bid w/ GI/CNS SEs **Caution:** [C, +/–] **Contra:** Cerebral/retinal hemorrhage **Disp:** Tabs CR 400 mg; Tabs ER 400 mg **SE:** Dizziness, HA, GI upset

Pergolide (Permax) Uses: *Parkinson Dz* **Action:** Centrally active dopamine receptor agonist **Dose:** Initial, 0.05 mg PO tid, titrated q2–3d to effect; maint 2–3 mg/d in ÷ doses **Caution:** [B, ?/–] **Contra:** Ergot sensitivity **Disp:** Tabs 0.05, 0.25, 1.0 mg **SE:** Dizziness, somnolence, confusion, nausea, constipation, dyskinesia, rhinitis, MI **Notes:** May ↓ BP during start of therapy

Perindopril Erbumine (Aceon) Uses: *HTN,* CHF, DN, post-MI **Action:** ACE inhibitor **Dose:** 4–8 mg/d; avoid w/ food; ↓ in elderly/renal impair **Caution:** [C (1st tri), D 2nd & 3rd tri), ?/–] ACE-inhibitor-induced angioedema **Contra:** Bilateral renal artery stenosis, primary hyperaldosteronism **Disp:** Tabs 2, 4, 8 mg **SE:** HA, ↓ BP, dizziness, GI upset, cough **Notes:** OK w/ diuretics

Permethrin (Nix, Elimite) [OTC] Uses: *Eradication of lice/scabies* **Action:** Pediculicide **Dose:** *Adults & Peds.* Saturate hair & scalp; allow 10 min before rinsing **Caution:** [B, ?/–] **Contra:** Allergy **Disp:** Topical lotion 1%; cream 5% **SE:** Local irritation **Notes:** Disinfect clothing, bedding, combs, & brushes

Perphenazine (Trilafon) Uses: *Psychotic disorders, severe nausea,* intractable hiccups **Action:** Phenothiazine; blocks brain dopaminergic receptors **Dose:** *Antipsychotic:* 4–16 mg PO tid; max 64 mg/d. *Hiccups:* 5 mg IM q6h PRN or 1 mg IV at intervals not <1–2 mg/min, 5 mg max. **Peds.** 1–6 y: 4–6 m/d PO in ÷ doses. *6–12 y:* 6 mg/d PO in ÷ doses. >12 y: 4–16 mg PO bid–qid; ↓ in hepatic insuff **Caution:** [C, ?/–] NA glaucoma, severe ↑ /↓ BP **Contra:** Phenothiazine sensitivity, BM depression, severe liver or cardiac Dz **Disp:** Tabs 2, 4, 8, 16 mg; PO conc 16 mg/5 mL; inj 5 mg/mL **SE:** ↓ BP, tachycardia, bradycardia, EPS, drowsiness, Szs, photosensitivity, skin discoloration, blood dyscrasias, constipation

Phenazopyridine (Pyridium, others) Uses: *Lower urinary tract irritation* **Action:** Local anesthetic on urinary tract mucosa **Dose:** **Adults.** 100–200 mg PO tid. *Peds 6–12 y.* 12 mg/kg/24 h PO in 3 ÷ doses; ↓ in renal insuff **Caution:** [B, ?] Hepatic Dz **Contra:** Renal failure **Disp:** Tabs 95mg, 97.2, 100, 200 mg; **SE:** GI disturbances; red-orange urine color (can stain clothing); HA, dizziness, acute renal failure, methemoglobinemia

Phenelzine (Nardil) WARNING: Antidepressants increase the risk of suicidal thinking and behavior in children and adolescents w/major depressive disorder and other psychiatric disorders **Uses:** *Depression* **Action:** MAOI **Dose:** 15 mg PO tid. **Elderly:** 15–60 mg/d ÷ doses **Caution:** [C, –] Interacts w/ SSRI, ergots, triptans **Contra:** CHF, Hx liver Dz **Disp:** Tabs 15 mg **SE:** Postural ↓ BP; edema, dizziness, sedation, rash, sexual dysfunction, xerostomia, constipation, urinary retention **Notes:** May take 2–4 wk for effect; avoid tyramine-containing foods (eg, cheeses)

Phenobarbital [C-IV] Uses: *Sz disorders,* insomnia, anxiety **Action:** Barbiturate **Dose:** **Adults.** Sedative–hypnotic: 30–120 mg/d PO or IM PRN. *Anticonvulsant:* Load 10–12 mg/kg in 3 ÷ doses, then 1–3 mg/kg/24 h PO, IM, or IV. **Peds.** Sedative–hypnotic: 2–3 mg/kg/24 h PO or IM hs PRN. *Anticonvulsant:* Load 15–20 mg/kg + in 2 equal doses 1 h apart, then 3–5 mg/kg/24h PO ÷ in 2–3 doses **Caution:** [D, M] **Contra:** Porphyria, liver dysfunction **Disp:** Tabs 8, 15, 16, 30, 32, 60, 65, 100 mg; elixir 15, 20 mg/5 mL; inj 30, 60, 65, 130 mg/mL **SE:** Bradycardia, ↓ BP, hangover, Stevens–Johnson syndrome, blood dyscrasias, resp depression **Notes:** Tolerance develops to sedation; paradoxic hyperactivity seen in ped pts; long half-life allows single daily dosing (Table 2)

Phenylephrine, nasal (Neo-Synephrine Nasal) (OTC) Uses: *Nasal congestion* **Action:** α-adrenergic agonist **Dose:** **Adults.** 2–3 drops or 1–2 sprays/nostril q4h (usual 0.25%) PRN. **Peds.** 6 mo–2 yr: 0.125% 1–2 drops/nostril q3-4h, *2–6 yr:* 0.125% 2–3 drops/nostril q3–4h *6-12 yr:* 1–2 sprays/nostril q4h or 0.125% 2–3 drops/nostril q4h or 0.25% 2–3 drops **Caution:** [C, +/–] HTN, acute pancreatitis, hepatitis, coronary Dz, NA glaucoma, hyperthyroidism **Contra:** Bradycardia, arrhythmias **Disp:** Nasal soln 0.125, 0.25, 0.5, 1%; Liquid 7.5 mg/5 mL; drops 2.5 mg/mL; tabs 10 mg; chew tabs 10 mg; tabs OD 10 mg; strips 10 mg. **SE:** Arrhythmias, HTN, nasal irritation, dryness, sneezing, rebound congestion w/ prolonged use, HA **Notes:** Do not use >3 days

Phenylephrine, ophthalmic (Neo-Synephrine Ophthalmic, AK-Dilate, Zincfrin [OTC]) Uses: * Mydriasis, ocular redness [OTC], periop mydriasis, posterior synechiae, uveitis w/posterior Synechiae* **Action:** α-

Adrenergic agonist **Dose:** *Adults.* Redness: 1 gtt 0.12% Q 3–4h PRN; *Exam mydriasis:* 1 gtt 2.5% (15 min–1 h for effect); Preop 1 gtt 2.5–10% 30–60 min preop; *Ocular disorders:* 1 gtt 2.5–10% QD-TID **Peds.** As adult, only use 2.5% for exam, preop and ocular conditions **Caution:** [C] may cause late-term fetal anoxia/bradycardia, +/–] HTN, w/ elderly w/ CAD, **Contra:** Narrow-angle glaucoma **Disp:** Ophth soln 0.12% (Zincfrin OTC), 2.5,10%; **SE:** Tearing, HA, irritation, eye pain, photophobia, arrhythmia, tremor

Phenylephrine, oral (Sudafed PE, SudoGest PE, Nasop, Lusonal, AH-chew D, Sudafed PE quick dissolve)(OTC) **Uses:**
Nasal congestion **Action:** α-adrenergic agonist **Dose:** *Adults.* 10 mg PO Q4H PRN, Max 60 mg/d **Peds.** 10 mg PO q4h prn, max 60 mg/day **Caution:** [C, +/–] HTN, acute pancreatitis, hepatitis, coronary Dz, NA glaucoma, hyperthyroidism **Contra:** MAOI w/in 14 d, narrow-angle glaucoma, severe ↑ (BP or CAD, urinary retention **Disp:** Liquid 7.5 mg/5 mL; drops 2.5 mg/mL; tabs 10 mg; chew tabs 10 mg; tabs OD 10 mg; strips 10 mg. **SE:** Arrhythmias, HTN, HA, agitation, anxiety, tremor, palpitations

Phenylephrine, systemic (Neo-Synephrine) **Uses:** *Vascular failure in shock, allergy, or drug-induced* ↓BP* **Action:** Stimulates α-adrenergic agonist **Dose:** *Adults.* Mild–moderate ↓BP: 2–5 mg IM or SQ ↑ BP for 2 h; 0.1–0.5 mg IV elevates BP for 15 min. *Severe ↓ BP/shock:* Cont inf at 100–180 mg/min; after BP stabilized, maint 40–60 mg/min **Peds.** ↓ BP: 5–20 mcg/kg/dose IV q10–15 min or 0.1–0.5 mg/kg/min IV inf, titrate to effect. **Caution:** [C, +/–] HTN, acute pancreatitis, hepatitis, coronary Dz, NA glaucoma, hyperthyroidism **Contra:** Bradycardia, arrhythmias **Disp:** Inj 10 mg/mL **SE:** Arrhythmias, HTN, peripheral vasoconstriction ↑ (w/oxytocin, MAOIs, & TCAs; HA, weakness, necrosis, ↓ renal perfusion **Notes:** Restore blood volume if loss has occurred; use large veins to avoid extravasation; phentolamine 10 mg in 10–15 mL of NS for local inj to Rx extravasasion

Phenytoin (Dilantin) **Uses:** *Sz disorders* **Action:** ↓(Sz spread in the motor cortex **Dose:** *Load: Adults & Peds.* 15–20 mg/kg IV, 25 mg/min max or PO in 400-mg doses at 4-h intervals. *Maint: Adults.* Initial, 200 mg PO or IV bid or 300 mg hs; then follow levels. **Peds.** 4–7 mg/kg/24h PO or IV ÷ qd–bid; avoid PO susp (erratic absorption) **Caution:** [D, +] **Contra:** Heart block, sinus bradycardia **Disp:** Dilatin Infatab chew 50 mg; Dilantin/Phenytek capsules 100 mg; capsules, ER 30, 100, 200, 300 mg; suspension 125 mg/5 mL. **SE:** Nystagmus/ataxia early signs of tox; gum hyperplasia w/ long-term use. *IV:* ↓ BP, bradycardia, arrhythmias, phlebitis; peripheral neuropathy, rash, blood dyscrasias, Stevens–Johnson syndrome **Notes:** Follow levels Table 2; phenytoin albumin bound & levels reflect bound & free phenytoin; w/ ↓ albumin & azotemia, low levels may be therapeutic (nl free levels); do not change dosage at intervals <7–10 d

Physostigmine (Antilirium) **Uses:** *Antidote for TCA, atropine, & scopolamine OD; glaucoma* **Action:** Reversible cholinesterase inhibitor **Dose:**

Piperacillin **157**

Adults. 2 mg IV or IM q 20 min. *Peds.* 0.01–0.03 mg/kg/dose IV q15–30 min up to 2 mg total if needed **Caution:** [C, ?] **Contra:** GI/GU obstruction, CV Dz **Disp:** Inj 1 mg/mL **SE:** Rapid IV admin associated w/Szs; cholinergic side effects; sweating, salivation, lacrimation, GI upset, asystole, changes in heart rate **Notes:** Excessive readministration can result in cholinergic crisis; crisis reversed w/ atropine

Phytonadione [Vitamin K] (AquaMEPHYTON, others) **Uses:** *Coagulation disorders due to faulty formation of factors II, VII, IX, X*; hyperalimentation **Action:** Cofactor for production of factors II, VII, IX, & X **Dose:** *Adults & Children.* Anticoagulant-induced prothrombin deficiency; 1–10 mg PO or IV slowly. *Hyperalimentation:* 10 mg IM or IV qwk. *Infants.* 0.5–1 mg/dose IM, SQ, or PO **Caution:** [C, +] **Contra:** Allergy **Disp:** Tabs 5 mg; inj 2, 10 mg/mL **SE:** Anaphylaxis from IV dosage; give IV slowly; GI upset (PO), inj site Rxns **Notes:** W/ parenteral Rx, 1st change in PT usually seen in 12–24 h; use makes re-Coumadinization more difficult

Pimecrolimus (Elidel) **Uses:** *Atopic dermatitis* refractory, severe perianal itching **Action:** Inhibits T lymphocytes **Dose:** Apply bid; use at least 1 wk following resolution **Caution:** [C, ?/–] w/ local Infxn, lymphadenopathy; immunocompromise; avoid <2 yrs of age **Contra:** Allergy **Disp:** cream 1%, 30-g, 60-g, 100-g tubes **SE:** Phototox, local irritation/burning, flulike Sxs, may ↑ malignancy **Notes:** Apply to dry skin only; wash hands after use; theoretical cancer risk; second-line/short-term use only

Pindolol (Visken) **Uses:** *HTN* **Action:** β-adrenergic receptor blocker, β₁, β₂, ISA **Dose:** 5–10 mg bid, 60 mg/d max; ↓ in hepatic/renal failure **Caution:** [B (1st tri; D if 2nd or 3rd tri), +/–] **Contra:** Uncompensated CHF, cardiogenic shock, bradycardia, heart block, asthma, COPD **Disp:** Tabs 5, 10 mg **SE:** Insomnia, dizziness, fatigue, edema, GI upset, dyspnea; fluid retention may exacerbate CHF

Pioglitazone/Metformin (ActoPlus Met) **WARNING:** Can cause lactic acidosis, which is fatal in 50% of cases **Uses:** *Type 2 DM as adjunct to diet and exercise* **Action:** Combined ↑ insulin sensitivity w/ ↓ hepatic glucose release **Dose:** Initial 1 tab PO qd or titrate; max daily pioglitazone 45 mg & metformin 2550 mg **Caution:** [C, –] stop w/ radiologic contrast agents **Contra:** Renal impair, acidosis **Disp:** Tabs pioglitazone mg/metformin mg: 15/500, 15/850 **SE:** Lactic acidosis, hypoglycemia, edema, weight gain, URI, HA, GI upset, liver damage **Notes:** Follow LFTs

Pioglitazone (Actos) **Uses:** *Type 2 DM* **Action:** ↓ Insulin sensitivity **Dose:** 15–45 mg/d PO **Caution:** [C, –] **Contra:** Hepatic impair **Disp:** Tabs 15, 30, 45 mg **SE:** Weight gain, URI, HA, hypoglycemia, edema

Piperacillin (Pipracil) **Uses:** *Infxns of skin, bone, resp &, urinary tract, abdomen, sepsis* **Action:** 4th-gen PCN; bactericidal; ↓ cell wall synthesis. *Spectrum:* Primarily gram(+), better *Enterococcus, H. influenza*, not staph; gram(–) *E. coli, Proteus, Shigella, Pseudomonas*, not β-lactamase-producing **Dose:** *Adults.* 3 g IV q4–6h. *Peds.* 200–300 mg/kg/d IV ÷ q4–6h; ↓ in renal failure **Caution:** [B,

M] PCN sensitivity **Disp:** Powder for inj: 2, 3, 4, 40-g **SE:** ↓ Plt aggregation, interstitial nephritis, renal failure, anaphylaxis, hemolytic anemia **Notes:** Often used w/ aminoglycoside

Piperacillin–Tazobactam (Zosyn) **Uses:** *Infxns of skin, bone, resp & urinary tract, abdomen, sepsis * **Action:** PCN plus β-lactamase inhibitor; bactericidal; ↓ cell wall synthesis. *Spectrum:* Good gram(+), excellent gram(–); covers anaerobes & β-lactamase producers **Dose:** *Adults.* 3.375–4.5 g IV q6h; ↓ in renal insuff **Caution:** [B, M] PCN or β-lactam sensitivity **Disp:** Powder for inj: 2.23, 3.373, 4.5g, inj 2.35, 3.375, 4.5g **SE:** D, HA, insomnia, GI upset, serum sickness-like reaction, pseudomembranous colitis **Notes:** Often used in combo w/ aminoglycoside

Pirbuterol (Maxair) **Uses:** *Prevention & Rx reversible bronchospasm* **Action:** β2-Adrenergic agonist **Dose:** 2 inhal q4–6h; max 12 inhal/d **Caution:** [C, ?/–] **Disp:** Aerosol 0.2 mg/actuation **SE:** Nervousness, restlessness, trembling, HA, taste changes, tachycardia

Piroxicam (Feldene) WARNING: May ↑risk of cardiovascular events & GI bleeding **Uses:** *Arthritis & pain* **Action:** NSAID; ↓ prostaglandins **Dose:** 10–20 mg/d **Caution:** [B (1st tri; D if 3rd tri or near term), +] GI bleeding **Contra:** ASA/NSAID sensitivity **Disp:** Caps 10, 20 mg **SE:** Dizziness, rash, GI upset, edema, acute renal failure, peptic ulcer

Plasma Protein Fraction (Plasmanate, others) **Uses:** *Shock & ↓ BP* **Action:** Plasma volume expander **Dose:** Initial, 250–500 mL IV (not >10 mL/min); subsequent inf based on response. *Peds.* 10–15 mL/kg/dose IV; subsequent inf based on response **Caution:** [C, +] **Contra:** Renal insuff, CHF **Disp:** Inj 5% **SE:** ↓ BP w/ rapid inf; hypocoagulability, metabolic acidosis, PE **Notes:** 130–160 mEq Na/L; not substitute for RBC

Pneumococcal 7-Valent Conjugate Vaccine (Prevnar) **Uses:** *Immunization against pneumococcal Infxns in infants & children* **Action:** Active immunization **Dose:** 0.5 mL IM/dose; series of 3 doses; 1st dose 2 mo of age w/ subsequent doses q2mo **Caution:** [C, +] Thrombocytopenia **Contra:** Diphtheria toxoid sensitivity, febrile illness **Disp:** Inj **SE:** Local reactions, arthralgia, fever, myalgia

Pneumococcal Vaccine, Polyvalent (Pneumovax-23) **Uses:** *Immunization against pneumococcal Infxns in pts at high risk (eg, all = 65 y of age)* **Action:** Active immunization **Dose:** 0.5 mL IM. **Caution:** [C, ?] **Contra:** *Do not* vaccinate during immunosuppressive therapy **Disp:** Inj 0.5 mL **SE:** Fever, inj site Rxn, hemolytic anemia, thrombocytopenia, anaphylaxis

Podophyllin (Podocon-25, Condylox Gel 0.5%, Condylox) **Uses:** *Topical therapy of benign growths (genital & perianal warts [condylomata acuminata],* papillomas, fibromas) **Action:** Direct antimitotic effect; exact mechanism unknown **Dose:** *Condylox gel & Condylox:* Apply 3 consecutive d/wk for 4 wk. *odocon-25:* Use sparingly on the lesion, leave on for 1–4 h, thoroughly wash off **Caution:** [C, ?] Immunosuppression **Contra:** DM, bleeding lesions **Disp:**

Podocon-25 (w/ benzoin) 15-mL bottles; Condylox gel 0.5% 35 g clear gel; Condylox soln 0.5% 35 g clear **SE:** Local reactions, significant absorption; anemias, tachycardia, paresthesias, GI upset, renal/hepatic damage **Notes:** Podocon-25 applied only by the clinician; do not dispense directly to patient

Polyethylene Glycol [PEG]–Electrolyte Solution (GoLYTELY, CoLyte) Uses: *Bowel prep prior to examination or surgery* Action: Osmotic cathartic **Dose:** *Adults.* Following 3–4-h fast, drink 240 mL of soln q10min until 4 L consumed. *Peds.* 25–40 mL/kg/h for 4–10 h **Caution:** [C, ?] **Contra:** GI obstruction, bowel perforation, megacolon, ulcerative colitis **Disp:** Powder for reconstitution to 4 L **SE:** Cramping or nausea, bloating **Notes:** 1st BM should occur in approximately 1 h

Polyethylene Glycol [PEG] 3350 (MiraLax) Uses: *Occasional constipation* **Action:** Osmotic laxative **Dose:** 17 g powder (1 heaping Tbsp) in 8 oz (1 cup) of H_2O & drink; max 14 d **Caution:** [C, ?] R/O bowel obstruction before use **Contra:** GI obstruction, allergy to PEG **Disp:** Powder for reconstitution; bottle cap holds 17 g **SE:** Upset stomach, bloating, cramping, gas, severe D, hives **Notes:** Can add to H_2O, juice, soda, coffee, or tea

Polymyxin B & Hydrocortisone (Otobiotic Otic) Uses: *Superficial bacterial Infxns of external ear canal* **Action:** Antibiotic/anti-inflammatory combo **Dose:** 4 gtt in ear(s) tid–qid **Caution:** [B, ?] **Disp:** Soln polymyxin B 10,000 units/hydrocortisone 0.5%/mL **SE:** Local irritation **Notes:** Useful in neomycin allergy

Potassium Citrate (Urocit-K) Uses: *Alkalinize urine, prevention of urinary stones (uric acid, calcium stones if hypocitraturic)* **Action:** Urinary alkalinizer **Dose:** 10–20 mEq PO tid w/ meals, max 100 mEq/d **Caution:** [A, +] **Contra:** Severe renal impair, dehydration, ↑ K^+, peptic ulcer; use of K^+-sparing diuretics or salt substitutes **Disp:** 540-, 1080-mg tabs **SE:** GI upset, ↓ Ca^{2+}, ↑ K^+, metabolic alkalosis **Notes:** Tabs 540 mg = 5 mEq, 1080 mg = 10 mEq

Potassium Citrate & Citric Acid (Polycitra-K) Uses: *Alkalinize urine, prevent urinary stones (uric acid, Ca stones if hypocitraturic)* **Action:** Urinary alkalinizer **Dose:** 10–20 mEq PO tid w/ meals, max 100 mEq/d **Caution:** [A, +] **Contra:** Severe renal impair, dehydration, ↑ K^+, peptic ulcer; use of K^+-sparing diuretics or salt substitutes **Disp:** Soln 10 mEq/5 mL; powder 30 mEq/packet **SE:** GI upset, ↓ Ca^{2+}, ↑ K^+, metabolic alkalosis

Potassium Iodide [Lugol Solution] (SSKI, Thyro-Block) Uses: *Thyroid storm,* ↓ *vascularity before thyroid surgery, block thyroid uptake of radioactive iodine, thin bronchial secretions* **Action:** Iodine supl **Dose:** *Adults & Peds >2 y.* Preop thyroidectomy: 50–250 mg PO tid (2–6 gtt strong iodine soln); give 10 d preop. *Peds 1 y.* Thyroid crisis: 300 mg (6 gtt SSKI q8h). *Peds <1 y:* ½ adult dose **Caution:** [D, +] ↑ K^+, TB, PE, bronchitis, renal impair **Contra:** Iodine sensitivity **Disp:** Tabs 130 mg; soln (SSKI) 1 g/mL; Lugol soln, strong iodine 100 mg/mL; syrup 325 mg/5 mL **SE:** Fever, HA, urticaria, angioedema, goiter, GI upset, eosinophilia

Potassium Supplements (Kaon, Kaochlor, K-Lor, Slow-K, Micro-K, Klorvess, others) Uses: *Prevention or Rx of ↓ K⁺* (eg, diuretic use) Action: K⁺ supl Dose: *Adults.* 20–100 mEq/d PO ÷ qd–bid; IV 10–20 mEq/h, max 40 mEq/h & 150 mEq/d (monitor K⁺ levels frequently w/ high-dose IV). *Peds.* Calculate K⁺ deficit; 1–3 mEq/kg/d PO ÷ qd–qid; IV max dose 0.5–1 mEq/kg/h Caution: [A, +] Renal insuff, use w/ NSAIDs & ACE inhibitors Contra: ↑ K⁺ Disp: PO forms (Table 8, page 225); injectable forms SE: Can cause GI irritation; bradycardia, ↑ K⁺, heart block Notes: Mix powder & liq w/ beverage (unsalted tomato juice, etc); follow K⁺; Cl– salt OK w/ alkalosis; w/ acidosis use acetate, bicarbonate, citrate, or gluconate salt

Pramipexole (Mirapex) Uses: *Parkinson Dz* Action: Dopamine agonist Dose: 1.5–4.5 mg/d PO, initial 0.375 mg/d in 3 ÷ doses; titrate slowly Caution: [C, ?/–] Contra: Component allergy Disp: Tabs 0.125, 0.25, 0.5, 1, 1.5 mg SE: Postural ↓ BP, asthenia, somnolence, abnormal dreams, GI upset, EPS

Pramoxine (Anusol Ointment, ProctoFoam-NS, others) Uses: *Relief of pain & itching from hemorrhoids, anorectal surgery*; topical for burns & dermatosis Action: Topical anesthetic Dose: Apply freely to anal area q3h Caution: [C, ?] Disp: [OTC] All 1%; foam (Proctofoam-NS), cream, oint, lotion, gel, pads, spray SE: Contact dermatitis, mucosal thinning w/ chronic use

Pramoxine + Hydrocortisone (Enzone, Proctofoam-HC) Uses: *Relief of pain & itching from hemorrhoids* Action: Topical anesthetic, anti-inflammatory Dose: Apply freely to anal area tid–qid Caution: [C, ?/–] Disp: Cream pramoxine 1% acetate 0.5/1%; foam pramoxine 1% hydrocortisone 1%; lotion pramoxine 1% hydrocortisone 0.25/1/2.5%, pramoxine 2.5% & hydrocortisone 1% SE: Contact dermatitis, mucosal thinning with chronic use

Pravastatin (Pravachol) Uses: *↓ Cholesterol* Action: HMG-CoA reductase inhibitor Dose: 10–80 mg PO hs; ↓ in significant renal/hepatic impair Caution: [X -] w/ gemfibrozil Contra: Liver Dz or persistent LFT ↑ Disp: Tabs 10, 20, 40, 80 mg SE: Use caution w/ concurrent gemfibrozil; HA, GI upset, hepatitis, myopathy, renal failure

Prazosin (Minipress) Uses: *HTN* Action: Peripherally acting α-adrenergic blocker Dose: *Adults.* 1 mg PO tid; can ↑ to 20 mg/d max PRN. *Peds.* 5–25 mcg/kg/dose q6h, to 25 mcg/kg/dose max Caution: [C, ?] Contra: Component allergy Disp: Caps 1, 2, 5 mg; Tabs ER 2.5, 5 mg extended release SE: Dizziness, edema, palpitations, fatigue, GI upset Notes: Can cause orthostatic ↓ BP, take the 1st dose hs; tolerance develops to this effect; tachyphylaxis may result

Prednisolone [See Steroids page 175 and Table 4, page 216],

Prednisone [See Steroids page 175 and Table 4, page 216]

Pregabalin (Lyrica) Uses: *DM peripheral neuropathy pain; postherpetic neuralgia; adjunct Rx adult partial onset seizures* Action: Nerve transmission modulator, antinociceptive and antiseizure effect; mechanism ? Dose: *Neuropathic*

pain: 50 mg PO tid, ↑ to 300 mg/d w/in 1 wk based on response (300 mg/d max) *Postherpetic neuralgia:* 75–150 mg bid, or 50–100 mg tid; start 75 mg bid or 50 mg tid; ↑ to 300 mg/d w/in 1 wk based on response; if pain persists after 2–4 wk, ↑ to 600 mg/d; *Epilepsy:* Start 150 mg/d (75 mg bid or 50 mg tid) may ↑ to max 600 mg/d; ↓ w/ renal insuffic; w/ or w/o food **Caution:** [X, –] w/ significant renal impair, see insert, w/ elderly, severe CHF, avoid abrupt D/C **Contra:** PRG **Disp:** Caps 25, 50, 75, 100, 150, 200, 225, 300 mg **SE:** Dizziness, drowsiness, xerostomia, peripheral edema, blurred vision, weight gain, difficulty concentrating **Notes:** Related to gabapentin; w/ D/C, taper over at least 1 wk

Probenecid (Benemid, others) Uses: *Prevent gout & hyperuricemia; prolongs levels of PCNs & cephalosporins* **Action:** Uricosuric, Renal tubular blocking for organic anions **Dose:** *Adults.* Gout: 250 mg bid × 1 × 1 wk, then 0.5 g PO bid; can ↑ by 500 mg/mo up to 2–3 g/d. *Antibiotic effect:* 1–2 g PO 30 min before dose. *Peds >2 y.* 25 mg/kg, then 40 mg/kg/d PO ÷ qid **Caution:** [B, ?] **Contra:** High-dose ASA, moderate–severe renal impair, age <2 y **Disp:** Tabs 500 mg **SE:** IIA, GI upset, rash, pruritus, dizziness, blood dyscrasias **Notes:** Do not use during acute gout attack

Procainamide (Pronestyl, Procan) Uses: *Supraventricular/ventricular arrhythmias* **Action:** Class 1A antiarrhythmic **Dose:** *Adults.* Recurrent VF/VT: 20 mg/min IV (total 17 mg/kg max). *Maint:* 1–4 mg/min. *Stable wide-complex tachycardia of unknown origin, AF w/ rapid rate in WPW:* 20 mg/min IV until arrhythmia suppression, ↓ BP, or QRS widens >50%, then 1–4 mg/min. *Chronic dosing:* 50 mg/kg/d PO in ÷ doses q4–6h. *Peds.* Chronic maint: 15–50 mg/kg/24 h PO ÷ q3–6h, ↓ in renal/hepatic impair **Caution:** [C, +] **Contra:** Complete heart block, 2nd- or 3rd-degree heart block w/o pacemaker, torsades de pointes, SLE **Disp:** Tabs & caps 250, 375, 500 mg; SR tabs 250, 500, 750, 1000 mg; inj 100, 500 mg/mL **SE:** ↓ BP, lupus-like syndrome, GI upset, taste perversion, arrhythmias, tachycardia, heart block, angioneurotic edema **Notes:** Follow levels (Table 2, page 210)

Procarbazine (Matulane) WARNING: Highly toxic; handle w/ care Uses: *Hodgkin Dz,* NHL, brain & lung tumors **Action:** Alkylating agent; ↓ DNA & RNA synthesis **Dose:** Per protocol **Caution:** [D, ?] W/ EtOH ingestion **Contra:** Inadequate BM reserve **Disp:** Caps 50 mg **SE:** Myelosuppression, hemolytic reactions (w/ G6PD deficiency), N/V/D; disulfiram-like Rxn; cutaneous & constitutional Sxs, myalgia, arthralgia, CNS effects, azoospermia, cessation of menses

Prochlorperazine (Compazine) Uses: *N/V, agitation, & psychotic disorders* **Action:** Phenothiazine; blocks postsynaptic dopaminergic CNS receptors **Dose:** *Adults.* Antiemetic: 5–10 mg PO tid–qid or 25 mg PR bid or 5–10 mg deep IM q4–6h. *Antipsychotic:* 10–20 mg IM acutely or 5–10 mg PO tid–qid for maint; ↑ doses may be required for antipsychotic effect. *Peds.* 0.1–0.15 mg/kg/dose IM q4–6h or 0.4 mg/kg/24 h PO ÷ tid–qid **Caution:** [C, +/–] NA glaucoma, severe liver/cardiac Dz **Contra:** Phenothiazine sensitivity; BM suppression **Disp:** Tabs 5, 10, 25 mg; SR caps 10, 15 mg; syrup 5 mg/5 mL; supp 2.5, 5, 25 mg; inj 5 mg/mL **SE:** EPS common; Rx w/ diphenhydramine

Promethazine (Phenergan) Uses: *N/V, motion sickness* **Action:** Phenothiazine; blocks CNS postsynaptic mesolimbic dopaminergic receptors **Dose:** *Adults.* 12.5–50 mg PO, PR, or IM bid–qid PRN. *Peds.* 0.1–0.5 mg/kg/dose PO or IM q2–6h PRN **Caution:** [C, +/–] use w/ agents w/ respiratory depressant effects **Contra:** Component allergy, NA glaucoma, age <2 yrs **Disp:** Tabs 12.5, 25, 50 mg; syrup 6.25 mg/5 mL, 25 mg/5 mL; supp 12.5, 25, 50 mg; inj 25, 50 mg/mL **SE:** Drowsiness, tardive dyskinesia, EPS, lowered Sz threshold, ↓ BP, GI upset, blood dyscrasias, photosensitivity, respiratory depression in children

Propafenone (Rythmol) Uses: *Life-threatening ventricular arrhythmias, AF* **Action:** Class IC antiarrhythmic (Table 12); **Dose:** *Adults.* 150–300 mg PO q8h. *Peds.* 8–10 mg/kg/d ÷ in 3–4 doses; may ↑ 2 mg/kg/d, to max of 20 mg/kg/d max **Caution:** [C, ?] w/ amprenavir, ritonavir **Contra:** Uncontrolled CHF, bronchospasm, cardiogenic shock, conduction disorders **Disp:** Tabs 150, 225, 300 mg, extended release caps 225, 325, 425 mg **SE:** Dizziness, unusual taste, 1st-degree heart block, arrhythmias, prolongs QRS & QT intervals; fatigue, GI upset, blood dyscrasias

Propantheline (Pro-Banthine) Uses: *PUD,* symptomatic Rx of small intestine hypermotility, spastic colon, ureteral spasm, bladder spasm, pylorospasm **Action:** Antimuscarinic **Dose:** *Adults.* 15 mg PO ac & 30 mg PO hs; ↓ in elderly. *Peds.* 2–3 mg/kg/24h PO ÷ tid–qid **Caution:** [C, ?] **Contra:** NA glaucoma, ulcerative colitis, toxic megacolon, GI/GU obstruction **Disp:** Tabs 7.5, 15 mg **SE:** Anticholinergic (eg, xerostomia, blurred vision)

Propofol (Diprivan) Uses: *Induction & maint of anesthesia; sedation in intubated pts* **Action:** Sedative–hypnotic; mechanism unknown **Dose:** *Adults.* Anesthesia: 2–2.5 mg/kg induction, then 0.1–0.2 mg/kg/min inf ICU sedation: 5 mcg/kg/min IV × 5 min, ↑ PRN 5–10 mcg/kg/min q5–10min 5–50 mcg/kg/min cont inf; ↓ in elderly, debilitated, ASA II/IV pts *Peds.* Anesthesia: 2.5–3.5 mg/kg induction; then 125–300 mcg/kg/min ↓ in elderly, debilitated, ASA II/IV pts **Caution:** [B, +] **Contra:** If general anesthesia contraindicated **Disp:** Inj 10 mg/mL **SE:** May ↑ triglycerides w/ extended dosing; ↓ BP, pain at site, apnea, anaphylaxis **Notes:** 1 mL of propofol has 0.1 g fat

Propoxyphene (Darvon); Propoxyphene & Acetaminophen (Darvocet); & Propoxyphene & Aspirin (Darvon Compound-65, Darvon-N + Aspirin) [C-IV] Uses: *Mild–moderate pain* **Action:** Narcotic analgesic **Dose:** 1–2 PO q4h PRN; ↓ in hepatic impair, elderly **Caution:** [C (D if prolonged use), M] Hepatic impair (APAP), peptic ulcer (ASA); severe renal impair **Contra:** Allergy **Disp:** *Darvon:* Propoxyphene HCl caps 65 mg. *Darvon-N:* Propoxyphene napsylate 100-mg tabs. *Darvocet-N:*

Propoxyphene napsylate 50 mg/APAP 325 mg. *Darvocet-N 100:* Propoxyphene napsylate 100 mg/APAP 650 mg. *Darvon Compound-65:* Propoxyphene HCl caps 65-mg/ASA 389 mg/caffeine 32 mg. *Darvon-N w/ ASA:* Propoxyphene napsylate 100 mg/ASA 325 mg **SE:** OD can be lethal; ↓ BP, dizziness, sedation, GI upset, ↑ levels on LFTs

Propranolol (Inderal)
Uses: *HTN, angina, MI, hyperthyroidism, essential tremor, hypertrophic subaortic stenosis, pheochromocytoma; prevents migraines & atrial arrhythmias* **Action:** β-adrenergic receptor blocker, $β_1$, $β_2$; only β-blocker to block conversion of T_4 to T_3 **Dose:** *Adults.* Angina: 80–320 mg/d PO ÷ bid–qid or 80–160 mg/d SR. *Arrhythmia:* 10–80 mg PO tid–qid or 1 mg IV slowly, repeat q5min, 5 mg max. *HTN.* 40 mg PO bid or 60–80 mg/d SR, ↑ weekly to max 640 mg/d. *Hypertrophic subaortic stenosis:* 20–40 mg PO tid–qid. *MI:* 180–240 mg PO ÷ tid–qid. *Migraine prophylaxis:* 80 mg/d ÷ qid–tid, ↑ weekly 160–240 mg/d ÷ tid–qid max; wean if no response in 6 wk. *Pheochromocytoma:* 30–60 mg/d ÷ tid–qid. *Thyrotoxicosis:* 1–3 mg IV × 1; 10–40 mg PO q6h. *Tremor:* 40 mg PO bid, ↑ PRN 320 mg/d max. **Peds.** Arrhythmia: 0.5–1.0 mg/kg/d ÷ tid–qid, ↑ PRN q3–7d to 60 mg/d max; 0.01–0.1 mg/kg IV over 10 min, 1 mg max. *HTN:* 0.5–1.0 mg/kg ÷ bid–qid, ↑ PRN q3–7d to 2 mg/kg/d max; ↓ in renal impair **Caution:** [C (1st tri, D if 2nd or 3rd tri), +] **Contra:** Uncompensated CHF, cardiogenic shock, bradycardia, heart block, PE, severe resp Dz **Disp:** Tabs 10, 20, 40, 60, 80 mg; SR caps 60, 80, 120, 160 mg; oral soln 4, 8, 80 mg/mL; inj 1 mg/mL **SE:** Bradycardia, ↓ BP, fatigue, GI upset

Propylthiouracil [PTU]
Uses: *Hyperthyroidism* **Action:** ↓ Production of T_3 & T_4 & conversion of T_4 to T_3 **Dose:** *Adults.* Initial: 100 mg PO q8h (may need up to 1200 mg/d); after pt euthyroid (6–8 wk), taper dose by ⅓ q4–6wk to maint, 50–150 mg/2–3 h; can usually D/C in 2–3 y; ↓ in elderly *Peds.* Initial: 5–7 mg/kg/24 h PO ÷ q8h. *Main:* ⅓–⅔ of initial dose **Caution:** [D, −] **Contra:** Allergy **Disp:** Tabs 50 mg **SE:** Fever, rash, leukopenia, dizziness, GI upset, taste perversion, SLE-like syndrome **Notes:** Monitor pt clinically, check TFT

Protamine (generic)
Uses: *Reverse heparin effect* **Action:** Neutralize heparin by forming a stable complex **Dose:** Based on degree of heparin reversal; give IV slowly; 1 mg reverses approx. 100 units of heparin given in the preceding 3–4 h, 50 mg max **Caution:** [C, ?] **Contra:** Allergy **Disp:** Inj 10 mg/mL **SE:** Follow coags; anticoag effect if given w/o heparin; ↓ BP, bradycardia, dyspnea, hemorrhage

Pseudoephedrine (Sudafed, Novafed, Afrinol, others) [OTC]
Uses: *Decongestant* **Action:** Stimulates α-adrenergic receptors w/ vasoconstriction **Dose:** *Adults.* 30–60 mg PO q6–8h. *Peds.* 4 mg/kg/24 h PO ÷ qid; ↓ in renal insuff **Caution:** [C, +] **Contra:** Poorly controlled HTN or CAD, w/MAOIs **Disp:** Tabs 30, 60 mg; caps 60 mg; SR tabs 120, 240 mg; liq 7.5 mg/0.8 mL, 15, 30 mg/5 mL **SE:** HTN, insomnia, tachycardia, arrhythmias, nervousness, tremor **Notes:** Found in many OTC cough/cold preparations; OTC restricted distribution

Psyllium (Metamucil, Serutan, Effer-Syllium) Uses: *Constipation & colonic diverticular Dz * Action: Bulk laxative Dose: 1 tsp (7 g) in glass of H$_2$O PO qd–tid Caution: [B, ?] Effer-Syllium (effervescent Psyllium) usually contains K$^+$ caution w/ renal failure; phenylketonuria (in products w/ aspartame) Contra: Suspected bowel obstruction Disp: Granules 4, 25 g/tsp; powder 3.5 g/packet, Caps 0.52g (3 g/6 caps), wafers 3.4 g/dose SE: D, abdominal cramps, bowel obstruction, constipation, bronchospasm

Pyrazinamide (generic) Uses: *Active TB in combo w/ other agents* Action: Bacteriostatic; unknown mechanism Dose: Adults. 15–30 mg/kg/24 h PO ÷ tid–qid; max 2 g/d. Peds. 15–30 mg/kg/d PO ÷ qd–bid; ↓ w/ renal/hepatic impair Caution: [C, +/–] Contra: Severe hepatic damage, acute gout Disp: Tabs 500 mg SE: Hepatotox, malaise, GI upset, arthralgia, myalgia, gout, photosensitivity Notes: Use in combo w/ other anti-TB drugs; consult MMWR for latest TB recommendations; dosage regimen differs for "directly observed" therapy

Pyridoxine [Vitamin B$_6$] Uses: *Rx & prevention of vitamin B$_6$ deficiency* Action: Vitamin B$_6$ supl Dose: Adults. Deficiency: 10–20 mg/d PO. Drug-induced neuritis: 100–200 mg/d; 25–100 mg/d prophylaxis. Peds. 5–25 mg/d × 3 wk Caution: [A (C if doses exceed RDA), +] Contra: Component allergy Disp: Tabs 25, 50, 100 mg; inj 100 mg/mL SE: Allergic Rxns, HA, N

Quazepam (Doral) [C-IV] Uses: *Insomnia* Action: Benzodiazepine Dose: 7.5–15 mg PO hs PRN; ↓ in elderly & hepatic failure Caution: [X, ?/–] NA glaucoma Contra: PRG, sleep apnea Disp: Tabs 7.5, 15 mg SE: Sedation, hangover, somnolence, resp depression Notes: Do not D/C abruptly

Quetiapine (Seroquel) WARNING: ↑mortality in elderly with dementia-related psychosis Uses: *Acute exacerbations of schizophrenia* Action: Serotonin & dopamine antagonism Dose: 150–750 mg/d; initiate at 25–100 mg bid–tid; slowly ↑ dose; ↓ dose for hepatic & geriatric pts Caution: [C, –] Contra: Component allergy Disp: Tabs 25, 50, 100, 200, 300, 400 mg SE: Reports of confusion w/ nefazodone; HA, somnolence, weight gain, orthostatic ↓ BP, dizziness, cataracts, neuroleptic malignant syndrome, tardive dyskinesia, QT prolongation

Quinapril (Accupril) WARNING: ACE inhibitors used during the 2nd & 3rd tri of PRG can cause fetal injury & death Uses: *HTN, CHF, DN, post-MI* Action: ACE inhibitor Dose: 10–80 mg PO qd; ↓ in renal impair Caution: [D, +] Contra: ACE inhibitor sensitivity or angioedema Disp: Tabs 5, 10, 20, 40 mg SE: Dizziness, HA, ↓ BP, impaired renal Fxn, angioedema, taste perversion, cough

Quinidine (Quinidex, Quinaglute) Uses: *Prevention of tachydysrhythmias, malaria* Action: Class 1A antiarrhythmic Dose: Adults. AF/flutter conversion: After digitalization, 200 mg q2–3h × 8 doses; ↑ qd to 3–4 g max or nl rhythm. Peds. 15–60 mg/kg/24 h PO in 4–5 ÷ doses; ↓ in renal impair Caution: [C, +] w/ ritonavir Contra: Digitalis tox & AV block; conduction disorders Disp: Sulfate: Tabs 200, 300 mg; SR tabs 300 mg. Gluconate: SR tabs 324 mg; inj 80 mg/mL SE: Extreme ↓ BP w/ IV use; syncope, QT prolongation, GI upset, arrhythmias, fatigue, cinchonism (tinnitus, hearing loss, delirium, visual changes), fever, hemolytic anemia, thrombocytopenia, rash **Notes:** Check levels (Table 2); sulfate salt 83% quinidine; gluconate salt 62% quinidine; use w/ drug that slows AV conduction (eg, digoxin, diltiazem, β-blocker)

Quinupristin–Dalfopristin (Synercid) **Uses:** *Vancomycin-resistant Infxns due to E. faecium & other gram(+)* **Action:** ↓ ribosomal protein synthesis. *Spectrum:* Vancomycin-resistant *Enterococcus faecium*, methicillin-susceptible *Staphylococcus aureus*, *Streptococcus pyogenes;* not active against *Enterococcus faecalis* **Dose: Adults & Peds.** 7.5 mg/kg IV q8–12h (use central line if possible); incompatible w/ NS or heparin, flush IV w/ dextrose; ↓ in hepatic failure **Caution:** [B, M] Multiple drug interactions (eg, cyclosporine) **Contra:** Component allergy **Disp:** Inj 500 mg (150 mg quinupristin/350 mg dalfopristin) **SE:** Hyperbilirubinemia, inf site Rxns & pain, arthralgia, myalgia

Rabeprazole (AcipHex) **Uses:** *PUD, GERD, ZE* *H. pylori* **Action:** Proton-pump inhibitor **Dose:** 20 mg/d; may ↑ to 60 mg/d; *H. pylori* 20 mg PO bid × 7 days (w/amoxicillin and clarithromycin) do not crush tabs **Caution:** [B, ?/–] **Disp:** Tabs 20 mg delayed release **SE:** HA, fatigue, GI upset **Notes:** Do not crush/chew tabs

Raloxifene (Evista) **Uses:** *Prevent osteoporosis* **Action:** Partial antagonist of estrogen, behaves like estrogen **Dose:** 60 mg/d **Caution:** [X, –] **Contra:** Thromboembolism, PRG **Disp:** Tabs 60 mg **SE:** Chest pain, insomnia, rash, hot flashes, GI upset, hepatic dysfunction

Ramipril (Altace) **WARNING:** ACE inhibitors used during the 2nd & 3rd tri of PRG can cause fetal injury & death **Uses:** *HTN, CHF, DN, post-MI* **Action:** ACE inhibitor **Dose:** 2.5–20 mg/d PO ÷ qd–bid; ↓ in renal impair **Caution:** [D, +] **Contra:** ACE-inhibitor-induced angioedema **Disp:** Caps 1.25, 2.5, 5, 10 mg **SE:** Cough, HA, dizziness, ↓ BP, renal impair, angioedema **Notes:** OK in combo w/ diuretics

Ranitidine Hydrochloride (Zantac) **Uses:** *Duodenal ulcer, active benign ulcers, hypersecretory conditions, & GERD* **Action:** H$_2$-receptor antagonist **Dose: Adults.** Ulcer: 150 mg PO bid, 300 mg PO hs, or 50 mg IV q6–8h; or 400 mg IV/d cont inf, then maint of 150 mg PO hs. *Hypersecretion:* 150 mg PO bid, up to 600 mg/d. *GERD:* 300 mg PO bid; maint 300 mg PO hs. *Dyspepsia:* 75 mg PO qd–bid *Peds.* 0.75–1.5 mg/kg/dose IV q6–8h or 1.25–2.5 mg/kg/dose PO q12h; ↓ in renal insuff/failure **Caution:** [B, +] **Contra:** Component allergy **Disp:** Tabs 75 [OTC], 150, 300 mg; Caps 150, 300 mg; Effervescent tabs 150 mg; syrup 15 mg/mL; inj 25 mg/mL **SE:** Dizziness, sedation, rash, GI upset **Notes:** PO & parenteral doses differ

Ranolazine (Ranexa) **Uses:** *Chronic angina* **Action:** ↓ ischemia-related Na+ entry into myocardium **Dose: Adults.** 500 mg PO bid, to 1000 mg PO bid **Contra:** CYP3A inhibitors (Table 13); w/ agents that ↑ QT interval **Caution:** [C, ?/–] QT interval prolongation; hepatic impairment; HTN may develop w/renal impairment **Disp:** SR tabs 500 mg **SE:** Dizziness, HA, constipation, arrhythmias **Notes:** Must use w/amlodipine, nitrates, beta blockers

Rasagiline mesylate (Azilect) **Uses:** *Early Parkinson disease as monotherapy; levodopa adjunct in advanced dz* **Action:** MAO B inhibitor **Dose:** *Adults.* Early dz: 1 mg PO daily, start 0.5 mg PO daily w/levodopa; ↓ CYP1A2 inhibitors or hepatic impair **Contra:** MAOIs, sympathomimetic amines, meperidine, methadone, tramadol, propoxyphene, dextromethorphan, mirtazapine, cyclobenzaprine, St. John's wort, sympathomimetic vasoconstrictors, general anesthetics, SSRIs **Caution:** [C, ?] Avoid tyramine-containing foods; moderate/severe hepatic impairment **Disp:** Tabs 0.5, 1 mg **SE:** Arthralgia, indigestion, dyskinesia, hallucinations, ↓ weight, postural ↓ BP, N, V, constipation, xerostomia, rash, sedation, CV conduction disturbances **Notes:** Rare melanoma reported; do periodic dermatologic exams; d/c 14 days prior to elective surgery; initial ↓ levodopa dose recommended

Rasburicase (Elitek) **Uses:** *Reduce ↑ uric acid due to tumor lysis (peds)* **Action:** Catalyzes uric acid **Dose:** *Peds.* 0.15 or 0.20 mg/kg IV over 30 min, qd × 5 **Caution:** [C, ?/–] Falsely ↓ uric acid values **Contra:** Anaphylaxis, screen for G6PD deficiency to avoid hemolysis, methemoglobinemia **Disp:** 1.5 mg inj **SE:** Fever, neutropenia, GI upset, HA, rash

Repaglinide (Prandin) **Uses:** *Type 2 DM* **Action:** ↑ pancreatic insulin release **Dose:** 0.5–4 mg ac, PO start 1–2 mg, ↑ to 16 mg/d max; take pc **Caution:** [C, ?/–] **Contra:** DKA, type 1 DM **Disp:** Tabs 0.5, 1, 2 mg **SE:** HA, hyper-/hypoglycemia, GI upset

Reteplase (Retavase) **Uses:** *Post-AMI* **Action:** Thrombolytic agent **Dose:** 10 Units IV over 2 min, 2nd dose in 30 min, 10 units IV over 2 min **Caution:** [C, ?/–] **Contra:** Internal bleeding, spinal surgery/trauma, Hx CNS vascular malformations, uncontrolled ↓ BP, sensitivity to thrombolytics **Disp:** Inj 10.8 units/2 mL **SE:** Bleeding, allergic reactions

Ribavirin (Virazole, Copegus) **Uses:** *RSV Infxn in infants; hepatitis C (in combo w/ interferon alfa-2b Copegus)* **Action:** Unknown **Dose:** *RSV:* 6 g in 300 mL sterile H_2O, inhale over 12–18 h. *Hep C:* 600 mg PO bid in combo w/ interferon alfa-2b (see Rebetron, page 113) **Caution:** [X, ?] May accumulate on soft contact lenses **Contra:** PRG, autoimmune hepatitis, CrCl <50 mL/min **Disp:** Powder for aerosol 6 g; tabs 200, 400, 600 mg, caps 200 mg, solution 40 mg/mL, Tabs 200, 400, 600 mg **SE:** Fatigue, HA, GI upset, anemia, myalgia, alopecia, bronchospasm **Notes:** Aerosolized by a SPAG; monitor Hbg/Hct; PRG test monthly

Rifabutin (Mycobutin) **Uses:** *Prevent M. avium complex Infxn in AIDS pts w/ CD4 count <100** **Action:** ↓ DNA-dependent RNA polymerase activity **Dose:** *Adults.* 150–300 mg/d PO. *Peds.* 1 y: 15–25 mg/kg/d PO. *2–10 y:* 4.4–18.8 mg/kg/d PO. *14–16 y:* 2.8–5.4 mg/kg/d PO **Caution:** [B; ?/–] WBC <1000/mm³ or platelets <50,000/mm³; ritonavir **Contra:** Allergy **Disp:** Caps 150 mg **SE:** Discolored urine, rash, neutropenia, leukopenia, myalgia, ↑ LFTs **Notes:** SEs/interactions similar to rifampin

Rifampin (Rifadin) **Uses:** *TB & Rx & prophylaxis of *N. meningitidis, H. influenzae*, or *S. aureus* carriers*; adjunct for severe *S. aureus* **Action:** ↓ DNA-dependent RNA polymerase **Dose:** *Adults.* N. meningitidis & H. influenzae carrier: 600 mg/d PO for 4 d. *TB:* 600 mg PO or IV qd or 2 ×/wk w/ combo regimen. *Peds.* 10–20 mg/kg/dose PO or IV qd–bid; ↓ in hepatic failure **Caution:** [C, +] Amprenavir, multiple drug interactions **Contra:** Allergy, presence of active *N. meningitidis* Infxn, w/saquinavir/ritonavir **Disp:** Caps 150, 300 mg; inj 600 mg **SE:** Orange-red discoloration of bodily fluids, ↑ LFTs, flushing, HA **Notes:** Never use as single agent w/ active TB

Rifapentine (Priftin) **Uses:** *Pulmonary TB* **Action:** ↓ DNA-dependent RNA polymerase. *Spectrum: M. tuberculosis* **Dose:** *Intensive phase:* 600 mg PO 2 ×/wk for 2 mo; separate doses by 3 or more days *Continuation phase:* 600 mg/wk for 4 mo; part of 3–4 drug regimen **Caution:** [C, red-orange breast milk] ↓ protease inhibitor efficacy, antiepileptics, β-blockers, CCBs **Contra:** Allergy to rifamycins **Disp:** 150-mg tabs **SE:** Neutropenia, hyperuricemia, HTN, HA, dizziness, rash, GI upset, blood dyscrasias, ↑ LFTs, hematuria, discolored secretions **Notes:** Monitor LFTs

Rifaximin (Xifaxan) **Uses:** *Travelers' diarrhea (noninvasive strains of *E. coli*) in patients >12 y* **Action:** Not absorbed, derivative of rifamycin. *Spectrum: E. coli* **Dose:** 1 tab PO qd × 3 d **Caution:** [C, ?/–] Allergy (rash, angioedema, urticaria); pseudomembranous colitis **Contra:** Allergy to rifamycins **Disp:** Tabs 200 mg **SE:** Flatulence, HA, abdominal pain, GI distress, fever **Notes:** D/C if Sx worsen or persist >24–48 h, or w/ fever or blood in stool

Rimantadine (Flumadine) **Uses:** * Prophylaxis & Rx of influenza A viral Infxns* **Action:** Antiviral **Dose:** *Adults & Peds >9 y.* 100 mg PO bid. *Peds 1–9 y.* 5 mg/kg/d PO, 150 mg/d max; qd w/ severe renal/hepatic impair & elderly; initiate w/in 48 h of Sx onset **Caution:** [C, –] w/ cimetidine; avoid in PRG or breast-feeding **Contra:** Component & amantadine allergy **Disp:** Tabs 100 mg; syrup 50 mg/5 mL **SE:** Orthostatic ↓ BP, edema, dizziness, GI upset, ↓ Sz threshold

Rimexolone (Vexol Ophthalmic) **Uses:** *Postop inflammation & uveitis* **Action:** Steroid **Dose:** *Adults & Peds >2 y.* Uveitis: 1–2 gtt/h daytime & q2h at night, taper to 1 gtt q4h. *Postop.* 1–2 gtt qid ≤2 wk **Caution:** [C, ?/–] Ocular Infxns **Disp:** Susp 1% **SE:** Blurred vision, local irritation **Notes:** Taper dose

Risedronate (Actonel) **Uses:** *Paget Dz; treat/prevent glucocorticoid-induced/postmenopausal osteoporosis* **Action:** Bisphosphonate; ↓ osteoclast-mediated bone resorption **Dose:** *Paget Dz:* 30 mg/d PO for 2 mo. *Osteoporosis Rx/prevention:* 5 mg qd or 35 mg qwk; 30 min before 1st food/drink of the day; stay upright for at least 30 min after **Caution:** [C, ?/–] Ca supls & antacids ↓ absorption **Contra:** Component allergy, ↓ Ca²⁺, esophageal abnormalities, unable to stand/sit for 30 min, CrCl < 30 mL/min **Disp:** Tabs 5, 30, 35 mg **SE:** HA, D, abdominal pain, arthralgia; flu-like Sxs, rash, esophagitis, bone pain **Notes:** Monitor LFT, Ca^{2+}, PO_3^{+}, K^+

Risperidone (Risperdal) **WARNING:** ↑ mortality in elderly with dementia-related psychosis **Uses:** *Psychotic disorders (schizophrenia),* dementia of the elderly, bipolar disorder, mania, Tourette disorder, autism **Action:** Benzisoxazole antipsychotic **Dose:** *Adults.* 0.5–6 mg PO bid. *Peds/Adolescents.* 0.25 mg PO bid, ↑ q5–7d; ↓ start dose w/ elderly, renal/hepatic impair **Caution:** [C, –], ↑ BP w/ antihypertensives, clozapine **Contra:** Component allergy **Disp:** Tabs 0.25, 0.5, 1, 2, 3, 4, 5 mg; soln 1 mg/mL, orally disintegrating tabs 0.5, 1, 2, 3, 4 mg **SE:** Orthostatic ↓ BP, EPS w/ high dose, tachycardia, arrhythmias, sedation, dystonias, neuroleptic malignant syndrome, sexual dysfunction, constipation, xerostomia, blood dyscrasias, cholestatic jaundice, weight gain **Notes:** Several weeks for effect

Ritonavir (Norvir) **Uses:** *HIV* **Actions:** Protease inhibitor; ↓ maturation of immature noninfectious virions to mature infectious virus **Dose:** *Adults.* Initial 300 mg PO bid, titrate over 1 wk to 600 mg PO bid (titration will ↓ GI SE). *Peds > 1 mo.* 250 mg/m^2 titrate to 400 mg bid (adjust w/ amprenavir, indinavir, nelfinavir, & saquinavir); (w/ food) **Caution:** [B, +] w/ ergotamine, amiodarone, bepridil, flecainide, propafenone, quinidine, pimozide, midazolam, triazolam **Contra:** W/ ergotamine, amiodarone, bepridil, flecainide, propafenone, quinidine, pimozide, midazolam, triazolam, St. John's wort **Disp:** Caps 100 mg; soln 80 mg/mL **SE:** ↑ triglycerides, ↑ LFTs, N/V/D/C, abdominal pain, taste perversion, anemia, weakness, HA, fever, malaise, rash, paresthesias **Notes:** Refrigerate

Rivastigmine (Exelon) **Uses:** *Mild–moderate dementia in Alzheimer Dz* **Action:** Enhances cholinergic activity **Dose:** 1.5 mg bid; ↑ to 6 mg bid, w/ ↑ at 2-wk intervals (w/ food) **Caution:** [B, ?] β-Blockers, CCBs, smoking, neuromuscular blockade, digoxin **Contra:** Allergy to rivastigmine or carbamates **Disp:** Caps 1.5, 3, 4.5, 6 mg; soln 2 mg/mL **SE:** Dose-related GI effects, N/V/D; dizziness, insomnia, fatigue, tremor, diaphoresis, HA **Notes:** Swallow capsules whole, do not break, chew, or crush; avoid EtOH

Rizatriptan (Maxalt, Maxalt MLT) (See Table 11, page 228)

Rocuronium (Zemuron) **Uses:** *Skeletal muscle relaxation during rapid-sequence intubation, surgery, or mechanical ventilation* **Action:** Nondepolarizing neuromuscular blocker **Dose:** *Rapid sequence intubation:* 0.6–1.2 mg/kg IV. *Continuous inf:* 4–16 mcg/kg/min IV; ↓ in hepatic impair **Caution:** [C, ?] Aminoglycosides, vancomycin, tetracycline, polymyxins enhance blockade **Contra:** Component or pancuronium allergy **Disp:** Inj preservative free 10 mg/mL 5-, 10-mL vials **SE:** BP changes, tachycardia

Ropinirole (Requip) **Uses:** *Rx of Parkinson Dz* **Action:** Dopamine agonist **Dose:** Initial 0.25 mg PO tid, weekly ↑ 0.25 mg/dose, to 3 mg max **Caution:** [C, ?/–] Severe CV, renal, or hepatic impair **Contra:** Component allergy **Disp:** Tabs 0.25, 0.5, 1, 2, 3, 4, 5 mg **SE:** Syncope, postural ↓ BP, N/V, HA, somnolence, hallucinations, dyskinesias **Notes:** D/C w/ 7-d taper

Rosiglitazone (Avandia) Uses: *Type 2 DM* Action: ↑ insulin sensitivity Dose: 4–8 mg/d PO or in 2 ÷ doses (w/o regard to meals) Caution: [C, –] Not for DKA; w/ ESRD (renal elimination) Contra: Active liver Dz Disp: Tabs 2, 4, 8 mg SE: Weight gain, hyperlipidemia, HA, edema, fluid retention, exacerbated CHF, hyper-/hypoglycemia, hepatic damage

Rosuvastatin (Crestor) Uses: *Rx primary hypercholesterolemia & mixed dyslipidemia* Action: HMG-CoA reductase inhibitor Dose: 5–40 mg PO qd; max 5 mg/d w/ cyclosporine, 10 mg/d w/ gemfibrozil or CrCl <30 mL/min (avoid Al-/Mg-based antacids for 2 h after) Caution: [X,?/–] Contra: Active liver Dz or un explained ↑ LFT Disp: Tabs 5, 10, 20, 40 mg SE: Myalgia, constipation, asthenia, abdominal pain, nausea, myopathy, rarely rhabdomyolysis Notes: May ↑ warfarin effect; monitor LFTs at baseline, 12 wk, then q6mo; ↓dose in Asian patients

Rotavirus vaccine, live, oral, pentavalent (RotaTeq) Uses: *Prevent rotavirus gastroenteritis* Action: Active immunization Dose: Peds. Single dose PO at 2, 4, and 6 mo Caution: [?,?]Disp: Oral susp 2-mL single-use tubes SE: D, V, otitis Notes: Begin series by 12 wks and conclude by 32 wks of age

Salmeterol (Serevent) Uses: *Asthma, exercise-induced asthma, COPD* Action: Sympathomimetic bronchodilator, β_2-agonist Dose: Adults & Peds ≥ 12 y. 1 diskus-dose inhaled bid Caution: [C, ?/–] Contra: Acute asthma; w/in 14 d of MAOI Disp: Dry powder discus, metered dose inhaler SE: HA, pharyngitis, tachycardia, arrhythmias, nervousness, GI upset, tremors Notes: Not for acute attacks; also prescribe short-acting β-agonist

Saquinavir (Fortovase, Invirase) Uses: *HIV Infxn* Action: HIV protease inhibitor Dose: 1200 mg PO tid w/in 2 h pc (dose adjust w/ ritonavir, delavirdine, lopinavir, & nelfinavir) Caution: [B, +] w/ rifampin, ketoconazole, statins, sildenafil Contra: Allergy, sun exposure w/o sunscreen/clothing, triazolam, midazolam, ergots, rifampin Disp: Caps 200, Tabs 500 mg SE: Dyslipidemia, lipodystrophy, rash, hyperglycemia, GI upset, weakness, hepatic dysfunction Notes: Take 2 h after meal, avoid direct sunlight

Sargramostim [GM-CSF] (Leukine) Uses: *Myeloid recovery following BMT or chemo* Action: Recombinant GF, Activates mature granulocytes & macrophages Dose: Adults & Peds. 250 mcg/m²/d IV for 21 d (BMT) Caution: [C, ?/–] Lithium, corticosteroids Contra: >10% blasts, allergy to yeast, concurrent chemo/RT Disp: Inj 250, 500 mcg SE: Bone pain, fever, ↓ BP, tachycardia, flushing, GI upset, myalgia Notes: Rotate inj sites; use APAP PRN for pain

Scopolamine, Scopolamine Transdermal and ophthalmic (Scopace, Transderm-Scop) Uses: *Prevent N/V associated w/ motion sickness, anesthesia, opiates; mydriatic,* cycloplegic, Rx uveitisiridiocyclitis Action: Anticholinergic, inhibits iris and ciliary bodies, antiemetic Dose: 1 mg/ 72 hr, 1 patch behind ear q3d; apply >4 h before exposure; 0.4–0.8 PO, repeat PRN q4–6h; cycloplegic 1–2 gtt 1 h pre, uveitis 1–2 gtt up to QID max ↓ in elderly Caution: [C, +] w/APAP, levodopa, ketoconazole, digitalis, KCl Contra: NA glaucoma, GI or GU obstruction, thyrotoxicosis, paralytic ileus **Disp:** Patch 1.5 mg, tabs 0.4 mg, ophth 0.25% **SE:** Xerostomia, drowsiness, blurred vision, tachycardia, constipation **Notes:** Do not blink excessively after dose, wait 5 min before dosing other eye; anti-emetic activity w/ patch requires several hours

Secobarbital (Seconal) [C-II] Uses: *Insomnia, short-term use,* preanesthetic agent **Action:** Rapid-acting barbiturate **Dose:** *Adults.* Caps 50, 100 mg, 100–200 mg HS, 100–300 mg preop. *Peds.* 2–6 mg/kg/dose, 100 mg/max, ↓ in elderly **Caution:** [D, +] CYP2C9, 3A3/4, 3A5/–7 inducer (Table 13, page 230); ↑ tox w/ other CNS depressants **Contra:** Porphyria, PRG **Disp:** Caps 50, 100 mg **SE:** Tolerance in 1–2 wk; resp depression, CNS depression, porphyria, photosensitivity

Selegiline, oral (Eldepryl) Uses: * Parkinson Dz* **Action:** MAOI **Dose:** 5 mg PO bid; ↓ in elderly **Caution:** [C, ?] Meperidine, SSRI, TCAs **Contra:** w/ concurrent meperidine **Disp:** Tabs/caps 5 mg **SE:** Nausea, dizziness, orthostatic ↓ BP, arrhythmias, tachycardia, edema, confusion, xerostomia **Notes:** ↓ carbidopa/levodopa if used in combo; see transdermal form

Selegiline, transdermal (Emsam) Uses: *Depression* **Action:** MAOI **Dose:** *Adults.* Apply patch daily to upper torso, upper thigh, or outer upper arm **Contra:** Tyramine-containing foods w/ 9- or 12-mg doses; serotonin-sparing agents **Caution:** [C,–] ↑ carbamazepine and oxcarbazepine levels **Disp:** ER Patches 6, 9, 12 mg **SE:** Local reactions requiring topical steroids; HA, insomnia, orthostatic hypotension, serotonin syndrome, suicide risk **Notes:** Rotate site; see oral form

Selenium Sulfide (Exsel Shampoo, Selsun Blue Shampoo, Selsun Shampoo) Uses: *Scalp seborrheic dermatitis,* scalp itching & flaking due to *dandruff*; tinea versicolor **Action:** Antiseborrheic **Dose:** *Dandruff, seborrhea:* Massage 5–10 mL into wet scalp, leave on 2–3 min, rinse, repeat; use 2× wk, then once q1–4wk PRN. *Tinea versicolor:* Apply 2.5% qd × d on area & lather w/ small amounts of water; leave on 10 min, then rinse **Caution:** [C, ?] **Contra:** Open wounds **Disp:** Shampoo [OTC] 1, 2.5% **SE:** Dry or oily scalp, lethargy, hair discoloration, local irritation Notes: Do not use more than 2×/wk

Sertaconazole (Ertaczo) Uses: *Topical Rx interdigital tinea pedis* **Action:** Imidazole antifungal. **Spectrum:** *Trichophyton rubrum, T. mentagrophytes, Epidermophyton floccosum* **Dose:** Adults & Peds > 12. Apply between toes & immediate surrounding healthy skin bid × 4 wk **Caution:** [C, ?] **Contra:** Component allergy **Disp:** 2% cream **SE:** Contact dermatitis, dry/burning skin, tenderness **Notes:** Use in immunocompetent pts

Sertraline (Zoloft) **WARNING:** Closely monitor pts for worsening depression or emergence of suicidality, particularly in ped pts **Uses:** *Depression, panic disorders, obsessive–compulsive disorder (OCD), posttraumatic stress disorders (PTSD),* social anxiety disorder, eating disorders, premenstrual disorders **Action:**

↓ neuronal uptake of serotonin **Dose:** *Adults. Depression:* 50–200 mg/d PO. *PTSD:* 25 mg PO qd ∞1 wk, then 50 mg PO qd, 200 mg/d max. *Peds.* 6–12 y: 25 mg PO qd. *13–17 y:* 50 mg PO qd **Caution:** [C, ?/–] w/ haloperidol (serotonin syndrome), sumatriptan, linezolid, hepatic impair **Contra:** MAOI use w/in 14 d; concomitant pimozide **Disp:** Tabs 25, 50, 100 mg; 20 mg/mL oral **SE:** Can activate manic/hypomanic state; weight loss; insomnia, somnolence, fatigue, tremor, xerostomia, N/D, dyspepsia, ejaculatory dysfunction, ↓ libido, hepatotox

Sevelamer (Renagel) Uses: *↓ serum phosphorus in ESRD* **Action:** Binds intestinal PO_4^{3+} **Dose:** 2–4 capsules PO tid w/ meals; adjust based on PO_4^{3+}, max 4 g/dose **Caution:** [C, ?] **Contra:** Hypophosphatemia, Bowel obstruction **Disp:** Capsules 403 mg, Tabs 400, 800 mg **SE:** BP changes, N/V/D, dyspepsia, thrombosis **Notes:** Do not open/ or chew capsules; may ↓ fat-soluble vitamin absorption; give other meds 1h before or 3 h after 800 mg sevelamer = 667 mg Ca acetate

Sibutramine (Meridia) [C-IV] Uses: *Obesity* **Action:** Blocks uptake of norepinephrine, serotonin, dopamine **Dose:** 10 mg/d PO, may ↓ to 5 mg after 4 wk **Caution:** [C, –] SSRIs, lithium, dextromethorphan, opioids **Contra:** MAOI w/in 14 d, uncontrolled HTN, arrhythmias **Disp:** Caps 5, 10, 15 mg **SE:** HA, insomnia, xerostomia, constipation, rhinitis, tachycardia, HTN **Notes:** Use w/ low-calorie diet, monitor BP & HR

Sildenafil (Viagra, Revatio) Uses: *Viagra:* *Erectile dysfunction,* *Revatio:* *Pulmonary artery HTN* **Action:** ↓ Phosphodiesterase type 5 (responsible for cGMP breakdown); ↑ cGMP activity, causing smooth muscle relaxation & ↑ flow to the corpus cavernosum and pulmonary vasculature; ?possible antiproliferative effect on pulmonary artery smooth muscle **Dose:** *ED:* 25–100 mg PO 1 h before sexual activity, max 1 × d; ↓ if >65 y; avoid fatty foods w/ dose; *Revatio Pulm HTN:* 20 mg PO tid **Caution:** [B, ?] CYP3A4 inhibitors (Table 13) **Contra:** W/ nitrates; retinitis pigmentosa; hepatic/severe renal impair **Disp:** Tabs (Viagra) 25, 50, 100 mg, tabs (Revatio) 20 mg **SE:** HA; flushing; dizziness; blue haze visual disturbance (usually reversible) **Notes:** Cardiac events in absence of nitrates debatable

Silver Nitrate (Dey-Drop, others) Uses: *Removal of granulation tissue & warts; prophylaxis in burns* **Action:** Caustic antiseptic & astringent **Dose:** *Adults & Peds.* Apply to moist surface 2–3 × wk for several wks or until effect **Caution:** [C, ?] **Contra:** Do not use on broken skin **Disp:** Topical impregnated applicator sticks, soln 10, 25, 50%; ophth 1% amp **SE:** May stain tissue black, usually resolves; local irritation, methemoglobinemia **Notes:** D/C if redness or irritation develop; no longer used in US for newborn prevention of GC conjunctivitis

Silver Sulfadiazine (Silvadene, others) Uses: *Prevention & Rx of Infxn in 2nd- & 3rd-degree burns* **Action:** Bactericidal **Dose:** *Adults & Peds.* Aseptically cover the area w/ 1/16-in. coating bid **Caution:** [B unless near term,

?/–] **Contra:** Infants <2 mo, PRG near term **Disp:** Cream 1% **SE:** Itching, rash, skin discoloration, blood dyscrasias, hepatitis, allergy **Notes:** Systemic absorption w/ extensive application

Simethicone (Mylicon, others) [OTC]
Uses: Flatulence **Action:** Defoaming, alters gas bubble surface tension action **Dose:** *Adults & Peds.* 40–125 mg PO pc & hs PRN; 500 mg/D max *Peds.* <2 yr: 20 mg PO QID PRN, 2–12 yr 40 mg PO QID PRN , >12 yr–adult **Caution:** [C, ?] **Contra:** GI Intestinal perforation or obstruction **Disp:** [OTC] Tabs 80, 125 mg; caps 125 mg; Softgels 125, 166, 180 mg, suspension 40 mg/0.6 mL, Chew tabs 80, 125 mg **SE:** N/D **Notes:** Available in combo products OTC

Simvastatin (Zocor)
Uses: ↓ Cholesterol **Action:** HMG-CoA reductase inhibitor **Dose:** 5–80 mg PO; w/ meals; ↓ in renal insuff **Caution:** [X, –] Avoid concurrent use of gemfibrozil **Contra:** PRG, liver Dz **Disp:** Tabs 5, 10, 20, 40, 80 mg **SE:** HA, GI upset, myalgia, myopathy (muscle pain, tenderness or weakness with creatine kinase 10× ULN), hepatitis **Notes:** Follow LFTs

Sirolimus [Rapamycin] (Rapamune)
WARNING: Can cause immunosuppression & Infxns **Uses:** Prophylaxis of organ rejection **Action:** ↓ T-lymphocyte activation **Dose:** *Adults >40 kg.* 6 mg PO on day 1, then 2 mg/d PO. *Adults <40 kg & Peds ≥ 13 y.* 3 mg/m² load, then 1 mg/m²/d (in H₂O/orange juice; no grapefruit juice while on sirolimus); take 4 h after cyclosporine; ↓ in hepatic impair **Caution:** [C, ?/–] Grapefruit juice, ketoconazole **Contra:** Component allergy **Disp:** Soln 1 mg/mL, tab 1, 2 mg **SE:** HTN, edema, CP, fever, HA, insomnia, acne, rash, ↑ cholesterol, GI upset, ↑↓ K⁺, Infxns, blood dyscrasias, arthralgia, tachycardia, renal impair, hepatic artery thrombosis, graft loss & death in de novo liver transplant **Notes:** Level not needed except in liver failure (trough 9–17 ng/mL)

Smallpox Vaccine (Dryvax)
Uses: Immunization against smallpox **Action:** Active immunization (live attenuated vaccinia virus) **Dose:** *Adults (routine nonemergency) or all ages (emergency):* 2–3 punctures w/ bifurcated needle dipped in vaccine into deltoid, posterior triceps muscle; check site for Rxn in 6–8 d; if major Rxn, site scabs, & heals, leaving scar; if mild/equivocal Rxn, repeat w/ 15 punctures **Caution:** [X, N/A] **Contra:** *Nonemergency use:* Febrile illness, immunosuppression, Hx eczema & their household contacts. *Emergency:* No absolute contraindications **Disp:** Vial for reconstitution: 100 million pock-forming units/mL **SE:** Malaise, fever, regional lymphadenopathy, encephalopathy, rashes, spread of inoculation to other sites administered; Stevens–Johnson syndrome, eczema vaccinatum w/ severe disability **Notes:** Avoid infant contact for 14 d

Sodium Bicarbonate [NaHCO₃]
Uses: *Alkalinization of urine,* RTA, *metabolic acidosis,* ↑ K⁺, TCA OD* **Action:** Alkalinizing agent **Dose:** *Adults.* Cardiac arrest: Initiate ventilation, 1 mEq/kg/dose IV; repeat 0.5 mEq/kg in 10 min once or based on acid–base status. *Metabolic acidosis:* 2–5 mEq/kg IV over 8 h & PRN based on acid–base status. *Alkalinize urine:* 4 g (48 mEq) PO,

then 1–2 g q4h; adjust based on urine pH; 2 amp/1 L D₅W at 100–250 mL/h IV, monitor urine pH & serum bicarbonate. *Chronic renal failure:* 1–3 mEq/kg/d. *Distal RTA:* 1 mEq/kg/d PO. *Peds >1 y:* Cardiac arrest: See Adult dosage. *Peds <1 y:* ECC: Initiate ventilation, 1:1 dilution 1 mEq/mL dosed 1 mEq/kg IV; can repeat w/ 0.5 mEq/kg in 10 min ×1 or based on acid–base status. *Chronic renal failure:* See Adult dosage. *Distal RTA:* 2–3 mEq/kg/d PO. *Proximal RTA:* 5–10 mEq/kg/d; titrate based on serum bicarbonate. *Urine alkalinization:* 84–840 mg/kg/d (1–10 mEq/kg/d) in ÷ doses; adjust based on urine pH **Caution:** [C, ?] **Contra:** Alkalosis, ↑ Na⁺, severe pulmonary edema, ↓ Ca²⁺ **Disp:** Powder, tabs; 300 mg = 3.6 mEq; 325 mg – 3.8 mEq; 520 mg = 6.3 mEq; 600 mg – 7.3 mEq; 650 mg – 7.6 mEq; inj 1 mEq/1 mL, 4.2% (5 mEq/10 mL), 7.5% 8.92 mEq/mL, 8.4% (10 mEq/10 mL) vial or amp **SE:** Belching, edema, flatulence, ↑ Na⁺, metabolic alkalosis **Notes:** 1 g neutralizes 12 mEq of acid; 50 mEq bicarb = 50 mEq Na; can make 3 amps in 1 L D₅W or = D₅NS w/ 150 mEq bicarb

Sodium Citrate/Citric Acid (Bicitra)
Uses: *Chronic metabolic acidosis, alkalinize urine; dissolve uric acid & cysteine stones* **Action:** Urinary alkalinizer **Dose:** *Adults.* 2–6 tsp (10–30 mL) diluted in 1–3 oz H₂O pc & hs. *Peds,* 1–3 tsp (5–15 mL) diluted in 1–3 oz H₂O pc & hs; best after meals **Caution:** [C, +] **Contra:** Aluminum-based antacids; severe renal impair or Na-restricted diets **Disp:** 15- or 30-mL unit dose: 16 (473 mL) or 4 (118 mL) fl oz **SE:** Tetany, metabolic alkalosis, ↑ K⁺, GI upset; avoid use of multiple 50-mL amps; can cause ↑ Na⁺/hyperosmolality **Notes:** 1 mL = 1 mEq Na & 1 mEq bicarb

Sodium Oxybate (Xyrem) [C-III]
Uses: *Narcolepsy-associated cataplexy* **Action:** Inhibitory neurotransmitter **Dose:** *Adults & Peds ≥ 16 y:* 2.25 g PO qhs, second dose 2.5–4 h later; may ↑ 9 g/d max **Caution:** [B, ?/–] **Contra:** Succinic semialdehyde dehydrogenase deficiency; potentiates EtOH **Disp:** 500 mg/mL 180 mL PO soln **SE:** Confusion, depression, ↓ diminished level of consciousness, incontinence, significant vomiting, resp depression, psychiatric Sxs **Notes:** May lead to dependence; synonym for γ-hydroxybutyrate (GHB), abused as a "date rape drug"; controlled distribution (prescriber & pt registration); must be administered when pt in bed

Sodium Phosphate (Visicol)
Uses: Bowel prep prior to colonoscopy **Action:** Hyperosmotic laxative **Dose:** 3 tabs PO w/ at least 8 oz clear liq every 15 min (20 tabs total night before procedure; 3–5 h before colonoscopy, repeat) **Caution:** [C, ?] Renal impair, electrolyte disturbances **Contra:** Megacolon, bowel obstruction, CHF, ascites, unstable angina, gastric retention, bowel perforation, colitis, hypomotility. **Disp:** Tablets 0.398, 1.102, 2 g **SE:** QT prolongation, D, ↑ Na⁺, flatulence, cramps

Sodium Polystyrene Sulfonate (Kayexalate)
Uses: *↑ K⁺* **Action:** Na⁺/K⁺ ion-exchange resin **Dose:** *Adults.* 15–60 g PO or 30–60 g PR based on serum K⁺. *Peds.* 1 g/kg/dose PO or PR q6h based on serum K⁺ (given w/ agent, eg, sorbitol, to promote movement through the bowel) **Caution:** [C, M]

Contra: ↑ Na⁺ **Disp:** Powder; susp 15 g/60 mL sorbitol **SE:** ↑ Na⁺, ↓ K⁺, Na retention, GI upset, fecal impaction **Notes:** Enema acts more quickly than PO; PO most effective

Solifenacin (VESIcare) **Uses:** OAB **Action:** Antimuscarinic, ↓ detrusor contractions **Dose:** 5 mg PO qd, 10 mg/d max; ↓ w/ renal/hepatic impair **Caution:** [C, ?/–] Bladder outflow or GI obstruction, ulcerative colitis, MyG, renal/hepatic impair, QT prolongation risk **Contra:** NA glaucoma, urinary/gastric retention **Disp:** Tabs 5, 10 mg **SE:** Constipation, xerostomia **Notes:** Interacts w/ azole antifungals; do not ↑ dose w/ severe renal/moderate hepatic impair

Sorafenib (Nexavar) **Uses:** *Advanced RCC* metastatic liver cancer **Action:** Kinase inhibitor **Dose:** *Adults.* 400 mg PO bid on empty stomach **Caution:** [D,–] w/irinotecan or doxorubicin **SE:** Hand–foot syndrome; treatment-emergent hypertension; bleeding, ↑ INR, cardiac infarction/ischemia; ↑ pancreatic enzymes, hypophosphatemia, lymphopenia, anemia, fatigue, alopecia, pruritus, D, GI upset, HA, neuropathy **Notes:** Monitor BP during first 6 wks; may require ↓ dose (QD or every other day); impaired metabolism w/Asian descent; unknown effect on wound healing, d/c for major surgery

Sorbitol (generic) **Uses:** *Constipation* **Action:** Laxative **Dose:** 30–60 mL PO of a 20–70% soln PRN **Caution:** [B, +] **Contra:** Anuria **Disp:** Liq 70% **SE:** Edema, electrolyte losses, lactic acidosis, GI upset, xerostomia **Notes:** May be vehicle for many liq formulations (eg, zinc, Kayexalate)

Sotalol (Betapace) **WARNING:** Monitor pts for 1st 3 d of Rx to ↓ risks of arrhythmia **Uses:** *Ventricular arrhythmias, AF* **Action:** β-Adrenergic-blocking agent **Dose:** *Adults.* 80 mg PO bid; may be ↑ to 240–320 mg/d. *Peds.* Neonates: 9 mg/m² tid. *1–19 mo:* 20 mg/m² tid. *20–23 mo:* 29.1 mg/m² tid;. = > 2 y: 30 mg/m² tid; ↓ w/ renal insuffin **Caution:** [B (1st tri) (D if 2nd or 3rd tri), +] **Contra:** Asthma, bradycardia, ↑prolonged QT interval, 2nd- or 3rd-degree heart block w/o pacemaker, cardiogenic shock, uncontrolled CHF, CrCl <40 mL/min **Disp:** Tabs 80, 120, 160, 240 mg **SE:** Bradycardia, CP, palpitations, fatigue, dizziness, weakness, dyspnea **Notes:** Betapace should not be substituted for Betapace AF because of differences in labeling

Sotalol (Betapace AF) **WARNING:** To minimize risk of induced arrhythmia, pts initiated/reinitiated on Betapace AF should be placed for a minimum of 3 d (on their maint dose) in a facility that can provide cardiac resuscitation, continuous ECG monitoring, & calculations of CrCl; Betapace should not be substituted for Betapace AF because of labeling differences **Uses:** *Maintain sinus rhythm for symptomatic A fib/flutter* **Action:** β-Adrenergic-blocking agent **Dose:** *Adults.* Initial CrCl >60 mL/min: 80 mg PO q12h. *CrCl 40–60 mL/min:* 80 mg PO q2h; ↑ to 120 mg during hospitalization; monitor QT interval 2–4 h after each dose, w/ dose reduction or D/C if QT interval >500 ms. *Peds.* Neonates: 9 mg/m² tid. *1–19 mo:* 20 mg/m² tid. *20–23 mo:* 29.1 mg/m² tid. = 2 y: 30 mg/m² tid; can double all doses as max daily dose; allow ≅ 36 h between dosage titrations **Caution:** [B (1st tri; D if 2nd or 3rd tri), +] if converting from previous antiarrhythmic therapy **Contra:** Asthma, bradycardia, prolonged QT interval, 2nd- or 3rd-degree heart block w/o pacemaker, cardiogenic shock, uncontrolled CHF, CrCl <40 mL/min **Disp:** Tabs 80, 120, 160 mg **SE:** Bradycardia, CP, palpitations, fatigue, dizziness, weakness, dyspnea **Notes:** Follow renal Fxn & QT interval

Sparfloxacin (Zagam) **Uses:** *Community-acquired pneumonia, acute exacerbations of chronic bronchitis* **Action:** Quinolone; ↓ DNA gyrase **Dose:** 400 mg PO day 1, then 200 mg q24h × 1 ∞ 10 d; ↓ in renal impair **Caution:** [C, ?/–] W/ theophylline, caffeine, sucralfate, warfarin, antacids **Contra:** w/QT prolongation & drugs that prolong QT interval **Disp:** Tabs 200 mg **SE:** Phototox (even daylight through windows), N/V/D, rash, ruptured tendons, ↑ LFTs, sleep disorders, confusion, convulsions **Notes:** Protect from sunlight up to 5 d after last dose

Spironolactone (Aldactone) **Uses:** *Hyperaldosteronism, ascites from CHF or cirrhosis* **Action:** Aldosterone antagonist; K⁺-sparing diuretic **Dose:** *Adults.* 25–100 mg PO qid; CHF (NYHA class III–IV) 25–50 mg/d. *Peds.* 1–3.3 mg/kg/24 h PO ÷ bid–qid. *Neonates.* 0.5–1 mg/kg/dose q8h; w/ food **Caution:** [D, +] Contra: renal failure, anuria **Disp:** Tabs 25, 50, 100 mg **SE:** ↑ K⁺ & gynecomastia, arrhythmia, sexual dysfunction, confusion, dizziness

Stavudine (Zerit) **WARNING:** Lactic acidosis & severe hepatomegaly w/ steatosis & pancreatitis reported **Uses:** *Advanced HIV* **Action:** Reverse transcriptase inhibitor **Dose:** *Adults.* >60 kg: 40 mg bid. <60 kg: 30 mg bid. *Peds.* Birth 13 d: 0.5 mg/kg q12h >14 d & <30 kg: 1 mg/kg q12h. = 30 kg: Adult dose; ↓ in renal insuff failure **Caution:** [C, +] **Contra:** Allergy **Disp:** Caps 15, 20, 30, 40 mg, soln 1 mg/mL **SE:** Peripheral neuropathy, HA, chills, fever, malaise, rash, GI upset, anemias, lactic acidosis, ↑ LFTs, pancreatitis **Notes:** Take w/ plenty of H₂O

Steroids, Systemic (See also Table 4, page 216) The following relates only to the commonly used systemic glucocorticoids **Uses:** *Endocrine disorders* (adrenal insuff), *rheumatoid disorders,* collagen–vascular Dzs, dermatologic Dzs, allergic states, cerebral edema,* nephritis, nephrotic syndrome, immunosuppression for transplantation, ↑ Ca²⁺, malignancies (breast, lymphomas), preop (in any pt who has been on steroids in the previous year, known hypoadrenalism, preop for adrenalectomy); inj into joints/tissue **Action:** Glucocorticoid **Dose:** Varies w/ use & institutional protocols.

• *Adrenal insuff, acute: Adults.* Hydrocortisone: 100 mg IV; then 300 mg/d ÷ q6h; convert to 50 mg PO q8h × 6 doses, taper to 30–50 mg/d ÷ bid. *Peds.* Hydrocortisone: 1–2 mg/kg IV, then 150–250 mg/d ÷ tid.

• *Adrenal insuff, chronic (physiologic replacement):* May need mineralocorticoid supl such as Florinef. *Adults.* Hydrocortisone 20 mg PO qAM, 10 mg PO qPM; cortisone 0.5–0.75 mg/kg/d ÷ bid; cortisone 0.25–0.35 mg/kg/d IM; dexamethasone 0.03–0.15 mg/kg/d or 0.6–0.75 mg/m²/d ÷ q6–12h PO, IM, IV. *Peds.* Hydrocortisone: 0.5–0.75 mg/kg/d PO tid; hydrocortisone succinate 0.25–0.35 mg/kg/d IM.

- *Asthma, acute: Adults.* Methylprednisolone 60 mg PO/IV q6h or dexamethasone 12 mg IV q6h. *Peds.* Prednisolone 1–2 mg/kg/d or prednisone 1–2 mg/kg/d ÷ qd–bid for up to 5 d; methylprednisolone 2–4 mg/kg/d IV ÷ tid; dexamethasone 0.1–0.3 mg/kg/d divided q6h. *Congenital adrenal hyperplasia: Peds.* Initial hydrocortisone 30–36 mg/m²/d PO ÷ 1/3 dose qAM, 2/3 dose qPM; maint 20–25 mg/m²/d ÷ bid.

- *Extubation/airway edema: Adults.* Dexamethasone 0.5–1 mg/kg/d IM/IV ÷ q6h (start 24 h prior to extubation; continue × 4 more doses). *Peds.* Dexamethasone 0.1–0.3 mg/kg/d ÷ q6h × 3 3–5 d (start 48–72 h before extubation)

- *Immunosuppressive/antiinflammatory: Adults & Older Peds.* Hydrocortisone: 15–240 mg PO, IM, IV q12h; *methylprednisolone:* 4–48 mg/d PO, taper to lowest effective dose; *methylprednisolone Na succinate:* 10–80 mg/d IM. *Adults.* Prednisone or prednisolone: 5–60 mg/d PO ÷ qd–qid. *Infants & Younger Children.* Hydrocortisone 2.5–10 mg/kg/d PO ÷ q6–8h; 1–5 mg/kg/d IM/IV ÷ bid.

- *Nephrotic syndrome: Peds.* Prednisolone or prednisone 2 mg/kg/d PO tid–qid until urine is protein-free for 5 d, use up to 28 d; for persistent proteinuria, 4 mg/kg/dose PO qod max 120 mg/d for an additional 28 d; maint 2 mg/kg/dose qod for 28 d; taper over 4–6 wk (max 80 mg/d).

- *Septic shock (controversial): Adults.* Hydrocortisone 500 mg–1 g IM/IV q2–6h. *Peds.* Hydrocortisone 50 mg/kg IM/IV, repeat q4–24 h PRN. *Status asthmaticus: Adults & Peds.* Hydrocortisone 1–2 mg/kg/dose IV q6h; then ↓ by 0.5–1 mg/kg q6h.

- *Rheumatic Dz: Adults. Intraarticular:* Hydrocortisone acetate 25–37.5 mg large joint, 10–25 mg small joint; methylprednisolone acetate 20–80 mg large joint, 4–10 mg small joint. *Intrabursal:* Hydrocortisone acetate 25–37.5 mg. *Intraganglial:* Hydrocortisone acetate 25–37.5 mg. *Tendon sheath:* Hydrocortisone acetate 5–12.5 mg.

- *Periop steroid coverage:* Hydrocortisone 100 mg IV night before surgery, 1 h preop, intraop, & 4, 8, & 12 h postop; postop d #1 100 mg IV q6h; postop d #2 100 mg IV q8h; postop d #3 100 mg IV q12h; postop d #4 50 mg IV q12h; postop d #5 25 mg IV q12h; resume prior PO dosing if chronic use or D/C if only periop coverage required.

- *Cerebral edema:* Dexamethasone 10 mg IV; then 4 mg IV q4–6h

- **Caution:** [C, ?/–] **Contra:** Active varicella Infxn, serious Infxn except TB, fungal Infxns **Disp:** See Table 4, page 216. **SE:** All can cause ↑ appetite, hyperglycemia, ↓ K⁺, osteoporosis, nervousness, insomnia, "steroid psychosis," adrenal suppression **Notes:** Hydrocortisone succinate for systemic, acetate for intraarticular; never abruptly D/C steroids, taper dose

Streptokinase (Streptase, Kabikinase) Uses: *Coronary artery thrombosis, acute massive PE, DVT, & some occluded vascular grafts* **Action:**

Activates plasminogen to plasmin that degrades fibrin **Dose:** *Adults.* PE: Load 250,000 units peripheral IV over 30 min, then 100,000 units/h IV for 24–72 h. *Coronary artery thrombosis:* 1.5 million units IV over 60 min. *DVT or arterial embolism:* Load as w/ PE, then 100,000 units/h for 72 h. *Peds.* 3500–4000 units/kg over 30 min, followed by 1000–1500 units/kg/h. *Occluded catheter* (controversial): 10,000–25,000 units in NS to final volume of catheter (leave in place for 1 h, aspirate & flush catheter w/ NS) **Caution:** [C, +] **Contra:** Streptococcal Infxn or streptokinase in last 6 mo, active bleeding, CVA, TIA, spinal surgery, or trauma in last month, vascular anomalies, severe hepatic or renal Dz, endocarditis, pericarditis, severe uncontrolled HTN **Disp:** Powder for inj 250,000, 750,000, 1,500,000 units **SE:** Bleeding, ↓ BP, fever, bruising, rash, GI upset, hemorrhage, anaphylaxis **Notes:** If maint inf inadequate to maintain thrombin clotting time 2–5X control, see package for adjustments; antibodies remain 3–6 mo following dose

Streptomycin Uses: *TB,* streptococcal or enterococcal endocarditis **Action:** Aminoglycoside; interferes w/ protein synthesis **Dose:** *Adults.* Endocarditis: 1 g q12h 1–2 wk, then 500 mg q12h 1–4 wk; *TB:* 15 mg/kg/d (up to 1 g), directly observed therapy (DOT) 2×wk 20–30 mg/kg/dose (max 1.5 gm), DOT 3×wk 25–30 mg/kg/dose (max 1 g). *Peds.* 15 mg/kg/d; DOT 2×wk 20–40 mg/kg/dose (max 1 g); DOT 3×wk 25–30 mg/kg/dose (max 1 g); ↓ w/in renal failure insuff, either IM or IV over 30–60 min **Caution:** [D, +] **Contra:** PRG **Disp:** Inj 400 mg/mL (1-g vial) **SE:** ↑ incidence of vestibular & auditory tox neurotox, nephrotox **Notes:** Monitor levels: peak 20–30 mcg/mL, trough <5 mcg/mL; toxic peak > 50, trough > 10; IV over 30–60 min

Streptozocin (Zanosar) Uses: *Pancreatic islet cell tumors* & carcinoid tumors **Action:** DNA–DNA (interstrand) cross-linking; DNA, RNA, & protein synthesis inhibitor **Dose:** Per protocol; ↓ in renal failure **Caution:** W/renal failure [D, ?/] **Contra:** Caution, PRG **Disp:** Inj 1 g **SE:** N/V, duodenal ulcers; myelosuppression rare (20%) & mild; nephrotox (proteinuria & azotemia often heralded by hypophosphatemia) dose-limiting; hypo-/hyperglycemia; inj site Rxns **Notes:** Monitor Cr

Succimer (Chemet) Uses: *Lead poisoning (levels >45 mcg/mL)* **Action:** Heavy-metal chelating agent **Dose:** *Adults & Peds.* 10 mg/kg/dose q8h × 5 d, then 10 mg/kg/dose q12h for 14 d; ↓ in renal impair **Caution:** [C, ?] **Contra:** Allergy **Disp:** Caps 100 mg **SE:** Rash, fever, GI upset, hemorrhoids, metallic taste, drowsiness, ↑ LFTs **Notes:** Monitor lead levels, maintain hydration, may open capsules

Succinylcholine (Anectine, Quelicin, Sucostrin, others) **WARNING:** Risk of cardiac arrest from hyperkalemic rhabdomyolysis **Uses:** *Adjunct to general anesthesia to facilitate ET intubation & to induce skeletal muscle relaxation during surgery or mechanical ventilation* **Action:** Depolarizing neuromuscular blocking agent **Dose:** *Adults.* 1–1.5 mg/kg IV over 10–30 s, then followed by 0.04–0.07 mg/kg or 10–100 mcg/kg/min inf. *Peds.* 1–2 mg/kg/dose IV, then followed by 0.3–0.6 mg/kg/dose q5min use of CI not OK; ↓ w/ severe renal/hepatic impair **Caution:** See warning; [C, M] **Contra:** If rw/risk for malignant hyperthermia, myopathy, skeletal myopathy in children; recent major burn, multiple trauma, extensive skeletal muscle denervation, NAG, pseudo-cholinesterase deficiency **Disp:** Inj 20, 50, 100 mg/mL **SE:** May precipitate malignant hyperthermia, resp depression, or prolonged apnea; multiple drugs potentiate; observe for CV effects (arrhythmias, ↓ BP, brady/tachycardia); ↑ intraocular pressure, postop stiffness, salivation, myoglobinuria **Notes:** May be given IVP/inf/IM deltoid; hyperkalemic rhabdomyolysis in children with undiagnosed myopathy such as Duchenne muscular dystrophy

Sucralfate (Carafate) **Uses:** *Duodenal ulcers,* gastric ulcers, stomatitis, GERD, preventing stress ulcers, esophagitis **Action:** Forms ulcer-adherent complex that protects against acid, pepsin, & bile acid **Dose:** *Adults.* 1 g PO qid, 1 h prior to meals & hs. *Peds.* 40–80 mg/kg/d ÷ q6h; continue 4–8 wk unless healing demonstrated by x-ray or endoscopy; separate from other drugs by 2 h; on empty stomach ac **Caution:** [B, +] **Contra:** Component allergy **Disp:** Tabs 1 g; susp 1 g/10 mL **SE:** Constipation; D, dizziness, xerostomia **Notes:** Aluminum may accumulate in renal failure

Sulfacetamide (Bleph-10, Cetamide, Sodium Sulamyd) **Uses:** *Conjunctival Infxns* **Action:** Sulfonamide antibiotic **Dose:** 10% oint apply qid & hs; soln for keratitis apply q2–3h based on severity **Caution:** [C, M] **Contra:** Sulfonamide sensitivity; age <2 mo **Disp:** Oint 10%; soln 10, 15, 30% **SE:** Irritation, burning; blurred vision, brow ache, Stevens–Johnson syndrome, photosensitivity

Sulfacetamide & Prednisolone (Blephamide, others) **Uses:** *Steroid-responsive inflammatory ocular conditions w/ Infxn or a risk of Infxn* **Action:** Antibiotic & antiinflammatory **Dose:** *Adults & Peds >2 y.* Apply oint to lower conjunctival sac qd–qid; soln 1–3 gtt 2–3 h while awake **Caution:** [C, ?/–] Sulfonamide sensitivity; age <2 mon **Disp:** Oint sulfacetamide 10%/prednisolone 0.5%, sulfacetamide 10%/prednisolone 0.2%, sulfacetamide 10%/prednisolone 0.25%; susp sulfacetamide 10%/prednisolone 0.25%, sulfacetamide 10%/prednisolone 0.5%, sulfacetamide 10%/prednisolone 0.2% **SE:** Irritation, burning, blurred vision, brow ache, Stevens–Johnson syndrome, photosensitivity **Notes:** OK ophth susp use as otic agent

Sulfasalazine (Azulfidine, Azulfidine EN) **Uses:** *Ulcerative colitis, RA, juvenile RA,* active Crohn Dz, ankylosing spondylitis, psoriasis **Action:** Sulfonamide; actions unclear **Dose:** *Adults.* Initial, 1 g PO tid–qid; ↑ to a max of 8 g/d in 3–4 ÷ doses; maint 500 mg PO qid. *Peds.* Initial, 40–60 mg/kg/24 h PO ÷ q4–6h; maint, 20–30 mg/kg/24 h PO ÷ q6h. *RA >6 y:* 30–50 mg/kg/d in 2 doses, start w/ 1/4–1/3 maint dose, ↑ weekly until dose reached at 1 mo, 2 g/d max; ↓ in renal failure **Caution:** [B (D if near term), M] **Contra:** Sulfonamide or salicylate sensitivity, porphyria, GI or GU obstruction; avoid in hepatic impair **Disp:** Tabs 500 mg; EC Delayed release tabs 500 mg; PO susp 250 mg/5 mL **SE:** GI upset; discolors urine; dizziness, HA, photosensitivity, oligospermia, anemias, Stevens–Johnson syndrome **Notes:** May cause yellow-orange skin/contact lens discoloration; avoid sunlight exposure

Sulfinpyrazone (Anturane) Uses: *Acute & chronic gout* **Action:** ↓ renal tubular absorption of uric acid **Dose:** 100–200 mg PO bid for 1 wk, ↑ PRN to maint of 200–400 mg bid; max 800 mg/d; take w/ food or antacids, & plenty of fluids; avoid salicylates **Caution:** [C (D if near term), ?/–] **Contra:** Renal impair, avoid salicylates, peptic ulcer; blood dyscrasias, near term PRG, allergy **Disp:** Tabs 100 mg, caps 200 mg **SE:** N/V, stomach pain, urolithiasis, leukopenia **Notes:** Take w/ plenty of H$_2$O

Sulindac (Clinoril) **WARNING:** May ↑risk of cardiovascular events & GI bleeding Uses: *Arthritis & pain* **Action:** NSAID; ↓ prostaglandins **Dose:** 150–200 mg bid w/ food **Caution:** [B (D if 3rd tri or near term), ?] **Contra:** NSAID or ASA sensitivity, ulcer, GI bleeding **Disp:** Tabs 150, 200 mg **SE:** Dizziness, rash, GI upset, pruritus, edema, ↓ renal blood flow, renal failure (? fewer renal effects than other NSAIDs), peptic ulcer, GI bleeding

Sumatriptan (Imitrex) Uses: Rx acute migraine attacks **Action:** Vascular serotonin receptor agonist **Dose:** *Adults.* SQ: 6 mg SQ as a single dose PRN; repeat PRN in 1 h to a max of 12 mg/24 h. PO: 25 mg, repeat in 2 h, PRN, 100 mg/d max PO dose; max 300 mg/d. *Nasal spray:* 1 spray into 1 nostril, repeat in 2 h to 40 mg/24 h max. *Peds.* Nasal spray: 6–9 y: 5–20 mg/d. 12–17 y: 5–20 mg, up to 40 mg/d **Caution:** [C, M] **Contra:** Angina, Ischemic heart Dz, uncontrolled HTN, ergot use, MAOI use w/in 14 d **Disp:** OD tabs 25, 50, 100 mg; Inj 6, 8, 12 mg/mL; OD tabs 25, 50, 100 mg, orally disintegrating tabs 25, 50, 100 mg; nasal spray 5, 10, 20 mg/spray **SE:** Pain & bruising at site, dizziness, hot flashes, paresthesias, CP, weakness, numbness, coronary vasospasm, HTN

Sunitinib (Sutent) Uses: *Advanced GI stromal tumor refractory/intolerant of imatinib; advanced RCC* **Action:** Kinase inhibitor **Dose:** *Adults.* 50 mg PO daily × 4 wks, followed by 2 wk holiday = 1 cycle; ↓ to 37.5 mg w/CYP3A4 inhibitors (Table 13), to ↑ 87.5 mg w/CYP3A4 inducers (PRN) **Caution:** [D,-] Multiple interactions require dose modification (eg, St. John's wort) **Disp:** Caps 12.5, 25, 50 mg **SE:** ↓ WBC & plt, bleeding, ↑ BP, ↓ ejection fraction, ↑ QT interval, pancreatitis, DVT, seizures, adrenal insufficiency, N, V, D, skin discoloration, oral ulcers, taste perversion, hypothyroidism **Notes:** Monitor CBC, platelets, chemistries at cycle onset; baseline cardiac fxn recommended, ↓ dose in 12.5-mg increments if not tolerated

Tacrine (Cognex) Uses: *Mild–moderate Alzheimer dementia* **Action:** Cholinesterase inhibitor **Dose:** 10–40 mg PO qid to 160 mg/d; separate doses from food **Caution:** [C, ?] **Contra:** Previous tacrine-induced jaundice **Disp:** Caps 10, 20, 30, 40 mg **SE:** ↑ LFT, HA, dizziness, GI upset, flushing, confusion, ataxia, myalgia, bradycardia **Notes:** Serum conc >20 ng/mL have more SE; monitor LFTs

Tacrolimus [FK 506] (Prograf, Protopic) Uses: *Prevent organ rejection,* eczema **Action:** Macrolide immunosuppressant **Dose:** *Adults.* IV: 0.05–0.1 mg/kg/d cont inf. *PO:* 0.15–0.3 mg/kg/d ÷ 2 doses. *Peds.* IV: 0.03–0.05 mg/kg/d as cont inf. *PO:* 0.15–0.2 mg/kg/d PO ÷ q 12 h. *Adults & Peds.* Eczema: Apply bid, continue 1 wk after clearing; ↓ in hepatic/renal impair **Caution:** [C, –] Do not use w/ cyclosporine; avoid topical if <2 yrs of age **Contra:** Component allergy **Disp:** Caps 1, 5 mg; inj 5 mg/mL; oint 0.03, 0.1% **SE:** Neurotox & nephrotox, HTN, edema, HA, insomnia, fever, pruritus, ↓/↑ K+, hyperglycemia, GI upset, anemia, leukocytosis, tremors, paresthesias, pleural effusion, Szs, lymphoma **Notes:** Monitor levels; reports of ↑cancer risk; topical use for short term/second line

Tadalafil (Cialis) Uses: *Erectile dysfunction* **Action:** PDE5 inhibitor, increases cGMP and NO levels; relaxes smooth muscles, dilates cavernosal arteries; Phosphodiesterase 5 inhibitor **Dose:** *Adults.* 10 mg PO before sexual activity w/o regard to meals (range 5–20 mg max); ↓ 5 mg (10 mg max) w/ renal/ & hepatic insuff **Caution:** [B, –] 1 dose/72h w/CYP3A4 inhibitor (Table 13) **Contra:** Nitrates, α-blockers (except tamsulosin), severe hepatic insuff **Disp:** 5-, 10-, 20-mg tabs **SE:** HA, flushing, dyspepsia, rhinitis, back pain, myalgia **Notes:** Longest acting of class (36 h)

Talc (Sterile Talc Powder) Uses: *↓ recurrence of malignant pleural effusions (pleurodesis)* **Action:** Sclerosing agent **Dose:** Mix slurry: 50 mL NS w/ 5-g vial, mix, distribute 25 mL into two 60-mL syringes, volume to 50 mL/syringe w/ NS. Infuse each into chest tube, flush w/ 25 mL NS. Keep tube clamped; have pt change positions q15min for 2 h, unclamp tube **Caution:** [X, –] **Contra:** Planned further surgery on site **Disp:** 5 g powder **SE:** Pain, Infxn **Notes:** May add 10–20 mL 1% lidocaine/syringe; must have chest tube placed, monitor closely while tube clamped (tension pneumothorax), not antineoplastic

Tamoxifen (Nolvadex) Warning: Cancer of the uterus, stroke, and blood clots can occur Uses: *Breast CA [postmenopausal, estrogen receptor(+)],↓ reduction of breast CA in high-risk women, metastatic male breast CA,* ductal carcinoma in situ, mastalgia, pancreatic CA, gynecomastia, ovulation induction **Action:** Nonsteroidal antiestrogen; mixed agonist–antagonist effect **Dose:** 20–40 mg/d (typically 10 mg bid or 20 mg/d) Prevention: 10 mg PO bid ×5y **Caution:** [D, –] leukopenia, thrombocytopenia, hyperlipidemia **Contra:** PRG, undiagnosed vag bleeding, Hx thromboemblolism **Disp:** Tabs 10, 20 mg **SE:** Uterine malignancy & thrombotic events noted in breast CA prevention trials; menopausal Sxs (hot flashes, N/V) in premenopausal pts; vaginal bleeding & menstrual irregularities; skin rash, pruritus vulvae, dizziness, HA, peripheral edema; acute flare of bone metastasis pain & ↑ Ca²+; retinopathy reported (high dose) **Notes:** ↑ risk of PRG in premenopausal women (induces ovulation); brand Nolvadex suspended in US

Tamsulosin (Flomax) Uses: *BPH* **Action:** Antagonist of prostatic α-receptors **Dose:** 0.4 mg/d PO; do not crush, chew, or open caps **Caution:** [B, ?] Con-

tra: Female gender **Disp:** Caps 0.4 mg **SE:** HA, dizziness, syncope, somnolence, ↓ libido, GI upset, retrograde ejaculation, rhinitis, rash, angioedema, IFIS **Notes:** Not for use as antihypertensive

Tazarotene (Tazorac) **Uses:** *Facial acne vulgaris; stable plaque psoriasis up to 20% body surface area* **Action:** Keratolytic **Dose:** *Adults & Peds >12 y. Acne:* Cleanse face, dry, & apply thin film qd hs on acne lesions. *Psoriasis:* Apply hs **Caution:** [X, ?/–] **Contra:** Retinoid sensitivity **Disp:** Gel 0.05, 0.1%; Cream 0.05%, 0.1% **SE:** Burning, erythema, irritation, rash, photosensitivity, desquamation, bleeding, skin discoloration **Notes:** D/C w/ excessive pruritus, burning, skin redness or peeling occur until SxS resolve

Tegaserod (Zelnorm) **WARNING:** Rare reports of ischemic colitis **Uses:** *Short term Rx of constipation-predominant IBS in women, chronic idiopathic constipation in pts <65 y* **Action:** 5HT4 serotonin agonist **Dose:** 6 mg PO bid pc for 4–6 wk; may continue for 2nd course **Caution:** Do not administer if D present, as GI motility ↑ [B, ?/–] **Contra:** Severe renal, moderate–severe hepatic impair, Hx of bowel obstruction, gallbladder Dz, sphincter of Oddi dysfunction, abdominal adhesions **Disp:** Tabs 2, 6 mg **SE:** Do not administer if D present, as GI motility ↑; D/C if abdominal pain worsens **Notes:** Maintain hydration

Telithromycin (Ketek) **WARNING:** May be associated with pseudomembranous colitis and hepatic failure **Uses:** *Acute bacterial exacerbations of chronic bronchitis, acute bacterial sinusitis; mild–moderate community-acquired pneumonia* **Action:** Unique macrolide, blocks ↓ protein synthesis; bactericidal. *Spectrum:* Staphylococcus aureus, Streptococcus pneumoniae, H. influenzae, M. catarrhalis, Chlamydophila pneumoniae, M. pneumoniae **Dose:** *Chronic bronchitis/sinusitis:* 800 mg (2 tabs) PO qd ×5; *Pneumonia:* 800 mg (2 tabs) PO qd × 7–10 d **Caution:** [C, M] pseudomembranous colitis, ↑ QTc interval, MyG exacerbations, visual disturbances, hepatic dysfunction; dosing in renal impair unknown **Contra:** Macrolide allergy, use w/ cisapride or pimozide **Disp:** Tabs 300, 400 mg **SE:** N/V/D, dizziness **Notes:** CYP450 inhibitor; multiple drug interactions

Telmisartan (Micardis) **Uses:** *HTN, CHF,* DN **Action:** Angiotensin II receptor antagonist **Dose:** 40–80 mg qd **Caution:** [C (1st tri; D 2nd & 3rd tri), ?/–] **Contra:** Angiotensin II receptor antagonist sensitivity **Disp:** Tabs 20, 40, 80 mg **SE:** Edema, GI upset, HA, angioedema, renal impair, orthostatic ↓ BP

Temazepam (Restoril) [C-IV] **Uses:** *Insomnia,* anxiety, depression, panic attacks **Action:** Benzodiazepine **Dose:** 15–30 mg PO hs PRN; ↓ in elderly **Caution:** [X, ?/–] Potentiates CNS depressive effects of opioids, barbs, EtOH, antihistamines, MAOIs, TCAs **Contra:** NA glaucoma **Disp:** Caps 7.5, 15, 30 mg **SE:** Confusion, dizziness, drowsiness, hangover **Notes:** Abrupt D/C after >10 d use may cause withdrawal

Tenecteplase (TNKase) **Uses:** *Restore perfusion & mortality w/ AMI* **Action:** Thrombolytic; TPA **Dose:** 30–50 mg; see table:

Tenecteplase Dosing

Weight (kg)	TNKase (mg)	TNKase[a] Volume (mL)
<60	30	6
60–69	35	7
70–79	40	8
80–89	45	9
≥90	50	10

[a]From one vial of reconstituted TNKase.
*Based on data in Haist SA and Robbins JB: *Internal Medicine on Call*, 4th ed, 2005 McGraw-Hill). See also www.fda.gov.

Caution: [C, ?], ↑ bleeding w/ NSAIDs, ticlopidine, clopidogrel, GPIIb/IIIa antagonists **Contra:** Bleeding, CVA, major surgery (intracranial, intraspinal) or trauma w/in 2 mo **Disp:** Inj 50 mg, reconstitute w/ 10 mL sterile H_2O **SE:** Bleeding, allergy **Notes:** Do not shake w/reconstitution; do *not* use w/D_5W

Tenofovir (Viread) **Uses:** *HIV Infxn* **Action:** Nucleotide RT inhibitor **Dose:** 300 mg PO qd w/ a meal **Caution:** [B, ?/–] Didanosine (separate admin times), lopinavir, ritonavir w/ known risk factors for liver Dz **Contra:** CrCl <60 mL/min; **Disp:** Tabs 300 mg **SE:** GI upset, metabolic syndrome, hepatotox; separate didanosine doses by 2 h **Notes:** Take w/ fatty meal; combo product w/emtricitabine known as Truvada

Tenofovir/Emtricitabine (Truvada) **WARNING:** Lactic acidosis & severe hepatomegaly with steatosis, including fatal cases, have been reported with the use of nucleoside analogs alone or in combo w/ other antiretrovirals. Not OK w/ chronic hepatitis; effects in patients co-infected with hepatitis B & HIV unknown **Uses:** *HIV Infxn* **Action:** Dual nucleotide RT inhibitor **Dose:** 300 mg PO qd w/ or w/o a meal **Caution:** W/ known risk factors for liver Dz [B, ?/–] **Contra:** CrCl <30 mL/min; **Disp:** Tabs: 200 mg emtricitabine/300 mg tenofovir **SE:** GI upset, metabolic syndrome, hepatotox **Notes:** Take w/ fatty meal

Terazosin (Hytrin) **Uses:** *BPH & HTN* **Action:** α1-Blocker (blood vessel & bladder neck/prostate) **Dose:** Initial, 1 mg PO hs; ↑ 20 mg/d max **Caution:** [C, ?] w/ BB, CCB, ACEI **Contra:** α-Antagonist sensitivity **Disp:** Tabs 1, 2, 5, 10 mg; caps 1, 2, 5, 10 mg **SE:** ↓ BP, & syncope following 1st dose; dizziness, weakness, nasal congestion, peripheral edema, palpitations, GI upset **Notes:** Caution w/ 1st dose syncope; if for HTN, combine w/ thiazide diuretic

Terbinafine (Lamisil) Uses: *Onychomycosis, athlete's foot, jock itch, ringworm,* cutaneous candidiasis, pityriasis versicolor **Action:** ↓ squalene epoxidase resulting in fungal death **Dose:** *PO:* 250 mg/d PO for 6–12 wk. *Topical:* Apply to area; ↓ in renal/hepatic impair **Caution:** [B, –] ↑ effects of drug metab by CYP2D6 **Contra:** Liver Dz/kidney failure **Disp:** Tabs 250 mg; cream, gel, soln 1%; **SE:** HA, dizziness, rash, pruritus, alopecia, GI upset, taste perversion, neutropenia, retinal damage, Stevens–Johnson syndrome **Notes:** Effect may take months due to need for new nail growth; do not use occlusive dressings

Terbutaline (Brethine) Uses: *Reversible bronchospasm (asthma, COPD); inhibits labor ()* **Action:** Sympathomimetic; tocolytic **Dose:** *Adults.* Bronchodilator: 2.5–5 mg PO qid or 0.25 mg SQ; may repeat in 15 min (max 0.5 mg in 4 h). *Met-dose inhaler:* 2 inhal q4–6h. *Premature labor:* Acutely 2.5–10 mg/min/IV, gradually ↑ as tolerated q10–20min; maint 2.5–5 mg PO q4–6h until term *Peds.* PO: 0.05–0.15 mg/kg/dose PO tid; max 5 mg/24h; ↓ in renal failure **Caution:** [B, +] ↑ tox w/ MAOIs, TCAs; diabetes, HTN, hyperthyroidism **Contra:** Tachycardia, component allergy **Disp:** Tabs 2.5, 5 mg; inj 1 mg/mL; met-dose inhaler **SE:** HTN, hyperthyroidism, β₁-adrenergic effects w/ high dose, nervousness, trembling, tachycardia, HTN, dizziness

Terconazole (Terazol 7) Uses: *Vaginal fungal Infxns* **Action:** Topical antifungal **Dose:** 1 applicatorful or 1 supp intravag hs × 3–7 d **Caution:** [C, ?] **Contra:** Component allergy **Disp:** Vaginal cream 0.4, 0.8%; vaginal supp 80 mg **SE:** Vulvar/vaginal burning **Notes:** Insert high into vagina

Teriparatide (Forteo) Uses: *Severe/refractory osteoporosis* **Action:** PTH (recombinant) **Dose:** 20 mcg SQ qd in thigh or abdomen **Caution:** [C, ?/–] **Contra:** w/ Paget Dz, prior radiation, bone metastases, ↑ Ca²⁺; caution in urolithiasis **Disp:** 3-mL prefilled device (discard after 28 d) **SE:** orthostatic ↓ BP on administration, N/D, ↑ Ca, leg cramps **Notes:** 2 yr max use; osteosarcoma in animals

Testosterone (AndroGel, Androderm, Striant, Testim, Testoderm) [CIII] Uses: *Male hypogonadism* **Action:** Testosterone replacement; ↑ lean body mass, libido **Dose:** All daily *AndroGel:* 5 g gel. *Androderm:* two 2.5-mg or one 5-mg patch qd. *Striant:* 30-mg buccal tabs bid. *Testim:* one 5-g gel tube. *Testoderm:* one 4- or 6-mg scrotal patch **Caution:** [N/A, N/A] **Disp:** *AndroGel, Testim:* 5-gm gel (50-mg test); *Androderm:* 2.5-, 5 -mg patches; *Striant:* 30 -mg buccal tabs; *Testoderm:* 4,- or 6 -mg scrotal patch **SE:** Site Rxns, acne, edema, weight gain, gynecomastia, HTN, ↑ sleep apnea, prostate enlargement **Notes:** Injectable testosterone enanthate (Delatestryl; Testro-L.A.) & cypionate (Depo-Testosterone) require inj every 14–28 d with highly variable serum levels; PO agents (methyltestosterone & oxandrolone) associated w/ hepatitis/hepatic tumors; transdermal/mucosal forms preferred

Tetanus Immune Globulin Uses: *Passive tetanus immunization* (suspected contaminated wound w/ unknown immunization status, see also Table 9, page 226) **Action:** Passive immunization **Dose:** *Adults & Peds.* 250–500 units IM (higher dose w/ delayed Rx) **Caution:** [C, ?] **Contra:** Thimerosal sensitivity **Disp:** Inj 250-unit vial or syringe **SE:** Pain, tenderness, erythema at inj site; fever, angioedema, muscle stiffness, anaphylaxis **Notes:** May begin active immunization series at different inj site if required

Tetanus Toxoid **Uses:** *Tetanus prophylaxis* (See also Table 9, page 226) **Action:** Active immunization **Dose:** Based on previous immunization, Table 9 **Action:** [C, ?] **Contra:** Chloramphenicol use, neurologic Sxs w/ previous use, active Infxn (for routine primary immunization) **Disp:** Inj tetanus toxoid, fluid, 4–5 Lf units/0.5 mL; tetanus toxoid, adsorbed, 5, 10 Lf units/0.5 mL **SE:** Local erythema, induration, sterile abscess; chills, fever, neurologic disturbances

Tetracycline (Achromycin V, Sumycin) **Uses:** *Broad-spectrum antibiotic* **Action:** Bacteriostatic; ↓ protein synthesis. *Spectrum:* Gram(+):*Staph, Strep.* Gram(−):*H. pylori.* Atypicals: *Chlamydia, Rickettsia, & Mycoplasma* **Dose:** *Adults.* 250–500 mg PO bid–qid. *Peds >8 y.* 25–50 mg/kg/24 h PO q6–12h; ↓ in renal/hepatic impair **Caution:** [D, +] **Contra:** PRG, antacids, w/dairy products; children ≤8 y **Disp:** Caps 100, 250, 500 mg; tabs 250, 500 mg; PO susp 250 mg/5 mL **SE** Photosensitivity, GI upset, renal failure, pseudotumor cerebri, hepatic impair **Notes:** Can stain tooth enamel & depress bone formation in children

Thalidomide (Thalomid) **Uses:** *Erythema nodosum leprosum (ENL),* graft-versus-host Dz, aphthous ulceration in HIV(+) pts **Action:** ↓ Neutrophil chemotaxis, ↓ monocyte phagocytosis **Dose:** *GVHD.* 100–1600 mg PO qd. *Stomatitis:* 200 mg bid for 5 d, then 200 mg qd up to 8 wk. *ENL:* 100–300 mg PO qhs **Cautions:** [X, −] May ↑ HIV viral load; Hx Szs **Contra:** PRG; sexually active males not using latex condoms, or females not using 2 forms of contraception **Disp:** 50, 100, 200 mg cap **SE:** Dizziness, drowsiness, rash, fever, orthostasis, Stevens–Johnson syndrome, peripheral neuropathy, Szs **Notes:** MD must register w/ STEPS risk management program; informed consent necessary; immediately D/C if rash develops

Theophylline (Theo24, TheoChron) **Uses:** *Asthma, bronchospasm* **Action:** Relaxes smooth muscle of the bronchi & pulmonary blood vessels **Dose:** *Adults.* 900 mg PO ÷ q6h; SR products may be ÷ q8–12h (maint). *Peds.* 16–22 mg/kg/24 h PO ÷ q6h; SR products may be ÷ q8–12h (maint); ↓ in hepatic failure **Caution:** [C, +] Multiple interactions (eg, caffeine, smoking, carbamazepine, barbiturates, β-blockers, ciprofloxacin, E-mycin, INH, loop diuretics) **Contra:** Arrhythmia, hyperthyroidism, uncontrolled Szs **Disp:** Elixir 80, 15 mL; Solution 80 mg/15 mL; Syrup 80, 150 mg/15 mL caps 100, 200, 250 mg; tabs 100, 125, 200, 250, 300 mg; SR caps 100, 125, 200, 250, 260, 300 mg; SR tabs 100, 200, 300, 400, 450, 600 mg **SE:** N/V, tachycardia, & Szs; nervousness, arrhythmias **Notes:** Follow See levels, Table 2

Thiamine [Vitamin B₁] **Uses:** *Thiamine deficiency (beriberi), alcoholic neuritis, Wernicke encephalopathy* **Action:** Dietary supl **Dose:** *Adults.* Deficiency: 100 mg/d IM for 2 wk, then 5–10 mg/d PO for 1 mo. *Wernicke encephalopathy:* 100 mg IV single dose, then 100 mg/d IM for 2 wk. **Peds.** 10–25 mg/d IM for 2 wk, then 5–10 mg/24 h PO for 1 mo **Caution:** [A (C if doses exceed RDA), +] **Contra:** Component allergy **Disp:** Tabs 5, 10, 25, 50, 100, 250, 500 mg; inj 100, 200 mg/mL **SE:** Angioedema, paresthesias, rash, anaphylaxis w/ rapid IV **Notes:** IV use associated w/ anaphylactic Rxn; give IV slowly

Thiethylperazine (Torecan) **Uses:** *N/V* **Action:** Antidopaminergic antiemetic **Dose:** 10 mg, PO, PR, or IM qd–tid; ↓ in hepatic failure **Caution:** [X, ?] **Contra:** Phenothiazine & sulfite sensitivity, PRG **Disp:** Tabs 10 mg; supp 10 mg; inj 5 mg/mL **SE:** EPS, xerostomia, drowsiness, orthostatic ↓ BP, tachycardia, contusion

6-Thioguanine [6-TG] (Tabloid) **Uses:** *AML, ALL, CML* **Action:** Purine-based antimetabolite (substitutes for natural purines interfering w/ nucleotide synthesis) **Dose:** 2–3 mg/kg/d; ↓ in severe renal/hepatic impair **Caution:** [D, –] **Contra:** Resistance to mercaptopurine **Disp:** Tabs 40 mg **SE:** Myelosuppression (leucopenia/thrombocytopenia), N/V/D, anorexia, stomatitis, rash, hyperuricemia, rare hepatotox

Thioridazine (Mellaril) **WARNING:** Dose-related QT prolongation **Uses:** *Schizophrenia,* psychosis **Action:** Phenothiazine antipsychotic **Dose:** *Adults.* Initial, 50–100 mg PO tid; maint 200–800 mg/24 h PO in 2–4 ÷ doses. *Peds >2 y.* 0.5–3 mg/kg/24 h PO in 2–3 ÷ doses **Caution:** [C, ?] Phenothiazines, QT_c-prolonging agents, aluminum **Contra:** Phenothiazine sensitivity **Disp:** Tabs 10, 15, 25, 50, 100, 150, 200 mg; PO conc 30, 100 mg/mL; **SE:** Low incidence of EPS; ventricular arrhythmias; ↓ BP, dizziness, drowsiness, neuroleptic malignant syndrome, Szs, skin discoloration, photosensitivity, constipation, sexual dysfunction, blood dyscrasias, pigmentary retinopathy, hepatic impair **Notes:** Avoid EtOH, dilute PO conc in 2–4 oz liq

Thiothixene (Navane) **Uses:** *Psychotic disorders* **Action:** Antipsychotic **Dose:** *Adults & Peds >12 y. Mild–moderate psychosis:* 2 mg PO tid, up to 20–30 mg/d. *Severe psychosis:* 5 mg PO bid; ↑ to max of 60 mg/24 h PRN. *IM use:* 16–20 mg/24 h ÷ bid–qid; max 30 mg/d. *Peds <12 y.* 0.25 mg/kg/24 h PO ÷ q6–12h **Caution:** [C, ?] **Contra:** Phenothiazine sensitivity **Disp:** Caps 1, 2, 5, 10, 20 mg; PO conc 5 mg/mL; inj 10 mg/mL **SE:** Drowsiness, EPS most common; ↓ BP, dizziness, drowsiness, neuroleptic malignant syndrome, Szs, skin discoloration, photosensitivity, constipation, sexual dysfunction, blood dyscrasias, pigmentary retinopathy, hepatic impair **Notes:** Dilute PO conc immediately before use

Tiagabine (Gabitril) **Uses:** *Adjunct in Rx of partial Szs,* bipolar disorder **Action:** Inhibition of GABA **Dose:** *Adults & Peds > 12 y.* Initial 4 mg/d PO, ↑ by 4 mg during 2nd wk; ↑ PRN by 4–8 mg/d based on response, 56 mg/d max **Caution:** [C, M] **Contra:** Component allergy **Disp:** Tabs 2, 4, 6, 8, 10, 12, 16 , 20 mg **SE:** Dizziness, HA, somnolence, memory impair, tremors **Notes:** Use gradual withdrawal; used in combo w/ other anticonvulsants

Ticarcillin (Ticar) Uses: Infxns due to gram(–) bacteria (*Klebsiella, Proteus, E. coli, Enterobacter, P. aeruginosa, & Serratia*) involving the skin, bone, resp & urinary tract, abdomen, sepsis Action: 4th-gen PCN, bactericidal; ↓ cell wall synthesis. *Spectrum:* Some gram(+) (strep, fair enterococcus, not MRSA), gram(–); enhanced w/aminoglycoside use, good anaerobes (*Bactericides*) Dose: *Adults.* 3 g IV q4–6h. *Peds.* 200–300 mg/kg/d IV ÷ q4–6h; ↓ w/in renal insuff failure Caution: [B, +] PCN sensitivity, renal impair, Sz hx, Na restriction Contra: Allergy to class Disp: Inj 1, 3, 6, 20, 30 g SE: Interstitial nephritis, anaphylaxis, bleeding, rash, hemolytic anemia Notes: Used in combo w/ aminoglycosides

Ticarcillin/Potassium Clavulanate (Timentin) Uses: *Infxns of the skin, bone, resp & urinary tract, abdomen, sepsis * Action: 4th-gen PCN; bactericidal; ↓ cell wall synthesis; clavulanic acid blocks β-lactamase. *Spectrum:* Good gram(+), not MRSA; good gram(–) & anaerobes Dose: *Adults.* 3.1 g IV q4–6h. *Peds.* 200–300 mg/kg/d IV ÷ q4–6h; ↓ in renal failure Caution: [B, +/–] PCN sensitivity Disp: Inj 3g/1g vial SE: Hemolytic anemia, false + proteinuria Notes: Often used in combo w/ aminoglycosides; penetrates CNS w/ meningeal irritation; see also ticarcillin

Ticlopidine (Ticlid) WARNING: Neutropenia/agranulocytosis, TTP, aplastic anemia reported Uses: *↓ risk of thrombotic stroke,* protect grafts status post CABG, diabetic microangiopathy, ischemic heart Dz, DVT prophylaxis, graft prophylaxis after renal transplant Action: Plt aggregation inhibitor Dose: 250 mg PO bid w/ food Caution: [B, ?/–], ↑ tox of ASA, anticoagulation, NSAIDs, theophylline Contra: Bleeding, hepatic impair, neutropenia, thrombocytopenia Disp: Tabs 250 mg SE: Bleeding, GI upset, rash, ↑ on LFTs Notes: Follow CBC 1st 3 mo

Tigecycline (Tygacil) Uses: *Rx complicated skin & soft tissue Infxns, & complicated intraabdominal Infxns* Action: New class: related to tetracycline; *Spectrum:* Broad gram(+), gram(–), anaerobic, some mycobacterial; *E. coli, Enterococcus faecalis (vanco-susceptible isolates), Staph aureus* (meth-susceptible/resistant), *Strep (agalactiae, anginosus grp, pyogenes), Citrobacter freundii, Enterobacter cloacae, B. fragilis* group, *C. perfringens, Peptostreptococcus* Dose: *Adults.* 100 mg, then 50 mg q12h IV over 30–60 min every 12 h Caution: [D, ?] hepatic impair, monotherapy w/ intestinal perf, not OK in peds Contra: Component sensitivity Disp: Inj 50 mg vial SE: N/V, inj site Rxn

Timolol (Blocadren) WARNING: Exacerbation of ischemic heart Dz w/ abrupt D/C Uses: *HTN & MI* Action: β-adrenergic receptor blocker, β₁, β₂ Dose: *HTN:* 10–20 mg bid, up to 60 mg/d. *MI:* 10 mg bid Caution: [C (1st tri; D if 2nd or 3rd tri), +] Contra: CHF, cardiogenic shock, bradycardia, heart block, COPD, asthma Disp: Tabs 5, 10, 20 mg SE: Sexual dysfunction, arrhythmia, dizziness, fatigue, CHF

Timolol, Ophthalmic (Timoptic) Uses: *Glaucoma* Action: β-Blocker Dose: 0.25% 1 gt bid; ↓ to qd when controlled; use 0.5% if needed; 1 gt/d gel Caution: [C (1st tri; D 2nd or 3rd), ?/+] Disp: Soln 0.25/0.5%; Timoptic XE (0.25, 0.5%) gel-forming soln SE: Local irritation

Tinidazole (Tindamax) **WARNING:** Off-label use discouraged (animal carcinogenicity w/ other drugs in class) **Uses:** *Adults/children >3 y.* * Trichomoniasis & giardiasis; intestinal amebiasis or amebic liver abscess * **Action:** Antiprotozoal nitroimidazole *Spectrum:* Trichomonas vaginalis, Giardia duodenalis, Entamoeba histolytica **Dose:** *Adults.* Trichomoniasis: 2 g PO; treat partner; *Giardiasis:* 2 g PO; *Amebiasis:* 2 g PO qd × 3; *Amebic liver abscess:* 2 g PO qd ×3–5; *Peds.* Trichomoniasis: 50 mg/kg PO, 2 g/day max; *Giardiasis:* 50 mg/kg PO, 2 g max; *Amebiasis:* 50 mg/kg PO qd ×3, 2 g/day max; *Amebic liver abscess:* 50 mg/kg PO qd ×3–5, 2 g/day max (w/food) **Caution:** [C, D in 1st trimester; –] May be cross-resistant with metronidazole; Sz/peripheral neuropathy may require D/C; w/CNS/hepatic impair **Contra:** Metronidazole allergy, 1st trimester PRG, w/ EtOH use **Disp:** Tabs 250, 500 **SE:** CNS disturbances; blood dyscrasias, taste disturbances, N/V, darkens urine **Notes:** D/C EtOH during & 3 d after Rx; potentiates warfarin & lithium; clearance ↓ w/other drugs; crush & disperse in cherry syrup for peds; removed by HD

Tinzaparin (Innohep) **Uses:** *Rx of DVT w/ or w/o PE* **Action:** LMW heparin **Dose:** 175 units/kg SQ qd at least 6 d until warfarin dose stabilized **Caution:** [B, ?] Pork allergy, active bleeding, mild–moderate renal dysfunction **Contra:** Allergy to sulfites, heparin, benzyl alcohol, HIT **Disp:** Inj 20,000 units/mL **SE:** Bleeding, bruising, thrombocytopenia, inj site pain, ↑ LFTs **Notes:** Monitor via Anti-Xa levels; no effect on: bleeding time, plt Fxn, PT, aPTT

Tioconazole (Vagistat) **Uses:** *Vaginal fungal Infxns* **Action:** Topical antifungal **Dose:** 1 applicatorful intravag hs (single dose) **Caution:** [C, ?] **Contra:** Component allergy **Disp:** Vaginal oint 6.5% **SE:** Local burning, itching, soreness, polyuria **Notes:** Insert high into vagina

Tiotropium (Spiriva) **Uses:** *Bronchospasm w/ COPD, bronchitis, emphysema* **Action:** Synthetic anticholinergic like atropine **Dose:** 1 cap/d inhaled using HandiHaler, *do not* use w/ spacer **Caution:** [C, ?/–] BPH, NA glaucoma, MyG, renal impair **Contra:** Acute bronchospasm **Disp:** Inhalation Caps 18 mcg **SE:** URI, xerostomia **Notes:** Monitor FEV_1 or peak flow

Tirofiban (Aggrastat) **Uses:** *Acute coronary syndrome* **Action:** Glycoprotein IIB/IIIa inhibitor **Dose:** Initial 0.4 mcg/kg/min for 30 min, followed 0.1 mcg/kg/min; use in combo w/ heparin; ↓ in renal insuff **Caution:** [B, ?/–] **Contra:** Bleeding, intracranial neoplasm, vascular malformation, stroke/surgery/trauma w/in last 30 d, severe HTN **Disp:** Inj 50, 250 mcg/mL **SE:** Bleeding, bradycardia, coronary dissection, pelvic pain, rash

Tobramycin (Nebcin) **Uses:** *Serious gram(–) Infxns* **Action:** Aminoglycoside, ↓ protein synthesis. *Spectrum:* Gram(–) bacteria (including *Pseudomonas*) **Dose:** *Adults.* 1–2.5 mg/kg/dose IV q8–24h. *Peds.* 2.5 mg/kg/dose IV q8h; ↓ w/ renal insuff **Caution:** [C, M] **Contra:** Aminoglycoside sensitivity **Disp:** Inj 10, 40 mg/mL **SE:** Nephrotox & ototox **Notes:** Follow CrCl & levels for dosage adjustments (Table 2)

Tobramycin Ophthalmic (AKTob, Tobrex) Uses: *Ocular bacterial Infxns* Action: Aminoglycoside Dose: 1–2 gtt q4h; oint bid–tid; if severe, use oint q3–4h, or 2 gtt q30–60min, then less frequently Caution: [C, M] Contra: Aminoglycoside sensitivity Disp: Oint & soln tobramycin 0.3% SE: Ocular irritation

Tobramycin & Dexamethasone Ophthalmic (TobraDex) Uses: *Ocular bacterial Infxns associated w/ significant inflammation* Action: Antibiotic w/ antiinflammatory Dose: 0.3% oint apply q3–8h or soln 0.3% apply 1–2 gtt q1–4h Caution: [C, M] Contra: Aminoglycoside sensitivity Disp: Oint & suspension 2.5, 5 & 10 mL tobramycin 0.3% & dexamethasone 0.1% SE: Local irritation/edema Notes: Use under ophthalmologist's direction

Tolazamide (Tolinase) Uses: *Type 2 DM* Action: Sulfonylurea; ↑ pancreatic insulin release; ↑ peripheral insulin sensitivity; ↓ hepatic glucose output Dose: 100–500 mg/d (no benefit >1 g/d) Caution: [C, +/–] Elderly, hepatic or renal impair Disp: Tabs 100, 250, 500 mg SE: HA, dizziness, GI upset, rash, hyperglycemia, photosensitivity, blood dyscrasias

Tolazoline (Priscoline) Uses: *Peripheral vasospastic disorders* Action: Competitively blocks α-adrenergic receptors Dose: *Adults.* 10–50 mg IM/IV/SQ qid. *Neonates.* 1–2 mg/kg IV over 10–15 min, then 1–2 mg/kg/h (adjust w/ ↓ renal Fxn) Caution: [C, ?] Contra: CAD Disp: Inj 25 mg/mL SE: ↓ BP, peripheral vasodilation, tachycardia, arrhythmias, GI upset & bleeding, blood dyscrasias, renal failure

Tolbutamide (Orinase) Uses: *Type 2 DM* Action: Sulfonylurea; ↑ pancreatic insulin release; ↑ peripheral insulin sensitivity; ↓ hepatic glucose output Dose: 500–1000 mg bid; ↓ in hepatic failure Caution: [C, +] Contra: Sulfonylurea sensitivity Disp: Tabs 250, 500 mg SE: HA, dizziness, GI upset, rash, photosensitivity, blood dyscrasias, hypoglycemia

Tolcapone (Tasmar) Uses: *Adjunct to carbidopa/levodopa in Parkinson Dz* Action: Catechol-*O*-methyltransferase inhibitor slows levodopa metabolism Dose: 100 mg PO w/ first daily levodopa/carbidopa dose, then dose 6 & 12 h later; ↓/w renal impair Caution: [C, ?] Contra: Hepatic impair; w/nonselective MAOI Disp: Tablets 100 mg, 200 mg SE: Constipation, xerostomia, vivid dreams, hallucinations, anorexia, N/D, orthostasis, liver failure Notes: Do not abruptly D/C or ↓ dose; monitor LFTs

Tolmetin (Tolectin) WARNING: May ↑risk of cardiovascular events & GI bleeding Uses: *Arthritis & pain* Action: NSAID; ↓ prostaglandins Dose: 200–600 mg PO tid; 2000 mg/d max Caution: [C (D in 3rd tri or near term), +] Contra: NSAID or ASA sensitivity Disp: Tabs 200, 600 mg; caps 400 mg SE: Dizziness, rash, GI upset, edema, GI bleeding, renal failure

Tolnaftate (Tinactin) [OTC] Uses: *Tinea pedis, cruris, corporis, manus, versicolor* Action: Topical antifungal Dose: Apply to area bid for 2–4 wk Caution: [C, ?] Contra: Nail & scalp Infxns Disp: OTC 1% liq; gel; powder; topical cream; ointment, powder, spray soln SE: Local irritation Notes: Avoid ocular contact, Infxn should improve in 7–10 d

Tolterodine (Detrol, Detrol LA) Uses: *OAB (frequency, urgency, incontinence)* Action: Anticholinergic Dose: Detrol 1–2 mg PO bid; Detrol LA 2–4 mg/d Caution: [C, ?/–] w/ CYP2D6 & 3A3/4 inhibitor (Table 13) Contra: Urinary retention, gastric retention, or uncontrolled NA glaucoma Disp: Tabs 1, 2 mg; Detrol LA tabs 2, 4 mg SE: Xerostomia, blurred vision

Topiramate (Topamax) Uses: *Adjunctive Rx for complex partial Szs & tonic–clonic Szs,* bipolar disorder, neuropathic pain, migraine prophylaxis Action: Anticonvulsant Dose: *Adults.* Seizures: Total dose 400 mg/d; see insert for 8-wk titration schedule. *Migraine prophylaxis:* titrate 100 m/d total *Peds 2–16 y:* Initial, 1–3 mg/kg/d PO qhs; titrate per insert to 5 9 mg/kg/d; ↓ w/ renal impair Caution: [C, ?/–] Contra: Component allergy Disp: Tabs 25, 50, 100, 200 mg; caps sprinkles 15, 25, 50 mg SE: Metabolic acidosis, kidney stones, fatigue, dizziness, psychomotor slowing, memory impair, GI upset, tremor, nystagmus, weight loss, acute secondary glaucoma requiring drug D/C Notes: Metabolic acidosis responsive to ↓ dose or D/C; D/C w/taper

Topotecan (Hycamtin) WARNING: Chemo precautions, BM suppression possible Uses: *Ovarian CA (cisplatin-refractory), small-cell lung CA,* sarcoma, ped non-small-cell lung CA Action: Topoisomerase I inhibitor; ↓DNA synthesis Dose: 1.5 mg/m^2/d as a 1-h IV inf ×5 days, repeat q3wk; ↓ w/renal impair Caution: [D, –] Contra: PRG, breast-feeding Disp: Inj 4-mg vials SE: Myelosuppression, N/V/D, drug fever, skin rash

Torsemide (Demadex) Uses: *Edema, HTN, CHF, & hepatic cirrhosis* Action: Loop diuretic; ↓ reabsorption of Na$^+$ & Cl$^-$ in ascending loop of Henle & distal tubule Dose: 5–20 mg/d PO or IV Caution: [B, ?] Contra: Sulfonylurea sensitivity Disp: Tabs 5, 10, 20, 100 mg; inj 10 mg/mL SE: Orthostatic ↓ BP, HA, dizziness, photosensitivity, electrolyte imbalance, blurred vision, renal impair Notes: 20 mg torsemide = 40 mg furosemide

Tramadol (Ultram) Uses: *Moderate–severe pain* Action: Centrally acting analgesic Dose: *Adults.* 50–100 mg PO q4–6h PRN, 400 mg/d max. *Peds.* 0.5–1 mg/kg PO q 4–6h PRN Caution: [C, ?/–] Contra: Opioid dependency; w/MAOIs; sensitivity to codeine Disp: Tabs 50 mg SE: Dizziness, HA, somnolence, GI upset, resp depression, anaphylaxis Notes: ↓ Sz threshold; tolerance or dependence may develop

Tramadol/Acetaminophen (Ultracet) Uses: *Short-term Rx acute pain (<5 d)* Action: Centrally acting analgesic; nonnarcotic analgesic Dose: 2 tabs PO q4–6h PRN; 8 tabs/d max. *Elderly/renal impair:* Lowest possible dose; 2 tabs q12h max if CrCl <30 Caution: [C, –] Szs, hepatic/renal impair, or Hx addictive tendencies Contra: Acute intox Disp: Tab 37.5 mg tramadol/325 mg APAP SE: SSRIs, TCAs, opioids, MAOIs ↑ risk of Szs; dizziness, somnolence, tremor, HA, N/V/D, constipation, xerostomia, liver tox, rash, pruritus, ↑ sweating, physical dependence Notes: Avoid EtOH

Trandolapril (Mavik) WARNING: Use in PRG in 2nd/3rd tri can result in fetal death **Uses:** *HTN,* CHF, LVD, post-AMI **Action:** ACE inhibitor **Dose:** *HTN:* 2–4 mg/d. *CHF/LVD:* 4 mg/d; ↓ w/severe renal/hepatic impair **Caution:** [D, +] ACE inhibitor sensitivity, angioedema w/ ACE inhibitors **Disp:** Tabs 1, 2, 4 mg **SE:** ↓ BP, bradycardia, dizziness, ↑ K+, GI upset, renal impair, cough, angioedema **Notes:** Afro-Americans, min. dose is 2 mg vs 1 mg in Caucasians

Trastuzumab (Herceptin) **Uses:** *Metastatic breast CAs that overexpress the HER2/neu overexpression protein* breast Ca adjuvant, w/ doxorubicin, cyclophosphamide, and paclitaxel if pt HER2/neu(+)**Action:** MoAb; binds human epidermal GF receptor 2 protein (HER2); mediates cellular cytotox **Dose:** Per protocol **Caution:** [B, ?] CV dysfunction, allergy/inf Rxns **Contra:** None known **Disp:** Inj form 21 mg/mL **SE:** Anemia, cardiomyopathy, nephrotic syndrome, pneumonitis **Notes:** Inf related Rxns minimized w/ acetaminophen, diphenhydramine, & meperidine

Trazodone (Desyrel) **Uses:** *Depression,* hypnotic, augment other antidepressants **Action:** Antidepressant; ↓ reuptake of serotonin & norepinephrine **Dose:** *Adults & Adolescents.* 50–150 mg PO qd–qid; max 600 mg/d. *Sleep:* 50 mg PO, qhs, PRN **Caution:** [C, ?/–] **Contra:** Component allergy **Disp:** Tabs 50, 100, 150, 300 mg **SE:** Dizziness, HA, sedation, nausea, xerostomia, syncope, confusion, tremor, hepatitis, EPS **Notes:** Takes 1–2 wk for symptom improvement; may interact with CYP3A4 inhibitors to ↑trazodone concentrations, carbamazepine to ↓trazodone concentrations

Treprostinil Sodium (Remodulin) **Uses:** *NYHA class II–IV pulmonary arterial HTN* **Action:** Vasodilation, inhibits plt aggregation **Dose:** 0.625–1.25 ng/kg/min inj cont inf **Caution:** [B, ?/–] **Contra:** Component allergy **Disp:** 1, 2.5, 5, 10 mg/mL inj **SE:** Additive effects w/ anticoagulants, antihypertensives; inf site Rxns **Notes:** Initiate in monitored setting; do not D/C or ↓ dose abruptly

Tretinoin, Topical [Retinoic Acid] (Retin-A, Avita, Renova) **Uses:** *Acne vulgaris, sun-damaged skin, wrinkles* (photo aging), some skin CAs **Action:** Exfoliant retinoic acid derivative **Dose:** *Adults & Peds >12 y.* Apply qd hs (w/ irritation, ↓ frequency). *Photoaging:* Start w/ 0.025%, ↑ to 0.1% over several months (apply only q3d if on neck area; dark skin may require bid use) **Caution:** [C, ?] **Contra:** Retinoid sensitivity **Disp:** Cream 0.02, 0.025, 0.05, 0.1%; gel 0.01, 0.025, microformulation gel 0.1, 0.04%; liq 0.05% **SE:** Avoid sunlight; edema; skin dryness, erythema, scaling, changes in pigmentation, stinging, photosensitivity

Triamcinolone (Azmacort) **Uses:** *Chronic asthma* **Actions:** Topical steroid **Dose:** Two inhalations tid–qid or 4 inhal bid **Caution:** [C, ?] **Contra:** Component allergy **Disp:** Aerosol, metered inhaler 100 mcg spray **SE:** Cough, oral candidiasis **Notes:** Instruct pts to rinse mouth after use; not for acute asthma

Triamcinolone & Nystatin (Mycolog-II) Uses: *Cutaneous candidiasis* Action: Antifungal & antiinflammatory Dose: Apply lightly to area bid; max 25 mg/d Caution: [C, ?] Contra: Varicella; systemic fungal Infxns Disp: Cream & oint 15, 30, 60, 120 mg SE: Local irritation, hypertrichosis, pigmentation changes Notes: For short-term use (<7 d)

Triamterene (Dyrenium) Uses: *Edema associated w/ CHF, cirrhosis* Action: K⁺-sparing diuretic Dose: *Adults.* 100–300 mg/24 h PO ÷ qd–bid. *Peds.* 2–4 mg/kg/d in 1–2 ÷ doses; ↓ w/renal/hepatic impair Caution: [B (manufacturer; D, cd, opinion), ?/–] Contra: ↑ K⁺, renal impair, DM; caution w/other K⁺-sparing diuretics Disp: Caps 50, 100 mg SE: ↓ K⁺, blood dyscrasias, liver damage, other Rxns

Triazolam (Halcion) [C-IV] Uses: *Short-term management of insomnia* Action: Benzodiazepine Dose: 0.125–0.25 mg/d PO hs PRN; ↓ in elderly Caution: [X, ?/–] Contra: NA glaucoma, cirrhosis; concurrent amprenavir, ritonavir, or nelfinavir Disp: Tabs 0.125, 0.25 mg SE: Tachycardia, CP, drowsiness, fatigue, memory impair, GI upset Notes: Additive CNS depression w/ EtOH & other CNS depressants

Triethanolamine (Cerumenex) [OTC] Uses: *Cerumen (ear wax) removal* Action: Ceruminolytic agent Dose: Fill ear canal & insert cotton plug; irrigate w/ H₂O after 15 min; repeat PRN Caution: [C, ?] Contra: Perforated tympanic membrane, otitis media Disp: Soln 10, 16, 12 mL SE: Local dermatitis, pain, erythema, pruritus

Triethylenetriphosphamide (Thio-Tepa, Tespa, TSPA) Uses: *Hodgkin Dz & NHLs; leukemia; breast, ovarian CA's), preparative regimens for allogeneic & ABMT w/ high doses, intravesical for bladder CA* Action: Polyfunctional alkylating agent Dose: 0.5 mg/kg q1–4wk, 6 mg/m² IM or IV × 4 d q2–4wk, 15–35 mg/m² by cont IV inf over 48 h; 60 mg into the bladder & retained 2 h q1–4wk; 900–125 mg/m² in ABMT regimens (highest dose w/o ABMT is 180 mg/m²); 1–10 mg/m² (typically 15 mg) IT 1 or 2 X/wk; 0.8 mg/kg in 1–2 L of soln may be instilled intraperitoneally; ↓ in renal failure Caution: [D, –] Contra: Component allergy Disp: Inj 15, 30 mg SE: Myelosuppression, N/V, dizziness, HA, allergy, paresthesias, alopecia Notes: Intravesical use in bladder Ca infrequent today

Trifluoperazine (Stelazine) Uses: *Psychotic disorders* Action: Phenothiazine; blocks postsynaptic CNS dopaminergic receptors Dose: *Adults.* 2–10 mg PO bid. *Peds 6–12 y.* 1 mg PO qd–bid initial, gradually ↑ to 15 mg/d; ↓ in elderly/debilitated pts Caution: [C, ?/–] Contra: Hx blood dyscrasias; phenothiazine sensitivity Disp: Tabs 1, 2, 5, 10 mg; PO conc 10 mg/mL; inj 2 mg/mL SE: Orthostatic ↓ BP, EPS, dizziness, neuroleptic malignant syndrome, skin discoloration, lowered Sz threshold, photosensitivity, blood dyscrasias Notes: PO conc must be diluted to 60 mL or more prior to administration; requires several weeks for onset of effects

Trifluridine Ophthalmic (Viroptic) Uses: *Herpes simplex keratitis & conjunctivitis* Action: Antiviral Dose: 1 gt q2h (max 9 gtt/d); ↓ to 1 gt q4h after healing begins; Rx up to 14 d Caution: [C, M] Contra: Component allergy Disp: Soln 1% SE: Local burning, stinging

Trihexyphenidyl (Artane) Uses: *Parkinson Dz* Action: Blocks excess acetylcholine at cerebral synapses Dose: 2–5 mg PO qd–qid Caution: [C, +] Contra: NA glaucoma, GI obstruction, MyG, bladder obstructions Disp: Tabs 2, 5 mg; SR caps 5 mg; elixir 2 mg/5 mL SE: Dry skin, constipation, xerostomia, photosensitivity, tachycardia, arrhythmias

Trimethobenzamide (Tigan) Uses: *N/V* Action: ↓ medullary chemoreceptor trigger zone Dose: Adults. 250 mg PO or 200 mg PR or IM tid–qid PRN. Peds. 20 mg/kg/24 h PO or 15 mg/kg/24 h PR or IM in 3–4 ÷ doses Caution: [C, ?] Contra: Benzocaine sensitivity Disp: Caps 100, 250 mg; supp 100, 200 mg; inj 100 mg/mL SE: Drowsiness, ↓ BP, dizziness; hepatic impair, blood dyscrasias, Szs, parkinsonian-like syndrome Notes: In the presence of viral Infxns, may mask emesis or mimic CNS effects of Reye's syndrome

Trimethoprim (Trimpex, Proloprim) Uses: *UTI due to susceptible gram(+) & gram(–) organisms;* suppression of UTI Action: ↓ dihydrofolate reductase. Spectrum: Many gram(+) & (–) except Bacteroides, Branhamella, Brucella, Chlamydia, Clostridium, Mycobacterium, Mycoplasma, Nocardia, Neisseria, Pseudomonas, & Treponema Dose: Adults. 100 mg/d PO bid or 200 m;g/d PO. Peds. 4 mg/kg/d in 2 ÷ doses; w/renal failure Caution: [C, +] Contra: Megaloblastic anemia due to folate deficiency Disp: Tabs 100, 200 mg; PO soln 50 mg/5 mL SE: Rash, pruritus, megaloblastic anemia, hepatic impair, blood dyscrasias Notes: Take w/ plenty of H₂O

Trimethoprim (TMP)–Sulfamethoxazole (SMX) [Co-Trimoxazole] (Bactrim, Septra) Uses: *UTI Rx & prophylaxis, otitis media, sinusitis, bronchitis* Action: SMX ↓ synthesis of dihydrofolic acid;, TMP ↓ dihydrofolate reductase to impair protein synthesis. Spectrum: Includes Shigella, P. jiroveci (formerly carinii), & Nocardia Infxns, Mycoplasma, Enterobacter sp, Staph, Strep, & more Dose: Adults. 1 DS tab PO bid or 5–20 mg/kg/24 h (based on TMP) IV in 3–4 ÷ doses. P. jiroveci: 15–20 mg/kg/d IV or PO (TMP) in 4 ÷ doses. Nocardia: 10–15 mg/kg/d IV or PO (TMP) in 4 ÷ doses. UTI prophylaxis: 1 PO qd. Peds. 8–10 mg/kg/24 h (TMP) PO ÷ into 2 doses or 3–4 doses IV; do not use in newborns; ↓ in renal failure; maintain hydration Caution: [B (D if near term), +] Contra: Sulfonamide sensitivity, porphyria, megaloblastic anemia w/ folate deficiency, significant hepatic impair Disp: Regular tabs 80 mg TMP/400 mg SMX; DS tabs 160 mg TMP/800 mg SMX; PO susp 40 mg TMP/200 mg SMX/5 mL; inj 80 mg TMP/ 400 mg SMX/5 mL SE: Allergic skin Rxns, photosensitivity, GI upset, Stevens–Johnson syndrome, blood dyscrasias, hepatitis Notes: Synergistic combo, interacts w/ warfarin

Trimetrexate (Neutrexin) WARNING: Must be used w/ leucovorin to avoid tox Uses: *Moderate–severe PCP* Action: ↓ dihydrofolate reductase Dose:

45 mg/m^2 IV q24h for 21 d; administer w/ leucovorin 20 mg/m^2 IV q6h for 24 d; ↓ in hepatic impair **Caution:** [D, ?/–] **Contra:** MTX sensitivity **Disp:** Inj 25, 200 mg/25 mg/vial **SE:** Sz, fever, rash, GI upset, anemias, ↑ LFTs, peripheral neuropathy, renal impair **Notes:** Use cytotoxic cautions; inf over 60 min

Triptorelin (Trelstar Depot, Trelstar LA) Uses: *Palliation of advanced CAP* **Action:** LHRH analog; ↓ GNRH w/ continuous dosing; transient ↑ in LH, FSH, testosterone, & estradiol 7–10 d after first dose; w/ chronic/continuous use (usually 2–4 wk), sustained ↓ LH & FSH w/ ↓ testicular & ovarian steroidogenesis similar to surgical castration **Dose:** 3.75 mg IM monthly or 11.25 mg IM q3mo **Caution:** [X, N/A] **Contra:** Not indicated in females **Disp:** Inj depot 3.75 mg; LA 11.25 mg **SE:** Dizziness, emotional lability, fatigue, HA, insomnia, HTN, D, vomiting, ED, retention, UTI, pruritus, anemia, inj site pain, musculoskeletal pain, osteoporosis, allergic Rxns

Trospium Chloride (Sanctura) Uses: *OAB* **Action:** Antimuscarinic, antispasmodic **Dose:** 20 mg PO bid, ↓ w/renal impair or >75 y; on empty stomach or 1 h ac **Caution:** [C, ?/–] BOO, GI obstruction, ulcerative colitis, MyG, renal/hepatic impair **Contra:** NA glaucoma, urinary/gastric retention **Disp:** Tabs 20 mg **SE:** Constipation, xerostomia

Trovafloxacin (Trovan) WARNING: Trovan has been associated w/ serious liver injury leading to need for liver transplantation &/or deaths Uses: *Life-threatening Infxns* including pneumonia, complicated intraabdominal, gynecologic/pelvic, or skin Infxns **Action:** Fluoroquinolone antibiotic; ↓ DNA gyrase. *Spectrum:* Broad spectrum gram(+) & gram(–), including anaerobes; TB typically resistant **Dose:** ↓ w/hepatic impair **Caution:** [C, –] in children **Contra:** Hepatic impair **Disp:** Inj 5 mg/mL in 40 & 60 mL; tabs 100, 200 mg **SE:** Liver failure, dizziness, HA, nausea, rash **Notes:** Use restricted to hospitals; hepatotox led to restricted availability

Urokinase (Abbokinase) Uses: *PE, DVT, restore patency to IV catheters* **Action:** Converts plasminogen to plasmin; causes clot lysis **Dose:** *Adults & Peds.* Systemic effect: 4,400 units/kg IV over 10 min, then 4,400–6,000 units/kg/h for 12 h. *Restore catheter patency:* Inject 5,000 units into catheter & aspirate **Caution:** [B, ↑] **Contra:** Do not use w/in 10 d of surgery, delivery, or organ biopsy; bleeding, CVA, vascular malformation **Disp:** Powder for inj, 250,000-unit vial **SE:** Bleeding, ↓ BP, dyspnea, bronchospasm, anaphylaxis, cholesterol embolism

Valacyclovir (Valtrex) Uses: *Herpes zoster; genital herpes* **Action:** Prodrug of acyclovir; ↓ viral DNA replication. *Spectrum:* Herpes simplex I & II **Dose:** 1 g PO tid. *Genital herpes:* 500 mg bid × 7 × 7 d. *Herpes prophylaxis:* 500–1000 mg/d; ↓ w/renal failure **Caution:** [B, +] **Disp:** Caplets 500, 1000 mg **SE:** HA, GI upset, dizziness, pruritus, photophobia

Valdecoxib (Bextra) Uses: *RA, osteoarthritis, primary dysmenorrhea* **Action:** COX-2 inhibition **Dose:** *Arthritis:* 10 mg PO qd. *Dysmenorrhea:* 20 mg

PO bid, PRN **Caution:** [C, ?] Asthma, urticaria, allergic-type reactions after ASA or NSAID ~~use Contra: Allergy Disp: Tabs 200 mg SE:~~ GI irritation or bleeding; dizziness, edema, HTN, HA, peptic ulcer, renal failure; serious allergic reactions have occurred, including Stevens–Johnson syndrome

Valganciclovir (Valcyte)   **Uses:** *CMV* **Action:** Ganciclovir prodrug; ↓ viral DNA synthesis **Dose:** Induction, 900 mg PO bid w/ food × 21 d, then 900 mg PO qd; ↓ in renal dysfunction **Caution:** [C, ?/–] Use w/ imipenem/cilastatin, nephrotoxic drugs **Contra:** Allergy to acyclovir, ganciclovir, valganciclovir; ANC < 500/mm²; plt <25 K; Hgb < 8 g/dL **Disp:** Tabs 450 mg **SE:** BM suppression **Notes:** Monitor CBC & Cr

Valproic Acid (Depakene, Depakote)   **Uses:** *Rx epilepsy, mania; prophylaxis of migraines,* Alzheimer behavior disorder **Action:** Anticonvulsant; ↑ availability of GABA **Dose:** *Adults & Peds.* Szs: 30–60 mg/kg/24 h PO ÷ tid (after initiation of 10–15 mg/kg/24 h). *Mania:* 750 mg in 3 ÷ doses, ↑ 60 mg/kg/d max. *Migraines:* 250 mg bid, ↑ 1000 mg/d max; ↓ w/ hepatic impair **Caution:** [D, +] **Contra:** Severe hepatic impair **Disp:** Caps 250 mg; syrup 250 mg/5 mL **SE:** Somnolence, dizziness, GI upset, diplopia, ataxia, rash, thrombocytopenia, hepatitis, pancreatitis, prolonged bleeding times, alopecia, weight gain, hyperammonemic encephalopathy reported in pts w/ urea cycle disorders **Notes:** Monitor LFTs & serum levels (Table 2); phenobarbital & phenytoin may alter levels

Valsartan (Diovan)   **WARNING:** Use during 2nd/3rd tri of PRG can cause fetal harm **Uses:** HTN, CHF, DN **Action:** Angiotensin II receptor antagonist **Dose:** 80–160 mg/d **Caution:** [C (1st tri); D 2nd & 3rd tri), ?/–] W/ K⁺-sparing diuretics or K⁺ supls **Contra:** Severe hepatic impair, biliary cirrhosis/obstruction, primary hyperaldosteronism, bilateral renal artery stenosis **Disp:** tabs 40, 80, 160, 320 mg **SE:** ↓ BP, dizziness

Vancomycin (Vancocin, Vancoled)   **Uses:** *Serious MRSA Infxns; enterococcal Infxns; PO Rx of C. difficile pseudomembranous colitis* **Action:** ↓ Cell wall synthesis. **Spectrum:** Gram(+) bacteria & some anaerobes (includes MRSA, *Staphylococcus* sp, *Enterococcus* sp, *Streptococcus* sp, *C. difficile*) **Dose:** *Adults.* 1 g IV q12h; for colitis 125–500 mg PO q6h. *Peds.* 40–60 mg/kg/24 h IV in ÷ doses q6–12 h. *Neonates.* 10–15 mg/kg/dose q12h; ↓ in renal insuff **Caution:** [C, M] **Contra:** Component allergy; w/ avoid in Hx hearing loss **Disp:** Caps 125, 250 mg; powder 250 mg/5 mL, 500 mg/6 mL for PO soln; powder for inj 500 mg, 1000 mg, 10 g/vial **SE:** Ototoxic & nephrotoxic, GI upset (PO), neutropenia **Notes:** See drug levels (Table 2, page 210); not absorbed PO, local effect in gut only; give IV dose slowly (over 1–3 h) to prevent "red-man syndrome" (red flushing of head, neck, upper torso); IV product may be given PO for colitis

Vardenafil (Levitra)   **WARNING:** May prolong QT_c interval **Uses:** *ED* **Action:** PDE5 inhibitor, increases cGMP and NO levels Relaxes smooth muscles, dilates cavernosal arteries **Dose:** 10 mg PO 60 min before sexual activity; 2.5 mg if administered w/ CYP3A4 inhibitors (Table 13); max × 1 ≤20 mg **Caution:** [B, –] W/ CV, hepatic, or renal Dz **Contra:** Nitrates, ↑ Qtc interval **Disp:** Tabs 2.5-, 5-, 10-, 20-mg tabs **SE:** ↓ BP, HA, dyspepsia, priapism **Notes:** Concomitant α-blockers may cause ↓ BP

Varenicline (Chantix) Uses: *Smoking cessation* **Action:** Nicotine receptor antagonist **Dose:** *Adults.* 0.5 mg PO daily × 3 d, 0.5 mg bid × 4 d, then 1 mg PO BID for 12 wks total; after meal w/ glass of water **Caution:** [C,?/–] ↓ dose w/renal impair **Disp:** Tabs 0.5, 1 mg **SE:** N, V, insomnia, flatulence, unusual dreams **Notes:** Slowly ↑ dose to ↓ N; initiate 1 wk before desired smoking cessation date

Varicella Virus Vaccine (Varivax) Uses: *Prevent varicella (chickenpox)* **Action:** Active immunization; live attenuated virus **Dose:** *Adults & Peds.* 0.5 mL SQ, repeat 4–8 wk **Caution:** [C, M] **Contra:** Immunocompromise; neomycin-anaphylactoid Rxn, blood dyscrasias; immunosuppressive drugs; avoid PRG for 3 mo after **Disp:** Powder for inj **SE:** Mild varicella Infxn; fever, local Rxns, irritability, GI upset **Notes:** OK for all children & adults who have not had chickenpox

Vasopressin [Antidiuretic Hormone, ADH] (Pitressin) Uses: *DI; Rx postop abdominal distension*; adjunct Rx of GI bleeding & esophageal varices; asystole and PEA pulseless VT & VF, adjunct systemic vasopressor (IV drip) **Action:** Posterior pituitary hormone, potent GI and peripheral vasoconstrictor **Dose:** *Adults & Peds.* DI: 2.5–10 units SQ or IM tid–qid. *GI hemorrhage.* 0.2–0.4 units/min; ↓ in cirrhosis; caution in vascular Dz. *VT/VF:* 40 units IVP X1. *Vasopressor:* 0.01–0.1 units/kg/min **Caution:** [B, +] **Contra:** Allergy **Disp:** Inj 20 units/mL **SE:** HTN, arrhythmias, fever, vertigo, GI upset, tremor **Notes:** Addition of vasopressor to concurrent norepinephrine or epi infs

Vecuronium (Norcuron) Uses: *Skeletal muscle relaxation during surgery or mechanical ventilation* **Action:** Nondepolarizing neuromuscular blocker **Dose:** *Adults & Peds.* 0.08–0.1 mg/kg IV bolus; maint 0.010–0.015 mg/kg after 25–40 min; additional doses q12–15 min PRN; ↓ in severe renal/hepatic impair **Caution:** [C, ?] Drug interactions cause ↑ effect (eg, aminoglycosides, tetracycline, succinylcholine) **Disp:** Powder for inj 10, 20 mg **SE:** Bradycardia, ↓ BP, itching, rash, tachycardia, CV collapse **Notes:** Fewer cardiac effects than pancuronium

Venlafaxine (Effexor) **WARNING:** Closely monitor for worsening depression or emergence of suicidality, particularly in ped pts Uses: *Depression, generalized anxiety,* social anxiety disorder; obsessive–compulsive disorder, chronic fatigue syndrome, ADHD, autism **Action:** Potentiation of CNS neurotransmitter activity **Dose:** 75–375 mg/d ÷ into 2–3 equal doses; ↓ w/renal/hepatic impair **Caution:** [C, ?/–] **Contra:** MAOIs **Disp:** Tabs 25, 37.5, 50, 75, 100 mg; ER caps 37.5, 75, 150 mg **SE:** HTN, ↑ HR, HA, somnolence, GI upset, sexual dysfunction; actuates mania or Szs **Notes:** Avoid EtOH

Verapamil (Calan, Isoptin) Uses: *Angina, HTN, PSVT, AF, atrial flutter,* migraine prophylaxis, hypertrophic cardiomyopathy, bipolar Dz **Action:** CCB **Dose:** *Adults. Arrhythmias:* 2nd line for PSVT w/ narrow QRS complex & adequate BP 2.5–5 mg IV over 1–2 min; repeat 5–10 mg in 15–30 min PRN (30 mg max). *Angina:* 80–120 mg PO tid, ↑ 480 mg/24 h max. *HTN:* 80–180 mg PO tid or SR tabs 120–240 mg PO qd to 240 mg bid. *Peds.* <1 y: 0.1–0.2 mg/kg IV over 2 min (may repeat in 30 min). *1–16 y:* 0.1–0.3 mg/kg IV over 2 min (may repeat in 30 min); 5 mg max. *PO:* *1–5 y:* 4–8 mg/kg/d in 3 ÷ doses. >5 y: 80 mg q6–8h; ↓ in renal/hepatic impair **Caution:** [C, +] Amiodarone/β-blockers/flecainide can cause bradycardia; statins, midazolam, tacrolimus, theophylline levels may be ↑ **Contra:** Conduction disorders, cardiogenic shock; caution w/ elderly pts **Disp:** Tabs 40, 80, 120 mg; SR tabs 120, 180, 240 mg; SR caps 120, 180, 240, 360 mg; inj 5 mg/2 mL **SE:** Gingival hyperplasia, constipation, ↓ BP, bronchospasm, heart rate or conduction disturbances

Vinblastine (Velban, Velbe) WARNING: Chemotherapeutic agent; handle w/ caution Uses: *Hodgkin Dz & NHLs, mycosis fungoides, CAs (testis, renal cell, breast, non-small-cell lung, AIDS-related Kaposi sarcoma,* choriocarcinoma), histiocytosis **Action:** ↓ microtubule assembly **Dose:** 0.1–0.5 mg/kg/wk (4–20 mg/m²); ↓ in hepatic failure **Caution:** [D, ?] **Contra:** Intrathecal use **Disp:** Inj 1 mg/mL in 10 mg vial **SE:** Myelosuppression (especially leukopenia), N/V, constipation, neurotox, alopecia, rash, myalgia, tumor pain

Vincristine (Oncovin, Vincasar PFS) WARNING: Chemotherapeutic agent; handle w/ caution; Fatal if administered intrathecally Uses: *ALL, breast & small-cell lung CA, sarcoma (eg, Ewing tumor, rhabdomyosarcoma), Wilms' tumor, Hodgkin Dz & NHLs, neuroblastoma, multiple myeloma* **Action:** Promotes disassembly of mitotic spindle, causing metaphase arrest **Dose:** 0.4–1.4 mg/m² (single doses 2 mg/max); ↓ in hepatic failure **Caution:** [D, ?] **Contra:** Intrathecal use **Disp:** Inj 1 mg/mL, 5 mg vial **SE:** Neurotox commonly dose limiting, jaw pain (trigeminal neuralgia), fever, fatigue, anorexia, constipation & paralytic ileus, bladder atony; no significant myelosuppression w/ standard doses; tissue necrosis w/ extravasation

Vinorelbine (Navelbine) WARNING: Chemotherapeutic agent; handle w/ caution Uses: *Breast & non-small-cell lung CA* (alone or w/ cisplatin) **Action:** ↓ polymerization of microtubules, impairing mitotic spindle formation; semisynthetic vinca alkaloid **Dose:** 30 mg/m²/wk; ↓ in hepatic failure **Caution:** [D, ?] **Contra:** Intrathecal use **Disp:** Inj 10 mg/mL **SE:** Myelosuppression (leukopenia), mild GI effects, infrequent neurotox (6–29%); constipation & paresthesias (rare); tissue damage from extravasation

Vitamin B₁ See Thiamine (page 184)
Vitamin B₆ See Pyridoxine (page 164)
Vitamin B₁₂ See Cyanocobalamin (page 65)
Vitamin K See Phytonadione (page 157)
Vitamin, multi See Multivitamins (Table 15, page 233)

Voriconazole (VFEND) Uses: *Invasive aspergillosis, serious fungal Infxns* Action: ↓ ergosterol synthesis. *Spectrum:* Several types of fungus: *Aspergillus, Scedosporium* sp, *Fusarium* sp Dose: *Adults & Peds ≥ 12 y. IV:* 6 mg/kg q12h × 2, then 4 mg/kg bid; may ↓ to 3 mg/kg dose. *PO:* <40 kg: 100 mg q12h, up to 150 mg; >40 kg: 200 mg q 12 h, up to 300 mg; ↓ w/mild–moderate hepatic impair; IV only one dose w/ renal impair (PO empty stomach) Caution: [D, ?/–] Contra: Severe hepatic impair Disp: Tabs 50, 200 mg; susp 200 mg/5 mL; 200 mg inj SE: Visual changes, fever, rash, GI upset, ↑ LFTs Notes: Screen for multiple drug interactions (eg, ↑ dose w/ phenytoin)

Warfarin (Coumadin) Uses: *Prophylaxis & Rx of PE & DVT, AF w/ embolization,* other postop indications Action: ↓ Vitamin K-dependent clotting factors in order: VII-IX-X-II Dose: *Adults.* Titrate, INR 2.0–3.0 for most; mechanical valves INR is 2.5–3.5. *ACCP guidelines:* 5 mg initial (unless rapid therapeutic INR needed), may use 7.5–10 mg; ↓ if pt elderly or w/has other bleeding risk factors. *Alternative:* 10 15 mg PO, IM, or IV qd for 1–3 d; maint 2–10 mg/d PO, IV, or IM; follow daily INR initial to adjust dosage (see Table 10, page 227). *Peds.* 0.05–0.34 mg/kg/24 h PO, IM, or IV; follow PT/INR to adjust dosage; monitor vitamin K intake; ↓ w/hepatic impair/elderly Caution: [X, +] Contra: Severe hepatic/renal Dz, bleeding, peptic ulcer, PRG Disp: Tabs 1, 2, 2.5, 3, 4, 5, 6, 7.5, 10 mg; inj SE: Bleeding due to overanticoagulation (PT >3× control or INR >5.0–6.0) or injury & INR w/in therapeutic range; bleeding, alopecia, skin necrosis, purple toe syndrome Notes: Monitor vitamin K intake as may ↓ effect; INR preferred test; to rapidly correct overanticoagulation, use vitamin K, FFP or both; highly teratogenic; do *not* use in PRG. Caution pt on taking w/ other meds, especially ASA *Common warfarin interactions:* Potentiated by: APAP, EtOH (w/ liver Dz), amiodarone, cimetidine, ciprofloxacin, cotrimoxazole, erythromycin, fluconazole, flu vaccine, isoniazid, itraconazole, metronidazole, omeprazole, phenytoin, propranolol, quinidine, tetracycline. *Inhibited by:* barbiturates, carbamazepine, chlordiazepoxide, cholestyramine, dicloxacillin, nafcillin, rifampin, sucralfate, high–vitamin K foods

Zafirlukast (Accolate) Uses: *Adjunctive Rx of asthma* Action: Selective & competitive inhibitor of leukotrienes Dose: Adults & Peds ≥ 12 y. 20 mg bid. Peds 5–11 y. 10 mg PO bid (empty stomach) Caution: [B, –] Interacts w/ warfarin, ↑ INR Contra: Component allergy Disp: Tabs 10, 20 mg SE: Hepatic dysfunction, usually reversible on D/C; HA, dizziness, GI upset; Churg–Strauss syndrome Notes: Not for acute asthma

Zalcitabine (Hivid) WARNING: Use w/ caution in pts w/ neuropathy, pancreatitis, lactic acidosis, hepatitis Uses: *HIV* Action: Antiretroviral agent Dose: *Adults.* 0.75 mg PO tid. *Peds.* 0.015–0.04 mg/kg PO q 6h; ↓ in renal failure Caution: [C, +] Contra: Component allergy Disp: Tabs 0.375, 0.75 mg SE: Peripheral neuropathy, pancreatitis, fever, malaise, anemia, hypo/hyperglycemia, hepatic impair Notes: May be used in combo w/ zidovudine

Zaleplon (Sonata) [C-IV] Uses: *Insomnia* Action: A nonbenzodiazepine sedative/hypnotic, a pyrazolopyrimidine Dose: 5–20 mg hs PRN; ↓ w/renal/hepatic insuff, elderly Caution: [C, ?/–] w/ mental/psychological conditions Contra: Component allergy Disp: Caps 5, 10 mg SE: HA, edema, amnesia, somnolence, photosensitivity Notes: Take immediately before desired onset

Zanamivir (Relenza) Uses: *Influenza A & B* Action: ↓ viral neuraminidase Dose: *Adults & Peds >7 y.* 2 inhal (10 mg) bid for 5 d; initiate w/in 48 h of Sxs Caution: [C, M] Contra: Pulmonary Dz Disp: Powder for inhal 5 mg SE: Bronchospasm, HA, GI upset Notes: Uses a Diskhaler for administration

Ziconotide (Prialt) WARNING: Psychiatric, cognitive, neurologic impair may develop over several weeks; monitor frequently; may necessitate D/C Uses: *IT Rx of severe, refractory, chronic pain* Action: N-type CCB in spinal cord Dose: 2.6 mcg/d IT at 0.1 mcg/h; may ↑ 0.8 mcg/h to total 19.2 mcg/d by day 21 Caution: [C, ?/–] Reversible psychiatric/neurologic impair Contra: Psychosis Disp: Inj 25, 100 mg/mL SE: Dizziness, N/V, confusion, abnormal vision; may require dosage adjustment Notes: May D/C abruptly; uses specific pumps; do not ↑ more frequently than 2–3 ×/wk

Zidovudine (Retrovir) WARNING: Neutropenia, anemia, lactic acidosis, & hepatomegaly w/ steatosis Uses: *HIV Infxn, prevention of maternal HIV transmission of HIV* Action: ↓ RT Dose: *Adults.* 200 mg PO tid or 300 mg PO bid or 1–2 mg/kg/dose IV q4h. *PRG:* 100 mg PO 5X/d until labor starts; during labor 2 mg/kg over 1 h followed by 1 mg/kg/h until clamping of the cord. *Peds.* 160 mg/m²/dose q8h; ↓ in renal failure Caution: [C, ?/–] Contra: Allergy Disp: Caps 100 mg; tabs 300 mg; syrup 50 mg/5 mL; inj 10 mg/mL SE: Hematologic tox, HA, fever, rash, GI upset, malaise

Zidovudine & Lamivudine (Combivir) WARNING: Neutropenia, anemia, lactic acidosis, & hepatomegaly w/ steatosis Uses: *HIV Infxn* Action: Combo of RT inhibitors Dose: *Adults & Peds >12 y.* 1 tab PO bid; ↓ in renal failure Caution: [C, ?/–] Contra: Component allergy Disp: Caps zidovudine 300 mg/lamivudine 150 mg SE: Hematologic tox, HA, fever, rash, GI upset, malaise, pancreatitis Notes: Combo product ↓ daily pill burden

Zileuton (Zyflo) Uses: *Chronic Rx of asthma* Action: Inhibitor of 5-lipoxygenase Dose: *Adults & Peds ≥ 12 y.* 600 mg PO qid Caution: [C, ?/–] Contra: Hepatic impair Disp: Tabs 600 mg SE: Hepatic damage, HA, GI upset, leukopenia Notes: Monitor LFTs every month × 3, then q2–3 mo; take on regular basis; not for acute asthma

Ziprasidone (Geodon) WARNING: ↑ mortality in elderly with dementia-related psychosis Uses: *Schizophrenia, acute agitation* Action: Atypical antipsychotic Dose: 20 mg PO bid, may ↑ in 2-d intervals up to 80 mg bid; agitation 10–20 mg IM PRN up to 40 mg/d; separate 10 mg doses by 2 h & 20 mg doses by 4h (w/ food) Caution: [C, –] w/ ↓ Mg²⁺, ↓ K⁺ Contra: QT prolongation, recent MI, uncompensated heart failure, meds that ↑ QT interval Disp: Caps 20, 40, 60,

80 mg; susp 10 mg/mL; Inj 20 mg/mL; suspension 10 mg/mL **SE:** Bradycardia; rash, somnolence, resp disorder, EPS, weight gain, orthostatic ↓ BP **Notes:** Monitor electrolytes

Zoledronic Acid (Zometa) Uses: *↑ Ca^{2+} of malignancy (HCM),* ↓ skeletal-related events in CAP, multiple myeloma, & metastatic bone lesions **Action:** Bisphosphonate; ↓ osteoclastic bone resorption **Dose:** *HCM:* 4 mg IV over at least 15 min; may retreat in 7 d if adequate renal Fxn. *Bone lesions/myeloma:* 4 mg IV over at least 15 min, repeat q3–4wk PRN; prolonged w/ Cr ↑ **Caution:** [C, ?/–] Loop diuretics, aminoglycosides; ASA-sensitive asthmatics; avoid invasive dental procedures in cancer patients; renal dysfunction **Contra:** Bisphosphonate allergy; w/dental procedures **Disp:** Vial 4 mg **SE:** all are adverse effects ↑ w/ renal dysfunction; fever, flulike syndrome, GI upset, insomnia, anemia; electrolyte abnormalities, osteonecrosis of jaw **Notes:** Requires vigorous prehydration; do not exceed recommended doses/inf duration to ↓ dose-related renal dysfunction; follow Cr; effect prolonged w/ Cr ↑; avoid oral surgery; dental examination recommended prior to therapy; ↓dose w/ renal dysfunction

Zolmitriptan (Zomig, Zomig XMT, Zomig Nasal) Uses: *Acute Rx migraine* **Action:** Selective serotonin agonist; causes vasoconstriction **Dose:** Initial 2.5 mg PO, may repeat after 2 h, 10 mg max in 24 h; nasal 5 mg; HA returns, repeated after 2 h 10 mg max 24 h **Caution:** [C, ?/–] **Contra:** Ischemic heart Dz, Prinzmetal angina, uncontrolled HTN, accessory conduction pathway disorders, ergots, MAOIs **Disp:** Tabs 2.5, 5 mg; Rapid tabs (ZMT) 2.5, 5 mg, nasal 5.0 mg. **SE:** Dizziness, hot flashes, paresthesias, chest tightness, myalgia, diaphoresis

Zolpidem (Ambien, Ambien CR) [C-IV] Uses: *Short-term Rx of insomnia* **Action:** Hypnotic agent **Dose:** 5–10 mg or 12.5 mg CR PO hs PRN; ↓ in elderly (use 6.25 mg CR), hepatic insuff **Caution:** [B, –] **Contra:** Breast-feeding **Disp:** Tabs 5, 10 mg; CR 6.25, 12.5 mg **SE:** HA, dizziness, drowsiness, nausea, myalgia **Notes:** May be habit-forming; CR delivers a rapid then a longer lasting dose

Zonisamide (Zonegran) Uses: *Adjunct Rx complex partial Szs* **Action:** Anticonvulsant **Dose:** Initial 100 mg/d PO; may ↑ to 400 mg/d **Caution:** [C, –] ↑ tox w/ CYP3A4 inhibitor; ↓ levels w/ concurrent carbamazepine, phenytoin, phenobarbital, valproic acid **Contra:** Allergy to sulfonamides; oligohydrosis & hypothermia in peds **Disp:** Caps 25, 50, 100 mg **SE:** Dizziness, drowsiness, confusion, ataxia, memory impair, paresthesias, psychosis, nystagmus, diplopia, tremor; anemia, leukopenia, GI upset, nephrolithiasis, Stevens–Johnson syndrome; monitor for ↓ sweating & ↑ body temperature **Notes:** Swallow capsules whole

Zoster vaccine, live (Zostavax) Uses: * Prevent varicella zoster in adults > 60 yrs* **Action:** Active immunization (live vaccine), to Herpes zoster **Dose:** *Adults.* 0.65 mL SQ **Contra:** Gelatin, neomycin anaphylaxis; untreated TB, immunocompromise **Caution:** [C,?/-] not for peds **Disp:** SDV **SE:** Inj site rxn, HA

NATURAL and HERBAL AGENTS

The following is a guide to some common herbal products. These may be sold separately or in combination with other products. According to the FDA: "manufacturers of dietary supplements can make claims about how their products affect the structure or function of the body, but they may not claim to prevent, treat, cure, mitigate, or diagnose a disease without prior FDA approval"[1]

Black Cohosh **Uses:** Sx of menopause (eg, hot flashes), PMS, hypercholesterolemia, peripheral arterial Dz; has anti-inflammatory & sedative effects **Efficacy:** May have short-term benefit on menopausal Sx **Dose:** 20–40 mg twice daily **Caution:** May further ↓ lipids &/or BP w/ prescription meds **Contra:** PRG (miscarriage, prematurity reports) **SE:** OD can cause N/V, dizziness, nervous system & visual changes, bradycardia, & (possibly) Szs, liver damage/failure

Chamomile **Uses:** Antispasmodic, sedative, anti-inflammatory, astringent, antibacterial. **Dose:** 10–15 g PO qd (3 g dried flower heads tid–qid between meals; can steep in 250 mL hot H_2O) **Caution:** w/ allergy to chrysanthemums, ragweed, asters (family Compositae) **SE:** Contact dermatitis; allergy, anaphylaxis **Interactions:** W/ anticoagulants, additive w/ sedatives (benzodiazepines); delayed ↓ gastric absorption of meds if taken together (↓ GI motility)

Cranberry (*Vaccinium macrocarpon*) **Uses:** Prevention & Rx UTI. **Efficacy:** Possibly effective **Dose:** 300–400 mg twice daily or 6 oz juice QID Tincture ½–1 tsp up to 3×/day, tea 2–3 tsps of dried flowers per cup; creams—apply topically 2–3 to 3 ×s/day PO **Caution:** May ↑ kidney stones in some susceptible individuals, vomiting **SE:** None known **Interactions:** None significant

Dong Quai (*Angelica polymorpha, sinensis*) **Uses:** Uterine stimulant; anemia, menstrual cramps, irregular menses, & menopausal Sx; anti-inflammatory, vasodilator, CNS stimulant, immunosuppressant, analgesic, antipyretic, antiasthmatic **Efficacy:** Possibly effective for menopausal Sx **Dose:** 3–15 gm daily, 9–12 g PO tab bid. **Caution:** Avoid in PRG & lactation. **SE:** D, photosensitivity, skin cancer. **Interactions:** Anticoagulants (↑ INR w/warfarin).

Echinacea (*Echinacea purpurea*) **Uses:** Immune system stimulant; prevention/Rx URI of colds, flu; supportive care in chronic infections of the resp/lower urinary tract **Efficacy:** Not established; may ↓ severity & duration of URI **Dose:** Cap 500 mg, 6–9 mL expressed juice or 2–5 g dried root PO **Caution:**

---

[1]Based on data in Haist SA and Robbins JB: *Internal Medicine on Call*, 4th ed, 2005 McGraw-Hill.

Do not use w/ progressive systemic or immune Dzs (eg, TB, collagen–vascular disorders, MS); may interfere with immunosuppressive therapy, not OK w/ PRG; do not use >8 consecutive wk; possible immunosuppression **SE:** N; rash **Interactions:** Anabolic steroids, amiodarone, MTX, corticosteroids, cyclosporine.

Ephedra/MaHuang
Uses: Stimulant, aid in weight loss, bronchial dilation. **Dose:** Not OK due to reported deaths. (>100 mg/d can be life-threatening). US sales banned by FDA in 2004 **Caution:** Adverse cardiac events, strokes, death **SE:** Nervousness, HA, insomnia, palpitations, V, hyperglycemia **Interactions:** Digoxin, antihypertensives, antidepressants, diabetic medications

Fish Oil Supplements (omega-3 polyunsaturated fatty acid):
Uses: CAD, hypercholesterolemia, hypertriglyceridemia, Type 2 DM, arthritis **Efficacy:** No definitive data on ↓ cardiac risk in general population; may ↓ lipids and help w/ secondary MI prevention **Dose:** One FDA approved (see Omacor, page 145); OTC 1500–3000 mg/d **Caution:** Mercury contamination possible, some studies suggest ↑ cardiac events, **SE:** ↑ bleed risk, dyspepsia, belching, aftertaste **Interactions:** Anticoagulants

Evening Primrose Oil
Uses: PMS, diabetic neuropathy, ADHD **Efficacy:** Possibly for PMS, not for menopausal Sx **Dose:** 2–4 g/d PO SE: Indigestion, N, soft stools, HA **Interactions:** ↑ Phenobarbital metabolism, ↓ Sz threshold

Feverfew (*Tanacetum parthenium*)
Uses: Prevent/Rx migraine; fever; menstrual disorders; arthritis; toothache; insect bites **Efficacy:** Weak for migraine prevention **Dose:** 125 mg PO of dried leaf (standardized to 0.2% of parthenolide) PO **Caution:** Do not use in PRG **SE:** Oral ulcers, gastric disturbance, swollen lips, abdominal pain; long-term SE unknown. **Interactions:** ASA, warfarin

Garlic (*Allium sativum*)
Uses: Antioxidant; hyperlipidemia; HTN; anti-infective (antibacterial, antifungal); tick repellant (oral) **Efficacy:** ↓ cholesterol by 4–6%; soln ↓ BP; possible ↓ GI/CAP risk **Dose:** 2–5 g, fresh garlic; 0.4–1.2 gm of dried powder; 2–5 mg oil; 300–1000 mg extract or other formulations = equal to 2–5 mg of allicin daily 400–1200 mg powder (2–5 mg allicin) PO **Caution:** Do not use in PRG (abortifacient); D/C 7 d preop (bleeding risk) **SE:** ↑ insulin levels, ↑ insulin/lipid/cholesterol levels, anemia, oral burning sensation, N/V/D **Interactions:** Warfarin & ASA (↓ plt aggregation), additive w/ DM agents (↑ hypoglycemia). CYP 450 3A4 inducer (may ↑ cyclosporine, HIV antivirals, oral contraceptives)

Ginger (*Zingiber officinale*)
Uses: Prevent motion sickness; N/V due to anesthesia **Efficacy:** Benefit in ↓ N/V w/motion or PRG; weak for postop or chemo **Dose:** 1–4 g rhizome or 0.5–2 g powder PO qd **Caution:** Pt w/ gallstones; excessive dose (↑ depression, & may interfere w/ cardiac Fxn or anticoagulants) **SE:** Heartburn **Interactions:** Excessive consumption may interfere with cardiac, DM, or anticoagulant meds (↓↓ plt aggregation) **Dose** Ginger powder tablets or capsules or fresh cut ginger in doses of 1–4 gms daily by mouth, divided into smaller doses

Ginkgo Biloba **Uses:** Memory deficits, dementia, anxiety, improvement Sx peripheral vascular Dz, vertigo, tinnitus, asthma/bronchospasm, antioxidant, premenstrual Sx (especially breast tenderness), impotence, SSRI-induced sexual dysfunction **Dose:** 60–80 mg standardized dry extract PO bid–tid **Efficacy:** Small cognition benefit w/ dementia; no other demonstrated benefit in healthy adults **Caution:** ↑ Bleeding risk (antagonism of plt-activating factor), concerning w/ antiplatelet agents (D/C 3 d preop); reports of ↑ Sz risk **SE:** GI upset, HA, dizziness, heart palpitations, rash **Interactions:** ASA, salicylates, warfarin

Ginseng **Uses:** "Energy booster," stress reduction, enhance brain activity & physical endurance (adaptogenic), antioxidant, aid in glucose control to type 2 diabetes **Efficacy:** Not established **Dose:** 1–2 g of root or 100–300 mg of extract (7% ginsenosides) PO TID **Caution:** w/ cardiac Dz, DM, hypotension, HTN, mania, schizophrenia, w/ corticosteroids; avoid in PRG; D/C 7 d preop (bleeding risk) **SE:** Controversial "ginseng abuse syndrome" w/ high dose (nervousness, excitation, HA, insomnia); palpitations, vaginal bleeding, breast nodules, hypoglycemia **Interactions:** Warfarin, antidepressants & caffeine (↑ stimulant effect), DM meds (↑ hypoglycemia)

Glucosamine Sulfate (Chitosamine) and Chondroitin Sulfate **Uses:** Osteoarthritis (glucosamine: rate-limiting step in glycosaminoglycan synthesis), ↑ cartilage rebuilding; chondroitin: biological polymer, flexible matrix between protein filaments in cartilage; draws fluids/nutrients into joint, "shock absorption") **Efficacy:** Controversial **Dose:** Glucosamine 500 PO tid, chondroitin 400 mg PO tid **Caution:** None known **SE:** ↑ Insulin resistance in DM; concentrated in cartilage, theoretically unlikely to cause toxic/teratogenic effects **Interactions:** *Glucosamine:* None. *Chondroitin:* Monitor anticoagulant therapy

Kava Kava (Kava Kava Root Extract, *Piper methysticum*) **Uses:** Anxiety, stress, restlessness, insomnia **Efficacy:** Possible mild anxiolytic **Dose:** Standardized extract (70% kavalactones) 100 mg PO bid–tid **Caution:** Hepatotox risk, banned in Europe/Canada. Not OK in PRG, lactation. D/C 24 h preop (may ↑ sedative effect of anesthetics) **SE:** Mild GI disturbances; rare allergic skin/rash reactions, may ↑ cholesterol; ↑ LFT /jaundice; vision changes, red eyes, puffy face, muscle weakness **Interactions:** Avoid w/ sedatives, alcohol, stimulants, barbiturates (may potentiate CNS effect)

Melatonin **Uses:** Insomnia, jet lag, antioxidant, immunostimulant **Efficacy:** Sedation most pronounced w/ elderly patients with ↑ endogenous melatonin levels; some evidence for jet lag **Dose:** 1–3 mg 20 min before HS (w/ CR 2 h before hs) **Caution:** Use synthetic rather than animal pineal gland, "heavy head," HA, depression, daytime sedation, dizziness **Interactions:** β-blockers, steroids, NSAIDs, benzodiazepines

Milk Thistle (*Silybum marianum*) **Uses:** Prevent/Rx liver damage (eg, from alcohol, toxins, cirrhosis, chronic hepatitis); preventive w/ chronic toxin exposure (painters, chemical workers, etc) **Efficacy:** Use before exposure more effective than use after damage has occurred **Dose:** 80–200 mg PO tid **SE:** GI intolerance **Interactions:** None

Saw Palmetto (*Serenoa repens*)
Uses: Rx BPH (weak 5-α-reductase inhibitor) **Efficacy:** Small–no significant benefit for prostatic Sx **Dose:** 320 mg qd **Caution:** Hormonal effects, avoid in PRG, w/ women of childbearing years **SE:** Mild GI upset, mild HA, D w/ large amounts **Interactions:** ↑ Iron absorption; ↑ estrogen replacement effects

St. John's Wort (*Hypericum perforatum*)
Uses: Mild–moderate depression, anxiety, gastritis, insomnia, vitiligo; anti-inflammatory; immune stimulant/anti-HIV/antiviral **Efficacy:** Variable; benefit w/ mild–moderate depression in several trials, but not always seen in clinically practice **Dose:** 2–4 g of herb or 0.2–1 mg of total hypericin (standardized extract) qd. Common preps: 300 mg PO tid (0.3% hypericin) **Caution:** Excessive doses may potentiate MAOI, cause allergic reaction, not OK in PRG **SE:** Photosensitivity, xerostomia, dizziness, constipation, confusion, fluctuating mood w/ chronic use **Interactions:** Do not use w/ prescription antidepressants, (especially MAOI); ↑ cyclosporine efficacy (may cause rejection), digoxin (may exacerbate CHF), protease inhibitors, theophylline, oral contraceptives; cytochrome P-450 3A4 enzyme inducer; potency can vary between products/batches

Valerian (*Valeriana officinalis*)
Uses: Anxiolytic, sedative, restlessness, dysmenorrheal **Efficacy:** Probably effective sedative (reduces sleep latency) **Dose:** 2–3 g in extract PO qd–bid added to ⅔ cup boiling H_2O, tincture 15–20 drops in H_2O, oral 400–900 mg at bedtime (combined w/ OTC sleep product Alluna) **Caution:** None known **SE:** Sedation, hangover effect, HA, cardiac disturbances, GI upset **Interactions:** Caution w/ other sedating agents (eg, alcohol, or prescription sedatives): may cause drowsiness w/ impaired Fxn

Yohimbine (*Pausinystalia yohimbe*)
Uses: Improve sexual vigor, Rx ED **Efficacy:** Variable **Dose:** 1 tablet = 5.4 mg PO tid (use w/ physician supervision) **Caution:** Do not use w/ renal/hepatic Dz; may exacerbate schizophrenia/mania (if pt predisposed). $α_2$-Adrenergic antagonist (↓ BP, abdominal distress, weakness w/ high doses), OD can be fatal; salivation, dilated pupils, arrhythmias **SE:** Anxiety, tremors, dizziness, high BP, ↑ heart rate **Interactions:** Do not use w/ antidepressants (eg, MAOIs, or similar agents)

Unsafe Herbs with Known Toxicity

Agent	Toxicities
Aconite	Salivation, N/V, blurred vision, cardiac arrhythmias
Aristolochic acid	Nephrotox
Calamus	Possible carcinogenicity
Chaparral	Hepatotox, possible carcinogenicity, nephrotox
"Chinese herbal mixtures"	May contain MaHuang or other dangerous herbs
Coltsfoot	Hepatotox, possibly carcinogenic
Comfrey	Hepatotox, carcinogenic
Ephedra/MaHuang	Adverse cardiac events, stroke, Sz
Juniper	High allergy potential, D, Sz, nephrotox
Kava kava	Hepatotox
Licorice	Chronic daily amounts (> 30 g/mo) can result in ↓ K⁺, Na/fluid retention w/HTN, myoglobinuria, hyporeflexia
Life root	Hepatotox, liver cancer
Mal luang/Ephedra	Adverse cardiac events, stroke, Sz
Pokeweed	GI cramping, N/D/V, labored breathing, ↓ BP, Sz
Sassafras	V, stupor, hallucinations, dermatitis, abortion, hypothermia, liver cancer
Usnic acid	Hepatotox
Yohimbine	Hypotension, abdominal distress, CNS stimulation (mania/& psychosis in predisposed individuals)

Tables

TABLE 1
Quick Guide to Dosing of Acetaminophen Based on the Tylenol Product Line

	Suspension[a] Drops and Original Drops 80 mg/0.8 mL Dropperful	Chewable[a] Tablets 80-mg tabs	Suspension[a] Liquid and Original Elixir 160 mg/5 mL	Junior[a] Strength 160-mg Caplets/ Chewables	Regular[b] Strength 325-mg Caplets/ Tablets	Extra Strength[b] 500-mg Caplets/ Gelcaps
Birth–3 mo/ 6–11 lb/ 2.5–5.4 kg	$\frac{1}{2}$ dppr[c] (0.4 mL)					
4–11 mo/ 12–17 lb/ 5.5–7.9 kg	1 dppr[c] (0.8 mL)		$\frac{1}{2}$ tsp			
12–23 mo/ 18–23 lb/ 8.0–10.9 kg	1$\frac{1}{2}$ dppr[c] (1.2 mL)		$\frac{3}{4}$ tsp			
2–3 y/24–35 lb/ 11.0–15.9 kg	2 dppr[c] (1.6 mL)	2 tab	1 tsp			
4–5 y/36–47 lb/ 16.0–21.9 kg		3 tab	1$\frac{1}{2}$ tsp			

208

6–8 y/48–59 lb/ 22.0–26.9 kg	4 tab	2 tsp	2 cap/tab
9–10 y/60–71 lb/ 27.0–31.9 kg	5 tab	2½ tsp	2½ cap/ tab
11 y/72–95 lb/ 32.0–43.9 kg	6 tab	4 tsp	3 cap/tab
Adults & children ≥ 12 y ≥ 96 lb ≥ 44.0 kg		4 cap/tab	1 or 2 caps/ tabs	2 caps/ gel

^a Doses should be administered 4 or 5 times daily. Do not exceed 5 doses in 24 h.

^b No more than 8 dosage units in any 24-h period. Not to be taken for pain for more than 10 days or for fever for more than 3 days unless directed by a physician.

^c Dropperful.

TABLE 2
Common Drug Levels[a]

Drug	When to Sample	Therapeutic Levels	Usual Half-Life	Potentially Toxic Levels
Antibiotics				
Gentamicin, Tobramycin	*Peak:* 30 min after 30-min infusion (peak level not necessary if extended-interval dosing: 6 mg/kg/dose) *Trough:* <0.5 h before next dose	*Peak:* 5–8 mcg/mL *Trough:* <2 mcg/mL <1.0 mcg/mL for extended intervals (6 mg/kg/dose) (peak levels not needed with extended-interval dosing)	2 h	Peak: >12 mcg/mL
Amikacin	Same as above *Peak:* 1 h after 1-h infusion	*Peak:* 20–30 mcg/mL	2 h	Peak: >35 mcg/mL
Vancomycin	*Trough:* <0.5 h before next dose	*Peak:* 30–40 mcg/mL	6–8 h	Peak: >50 mcg/mL Trough: >15 mcg/mL

Anticonvulsants

Carbamazepine	Trough: just before next oral dose	8–12 mcg/mL (monotherapy) 4–8 mcg/mL (polytherapy)	15–20 h	Trough: >12 mcg/mL
Ethosuximide	Trough: just before next oral dose	40–100 mcg/mL	30–60 h	Trough: >100 mcg/mL
Phenobarbital	Trough: just before next dose	15–40 mcg/mL	40–120 h	Trough: >40 mcg/mL
Phenytoin	May use free phenytoin to monitor[b] Trough: just before next dose	10–20 mcg/mL	Concentration-dependent	>20 mcg/mL
Primidone	Trough: just before next dose [primidone is metabolized to phenobarb; order levels separately]	5–12 mcg/mL	10–12 h	>12 mcg/mL
Valproic acid	Trough: just before next dose	50–100 mcg/mL	5–20 h	>100 mcg/mL

TABLE 2
(Continued)

Drug	When to Sample	Therapeutic Levels	Usual Half-Life	Potentially Toxic Levels
Bronchodilators				
Caffeine	*Trough:* just before next dose	Adults 5–15 mcg/mL Neonates 6–11 mcg/mL	Adults 3–4 h Neonates 30–140 h	20 mcg/mL
Theophylline (IV)	IV: 12–24 h after infusion started	5–15 mcg/mL	Nonsmoking adults 8 h Children and smoking adults 4 h	>20 mcg/mL
Theophylline (PO)	*Peak levels:* not recommended *Trough level:* just before next dose	5–15 mcg/mL		
Cardiovascular Agents				
Amiodarone	*Trough:* just before next dose	1–2.5 mcg/mL	30–100 days	>2.5 mcg/mL

Digoxin	Trough: just before next dose (levels drawn earlier than 6 h after a dose will be artificially elevated)	0.8–2.0 ng/mL	36 h	>2 ng/mL
Disopyramide	Trough: just before next dose	2–5 mcg/mL	4–10 h	>5 mcg/mL
Flecainide	Trough: just before next dose	0.2–1 mcg/mL	11–14 h	>1 mcg/mL
Lidocaine	Steady-state levels are usually achieved after 6–12 h	1.2–5 mcg/mL	1.5 h	>6 mcg/mL
Procainamide	Trough: just before next oral dose	4–10 mcg/mL NAPA + procaine: ≤30 mcg/mL	Procaine: 3–5 h NAPA: 6–10 h	>10 mcg/mL NAPA + procaine: >30 mcg/mL
Quinidine	Trough: just before next oral dose	2–5 mcg/mL	6 h	0.5 mcg/mL
Other Agents				
Amitriptyline plus nortriptyline	Trough: just before next dose	120–250 ng/mL		
Nortriptyline	Trough: just before next dose	50–140 ng/mL	18–20 h	
Lithium	Trough: just before next dose	0.5–1.5 mEq/mL		>1.5 mEq/mL

TABLE 2
(Continued)

Drug	When to Sample	Therapeutic Levels	Usual Half-Life	Potentially Toxic Levels
Imipramine plus desipramine	*Trough:* just before next dose	150–300 ng/mL		
Desipramine	*Trough:* just before next dose	50–300 ng/mL		
Methotrexate	By protocol	<0.5 mcmol/L after 48 h		
Cyclosporine	*Trough:* just before next dose	Highly variable *Renal:* 150–300 ng/mL (RIA) *Hepatic:* 150–300 ng/mL	Highly variable	
Doxepin	*Trough:* just before next dose	100–300 ng/mL		
Trazodone	*Trough:* just before next dose	900–2100 ng/mL		

ᵃResults of therapeutic drug monitoring *must* be interpreted in light of the complete clinical situation. For information on dosing or interpretation of drug levels contact the pharmacist or an order for a pharmacokinetic consult may be written in the patient's chart. Modified and reproduced with permission from the *Pharmacy and Therapeutics Committee Formulary*, 41st ed., Thomas Jefferson University Hospital, Philadelphia, PA.

ᵇMore reliable in cases of uremia and hypoalbuminemia.

TABLE 3
Local Anesthetic Comparison Chart for Commonly Used Injectable Agents

Agent	Proprietary Names	Onset	Duration	Maximum Dose mg/kg	Maximum Dose Volume in 70-kg Adult[a]
Bupivacaine	Marcaine	7–30 min	5–7 h	3	70 mL of 0.25% solution
Lidocaine	Xylocaine, Anestacon	5–30 min	2 h	4	23 mL of 1% solution
Lidocaine with epinephrine (1:200,000)		5–30 min	2–3 h	7	50 mL of 1% solution
Mepivacaine	Carbocaine	5–30 min	2–3 h	7	50 mL of 1% solution
Procaine	Novocaine	Rapid	30 min–1 h	10–15	70–105 mL of 1% solution

[a]To calculate the maximum dose if not a 70-kg adult, use the fact that a 1% solution has 10 mg of drug per milliliter.

215

TABLE 4
Comparison of Systemic Steroids

Drug	Relative Equivalent Dose (mg)	Mineralo- corticoid Activity	Duration (h)	Route
Betamethasone	0.75	0	36–72	PO, IM
Cortisone (Cortone)	25	2	8–12	PO, IM
Dexamethasone (Decadron)	0.75	0	36–72	PO, IV
Hydrocortisone (Solu-Cortef, Hydrocortone)	20	2	8–12	PO, IM, IV
Methylprednisolone acetate (Depo-Medrol)	4	0	36–72	PO, IM, IV
Methylprednisolone succinate (Solu-Medrol)	4	0	8–12	PO, IM, IV
Prednisone (Deltasone)	5	1	12–36	PO
Prednisolone (Delta-Cortef)	5	1	12–36	PO, IM, IV

TABLE 5
Topical Steroid Preparations

Agent	Common Trade Names	Potency	Apply
Alclometasone dipropionate	Aclovate, cream, oint 0.05%	Low	bid/tid
Amcinonide	Cyclocort, cream, lotion, oint 0.1%	High	bid/tid
Betamethasone			
Betamethasone valerate	Valisone cream, lotion 0.01%	Low	qd/bid
Betamethasone valerate	Valisone cream 0.01, 0.1%, oint, lotio- 0.1%	Intermediate	qd/bid
Betamethasone dipropionate	Diprosone cream 0.05%	High	qd/bid
Betamethasone dipropionate	Diprosone aerosol 0.1%	Ultrahigh	cd/bid
Betamethasone dipropionate, augmented	Diprolene oint, gel 0.5%		
Clobetasol propionate	Temovate cream, gel, oint, scalp, solr 0.5%	Ultrahigh	bid (2 wk max)
Clocortolone pivalate	Clocerm crem 0.1%	Intermediate	qd-qid
Desonide	DesOwen, cream, oint, lotion 0.05%	Low	bid-qid
Desoximetasone			
Desoximetasone 0.05%	Topicort LP cream, gel 0.05%	Intermediate	
Desoximetasone 0.25%	Topicort cream, oint	High	
Dexamethasone base	Aeroseb-Dex aerosol 0.01%	Low	bid-qid
	Decadron cream 0.1%		
Diflorasone diacetate	Psorcon oint 0.05%	Ultrahigh	bid/qid
Fluocinolone			
Fluocinolone acetonide 0.01%	Synalar cream, soln 0.01%	Low	bid/tid
Fluocinolone acetonide 0.025%	Synalar oint, cream 0.025%	Intermediate	bid/tid

(continued)

217

TABLE 5
(Continued)

Agent	Common Trade Names	Potency	Apply
Fluocinolone acetonide 0.2%	Synalar-HP cream 0.2%	High	bid/tid
Fluocinonide 0.05%	Lidex, anhydrous cream, gel, soln 0.05%	High	bid/tid oint
	Lidex-E aqueous cream 0.05%		
Flurandrenolide	Cordran cream, oint 0.025%	Intermediate	bid/tid
	cream, lotion, oint 0.05%	Intermediate	bid/tid
	tape, 4 mcg/cm²	Intermediate	
Fluticasone propionate	Cutivate cream 0.05%, oint 0.005%	Intermediate	qd
Halobetasol	Ultravate cream, oint 0.05%	Very high	bid
Halcinonide	Halog cream 0.025%, emollient base 0.1% cream, oint, sol 0.1%	High	qd/tid
Hydrocortisone			
Hydrocortisone	Cortizone, Caldecort, Hycort, Hytone, etc. aerosol 1%, cream 0.5, 1, 2.5%, gel 0.5% oint 0.5, 1, 2.5%, lotion 0.5, 1, 2.5%, paste 0.5%, soln 1%	Low	tid/qid
Hydrocortisone acetate	Corticaine cream, oint 0.5, 1%	Low	tid/qid
Hydrocortisone butyrate	Locoid oint, soln 0.1%	Intermediate	bid/tid
Hydrocortisone valerate	Westcort cream, oint 0.2%	Intermediate	bid/tid

Mometasone furoate	Elocon 0.1% cream, oint, lotion	Intermediate	qd
Prednicarbate	Dermatop 0.1% cream	Intermediate	b.d
Triamcinolone			
Triamcinolone acetonide 0.025%	Aristocort, Kenalog cream, oint, lotion 0.025%	Low	tid/qid
Triamcinolone acetonide 0.1%	Aristocort, Kenalog cream, oint, lotion 0.1%	Intermediate	tid/qid
	Aerosol 0.2-mg/2-sec spray		
Triamcinolone acetonide 0.5%	Aristocort, Kenalog cream, oint 0.5%	High	tid/qid

TABLE 6
Comparison of Insulins

Type of Insulin	Onset (h)	Peak (h)	Duration (h)
Ultra Rapid			
Apidra (glulisine)	Immediate	0.5–1.5	3–5
Humalog (lispro)	Immediate	0.5–1.5	3–5
NovoLog (insulin aspart)	Immediate	0.5–1.5	3–5
Rapid			
Regular Iletin II	0.25–0.5	2–4	5–7
Humulin R	0.5	2–4	6–8
Novolin R	0.5	2.5–5	5–8
Velosulin	0.5	2–5	6–8
Intermediate			
NPH Iletin II	1–2	6–12	18–24
Lente Iletin II	1–2	6–12	18–24
Humulin N	1–2	6–12	14–24
Novulin L	2.5–5	7–15	18–24
Novulin 70/30	0.5	7–12	24
Prolonged			
Ultralente	4–6	14–24	28–36
Humulin U	4–6	8–20	24–28
Lantus (insulin glargine)	4–6	No peak	24
Combination Insulins			
Humalog Mix (lispro protamine/ lispro)	0.25–0.5	1–4	24

TABLE 7
Commonly Used Oral Contraceptives[a]

Monophasics

Drug (Manufacturer)	Estrogen (mcg)	Progestin (mg)
Alesse 21, 28 (Wyeth)	Ethinyl estradiol (20)	Levonorgestrel (0.1)
Apri 28 (Barr)	Ethinyl estradiol (30)	Desogestrel (0.15)
Aviane 28 (Barr)	Ethinyl estradiol (20)	Levonorgestrel (0.1)
Brevicon 28 (Watson)	Ethinyl estradiol (35)	Norethindrone (0.5)
Cryselle 28 (Barr)	Ethinyl estradiol (30)	Norgestrel (0.3)
Demulen 1/35 21, 28 (Pfizer)	Ethinyl estradiol (35)	Ethynodiol diacetate (1)
Demulen 1/50 21, 28 (Pfizer)	Ethinyl estradiol (50)	Ethynodiol diacetate (1)
Desogen 28 (Organon)	Ethinyl estradiol (30)	Desogestrel (0.15)
Estrostep 28 (Warner-Chilcott)[b]	Ethinyl estradiol (20, 30, 35)	Norethindrone acetate (1)
Junel Fe 1/20 21, 28 (Barr)	Ethinyl estradiol (20)	Norethindrone acetate (1)
Junel Fe 1.5/30 21, 23 (Barr)	Ethinyl estradiol (30)	Norethindrone acetate (1.5)
Kariva 28 (Barr)	Ethinyl estradiol (20, 10)	Desogestrel (0.15)
Lessina 28 (Barr)	Ethinyl estradiol (20)	Levonorgestrel (0.1)
Levlen 28 (Berlex)	Ethinyl estradiol (30)	Levonorgestrel (0.15)
Levlite 28 (Berlex)	Ethinyl estradiol (20)	Levonorgestrel (0.1)
Levora 28 (Watson)	Ethinyl estradiol (30)	Levonorgestrel (0.15)
Loestrin Fe 1.5/30 21, 28 (Warner-Chilcott)	Ethinyl estradiol (30)	Norethindrone acetate (1.5)
Loestrin Fe 1/20 21, 28 (Warner-Chilcott)	Ethinyl estradiol (20)	Norethindrone acetate (1)
Lo/Ovral 21, 28 (Wyeth)	Ethinyl estradiol (30)	Norgestrel (0.3)
Low-Ogestrel 28 (Watson)	Ethinyl estradiol (30)	Norgestrel (0.3)
Microgestin Fe 1/20 21, 28 (Watson)	Ethinyl estradiol (20)	Norethindrone acetate (1)
Microgestin Fe 1.5/30 21, 28 (Watson)	Ethinyl estradiol (30)	Norethindrone acetate (1.5)

221

TABLE 7
(Continued)

Drug (Manufacturer)	Estrogen (mcg)	Progestin (mg)
Mircette 28 (Organon)	Ethinyl estradiol (20, 0, 10)	Desogestrel (0.15)
Modicon 28 (Ortho-McNeil)	Ethinyl estradiol (35)	Norethindrone (0.5)
MonoNessa 28 (Watson)	Ethinyl estradiol (35)	Norgestimate (0.25)
Necon 1/50 28 (Watson)	Mestranol (50)	Norethindrone (1)
Necon 0.5/35, 28 (Watson)	Ethinyl estradiol (35)	Norethindrone (0.5)
Necon 1/35 28 (Watson)	Ethinyl estradiol (35)	Norethindrone (1)
Nordette 21, 28 (King)	Ethinyl estradiol (30)	Levonorgestrel (0.15)
Nortrel 0.5/35 28 (Barr)	Ethinyl estradiol (35)	Norethindrone (0.5)
Nortrel 1/35 21, 28 (Barr)	Ethinyl estradiol (35)	Norethindrone (1)
Norinyl 1/35 28 (Watson)	Ethinyl estradiol (35)	Norethindrone (1)
Norinyl 1/50 28 (Watson)	Mestranol (50)	Norethindrone (1)
Ogestrel 28 (Watson)	Ethinyl estradiol (50)	Norgestrel (0.5)
Ortho-Cept 28 (Ortho-McNeil)	Ethinyl estradiol (30)	Desogestrel (0.15)
Ortho-Cyclen 28 (Ortho-McNeil)	Ethinyl estradiol (35)	Norgestimate (0.25)
Ortho-Novum 1/35 28 (Ortho-McNeil)	Ethinyl estradiol (35)	Norethindrone (1)
Ortho-Novum 1/50 28 (Ortho-McNeil)	Mestranol (50)	Norethindrone (1)
Ovcon 35 21, 28 (Warner-Chilcott)	Ethinyl estradiol (35)	Norethindrone (0.4)
Ovcon 50 28 (Warner-Chilcott)	Ethinyl estradiol (50)	Norethindrone (1)
Ovral 21, 28 (Wyeth-Ayerst)	Ethinyl estradiol (50)	Norgestrel (0.5)
Portia 28 (Barr)	Ethinyl estradiol (30)	Levonorgestrel (0.15)
Sprintec 28 (Barr)	Ethinyl estradiol (35)	Norgestimate (0.25)
Yasmin 28 (Berlex)	Ethinyl estradiol (30)	Drospirenone (3)
Zovia 1/50E 28 (Watson)	Ethinyl estradiol (50)	Ethynodiol diacetate (1)
Zovia 1/35E 28 (Watson)	Ethinyl estradiol (35)	Ethynodiol diacetate (1)

Multiphasics

Drug	Estrogen (mcg)	Progestin (mg)
Cyclessa 28 (Organon)	Ethinyl estradiol (25)	Desogestrel (0.1, 0.125, 0.15)
Enpresse 28 (Barr)	Ethinyl estradiol (30, 40, 30)	Levonorgestrel (0.05, 0.075, 0.125)
Necon 10/11 21, 28 (Watson)	Ethinyl estradiol (35)	Norethindrone (0.5, 1)
Necon 7/7/7 (Watson)	Ethinyl estradiol (35)	Norethindrone (0.5, 0.75, 1)
Nortrel 7/7/7 28 (Barr)	Ethinyl estradiol (35)	Norethindrone (0.5, 0.75, 1)
Ortho Tri-Cyclen 21, 28 (Ortho-McNeil)[b]	Ethinyl estradiol (25)	Norgestimate (0.18, 0.215, 0.25)
Ortho Tri-Cyclen lo 21, 28 (Ortho-McNei)	Ethinyl estradiol (35, 35, 35)	Norgestimate (0.18, 0.215, 0.25)
Ortho-Novum 10/11 21 (Ortho-McNeil)	Ethinyl estradiol (35, 35)	Norethindrone (0.5, 1.0)
Ortho-Novum 7/7/7 21 (Ortho-McNeil)	Ethinyl estradiol (35, 35, 35)	Norethindrone (0.5, 0.75, 1.0)
Tri-Levlen 28 (Berlex)	Ethinyl estradiol (30, 40, 30)	Levonorgestrel (0.05, 0.075, 0.125)
Tri-Nessa 28 (Watson)	Ethinyl estradiol (35)	Norgestimate (0.18, 0.215, 0.25)
Tri-Norinyl 21, 28 (Watson)	Ethinyl estradiol (35, 35, 35)	Norethindrone (0.5, 1.0, 0.5)
Triphasil 21, 28 (Wyeth)	Ethinyl estradiol (30, 40, 30)	Levonorgestrel (0.05, 0.075, 0.125)
Tri-Sprintec (Barr)	Ethinyl estradiol (35)	Norgestimate (0.18, 0.215, 0.25)
Trivora-28 (Watson)	Ethinyl estradiol (30, 40, 30)	Levonorgestrel (0.05, 0.075, 0.125)
Velivet (Barr)	Ethinyl estradiol (25)	Desogestrel (0.1, 0.125, 0.15)

223

TABLE 7
(Continued)

Progestin Only

Drug	Estrogen (mcg)	Progestin (mg)
Camila (Barr)	None	Norethindrone (0.35)
Errin (Barr)	None	Norethindrone (0.35)
Jolivette 28 (Watson)	None	Norethindrone (0.35)
Micronor (Ortho-McNeil)	None	Norethindrone (0.35)
Nor-QD (Watson)	None	Norethindrone (0.35)
Nora-BE 28 (Ortho-McNeil)	None	Norethindrone (0.35)
Ovrette (Wyeth-Ayerst)	None	Norgestrel (0.075)

Extended-Cycle Combination

Drug		
Seasonale (Duramed)	Ethinyl estradiol (30)	Levonorgestrel (0.15)

Based in part on data published in the *Medical Letter* Volume 2 (Issue 24) August 2004.

[a] The designations 21 and 28 refer to number of days in regimen available.

[b] Also approved for acne.

TABLE 8
Some Common Oral Potassium Supplements

Brand Name	Salt	Form	mEq Potassium/ Dosing Unit
Glu-K	Gluconate	Tablet	2 mEq/tablet
Kaochlor 10%	KCl	Liquid	20 mEq/15 mL
Kaochlor S-F 10% (sugar-free)	KCl	Liquid	20 mEq/15 mL
Kaochlor Eff	Bicarbonate/ KCl/citrate	Effervescent tablet	20 mEq/tablet
Kaon elixir	Gluconate	Liquid	20 mEq/15 mL
Kaon	Gluconate	Tablet	5 mEq/tablet
Kaon-Cl	KCl	Tablet, SR	6.67 mEq/tablet
Kaon-Cl 20%	KCl	Liquid	40 mEq/15 mL
KayCiel	KCl	Liquid	20 mEq/15 mL
K-Lor	KCl	Powder	15 or 20 mEq/packet
Klorvess	Bicarbonate/ KCl	Liquid	20 mEq/15 mL
Klotrix	KCl	Tablet, SR	10 mEq/tablet
K Lyte	Bicarbonate/ citrate	Effervescent tablet	25 mEq/tablet
K-Tab	KCl	Tablet, SR	10 mEq/tablet
Micro-K	KCl	Capsule, SR	8 mEq/capsule
Slow-K	KCl	Tablet, SR	8 mEq/tablet
Tri-K	Acetate/bicarbonate and citrate	Liquid	45 mEq/15 mL
Twin-K	Citrate/gluconate	Liquid	20 mEq/5 mL

SR = sustained release.

TABLE 9
Tetanus Prophylaxis

History of Absorbed Tetanus Toxoid Immunization	Clean, Minor Wounds		All Other Wounds[a]	
	Td[b]	TIG[c]	Td[d]	TIG[c]
Unknown or <3 doses	Yes	No	Yes	Yes
=3 doses	No[e]	No	No[f]	No

[a]Such as, but not limited to, wounds contaminated with dirt, feces, soil, saliva, etc; puncture wounds; avulsions and wounds resulting from missiles, crushing, burns, and frostbite.

[b]Td = tetanus-diphtheria toxoid (adult type), 0.5 mL IM.
- For children <7 y, DPT (DT, if pertussis vaccine is contraindicated) is preferred to tetanus toxoid alone.
- For persons >7 y, Td is preferred to tetanus toxoid alone.
- DT = diphtheria-tetanus toxoid (pediatric), used for those who cannot receive pertussis.

[c]TIG = tetanus immune globulin, 250 units IM.

[d]If only 3 doses of fluid toxoid have been received, then a fourth dose of toxoid, preferably an adsorbed toxoid, should be given.

[e]Yes, if >10 y since last dose.

[f]Yes, if >5 y since last dose.

Source: Based on guidelines from the Centers for Disease Control and Prevention and reported in MMWR.

TABLE 10
Oral Anticoagulant Standards of Practice

Thromboembolic Disorder	INR	Duration
Deep Venous Thrombosis & Pulmonary Embolism		
Treatment single episode		
Transient risk factor	2–3	3 mo
Idiopathic	2–3	6–12 mo
Recurrent systemic embolism	2–3	Indefinite
Prevention of Systemic Embolism		
Atrial fibrillation (AF)[a]	2–3	Indefinite
AF: cardioversion	2–3	3 wk prior; 4 wk post sinus rhythm
Valvular heart disease	2–3	Indefinite
Cardiomyopathy	2–3	Indefinite
Acute Myocardial Infarction		
High risk patients[c]	2–3 + low dose aspirin	3 mo
Prosthetic Valves		
Tissue heart valves	2–3	3 mo
Bileaflet mechanical valves in aortic position		2–3 mo Indefinite
Other mechanical prosthetic valves[h]	2.5–3.5	Indefinite

[a]With high-risk factors or multiple moderate risk factors.

[b]May add aspirin 81 mg to warfarin in patients with caged ball or caged disk valves or with additional risk factors.

[c]Large anterior MI, significant heart failure, intracardiac thrombus, and/or history of thromboembolic event

INR = international normalized ratio.

Source: Based on data published in *Chest* 2004 Sep; 126 (Suppl): 1635–6965.

TABLE 11
Serotonin 5-HT$_1$ Receptor Agonists

Drug	Initial Dose	Repeat Dose	Max. Dose/24h	Supplied
Almotriptan (Axert)	6.25 or 12.5 mg PO	× 1 in 2 h	25 mg	Tabs 6.25, 12.5 mg
Frovatriptan (Frova)	2.5 mg PO	in 2 h	7.5 mg	Tabs 2.5 mg
Naratriptan (Amerge)	1 or 2.5 mg PO[a]	in 4 h	5 mg	Tabs 1, 2.5 mg
Rizatriptan (Maxalt)	5 or 10 mg PO[b]	in 2 h	30 mg	Tabs 5, 10 mg Disintegrating tabs 5, 10 mg
Sumatriptan (Imitrex)	25, 50, or 100 mg PO	in 2 h	200 mg	Tabs 25, 50 mg
	5–20 mg intranasally	in 2 h	40 mg	Disintegrating tabs 25, 50 mg
	6 mg SQ	in 1 h	12 mg	Nasal spray 5, 20 mg Inj 12 mg/mL
Zolmitriptan (Zomig)	2.5 or 5 mg PO	in 2 h	10 mg	Tabs 2.5, 5 mg

Precautions/contraindications: [C, M]; ischemic heart disease, coronary artery vasospasm, Prinzmetal's angina, uncontrolled HTN, hemiplegic or basilar migraine, ergots, use of another serotonin agonist within 24 h, use with MAOI. Side effects: dizziness, somnolence, paresthesias, nausea, flushing, dry mouth, coronary vasospasm, chest tightness, HTN, GI upset.

[a]Reduce dose in mild renal and hepatic insufficiency (2.5 mg/d MAX); contraindicated with severe renal (CrCl <15 mL/min) or hepatic impairment.
[b]Initiate therapy at 5 mg PO (15 mg/d max) in patients receiving propranolol.

TABLE 12
Antiarrhythmics: Vaughn Williams Classification

Class I: Sodium Channel Blockade

A. **Class Ia:** Lengthens duration of action potential (↑ the refractory period in atrial and ventricular muscle, in SA and AV conduction systems, and Purkinje fibers)
   1. Amiodarone (also class II, III, IV)
   2. Disopyramide (Norpace)
   3. Imipramine (MAO inhibitor)
   4. Procainamide (Pronestyl)
   5. Quinidine
B. **Class Ib:** No effect on action potential
   1. Lidocaine (Xylocaine)
   2. Mexiletine (Mexitil)
   3. Phenytoin (Dilantin)
   4. Tocainide (Tonocard)
C. **Class Ic:** Greater sodium current depression (blocks the fast inward Na⁺ current in heart muscle and Purkinje fibers, and slows the rate of ↑ of phase 0 of the action potential)
   1. Flecainide (Tambocor)
   2. Propafenone

Class II: Beta blocker

D. Amiodarone (also class Ia, III, IV)
E. Esmolol (Brevibloc)
F. Sotalol (also class III)

Class III: Prolong refractory period via action potential

G. Amiodarone (also class Ia, II, IV)
H. Sotalol

Class IV: Calcium channel blocker

I. Amiodarone (also class Ia, II, III)
J. Diltiazem (Cardizem)
K. Verapamil (Calan)

TABLE 13
Cytochrome P-450 Isoenzymes and the Drugs They Metabolize, Inhibit, and Induce[a]

CYP1A2

Substrates:	Acetaminophen, caffeine, clozapine, imipramine, theophylline, propranolol
Inhibitors:	Most fluoroquinolone antibiotics, fluvoxamine, cimetidine
Inducers:	Tobacco smoking, charcoal-broiled foods, cruciferous vegetables, omeprazole

CYP2C9

Substrates:	Most NSAIDs (including COX-2), warfarin, phenytoin
Inhibitors:	Fluconazole
Inducers:	Barbiturates, rifampin

CYP2C19

Substrates:	Diazepam, lansoprazole, omeprazole, phenytoin, pantoprazole
Inhibitors:	Omeprazole, isoniazid, ketoconazole
Inducers:	Barbiturates, rifampin

CYP2D6

Substrates:	Most β-blockers, codeine, clomipramine, clozapine, codeine, encainide, flecainide, fluoxetine, haloperidol, hydrocodone, 4-methoxy-amphetamine, metoprolol, mexiletine, oxycodone, paroxetine, propafenone, propoxyphene, risperidone, selegiline (deprenyl), thioridazine, most tricyclic antidepressants, timolol
Inhibitors:	Fluoxetine, haloperidol, paroxetine, quinidine
Inducers:	Unknown

CYP3A

Substrates:	**Anticholinergics:** Darifenacin, oxybutynin, solifenacin, tolterodine **Benzodiazepines:** Alprazolam, midazolam, triazolam **Ca channel blockers:** Diltiazem, felodipine, nimodipine, nifedipine, nisoldipine, verapamil

(continued)

TABLE 13 (continued)
Cytochrome P-450 Isoenzymes and the Drugs They Metabolize, Inhibit, and Induce[a]

	Chemotherapy: Cyclophosphamide, erlotinib, ifosfamide, paclitaxel, tamoxifen, vinblastine, vincristine
	HIV protease inhibitors: Amprenavir, atazanavir, indinavir, nelfinavir, ritonavir, saquinavir
	HMG-CoA reductase inhibitors: Atorvastatin, lovastatin, simvastatin
	Immunosuppressive agents: Cyclosporine, tacrolimus
	Macrolide-type antibiotics: Clarithromycin, erythromycin, telithromycin, troleandomycin
	Opioids: Alfentanyl, cocaine, fentanyl, sufentanil
	Steroids: Budesonide, cortisol, 17-β-estradiol, progesterone
	Others: Acetaminophen, amiodarone, carbamazepine, delavirdine, efavirenz, nevirapine, quinidine, repaglinide, sildenafil, tadalafil, trazodone, vardenafil
Inhibitors:	Amiodarone, amprenavir, atazanavir, ciprofloxacin, cisapride, clarithromycin, diltiazem, erythromycin, fluconazole, fluvoxamine, grapefruit juice (in high ingestion), indinavir, itraconazole, ketoconazole, nefazodone, nelfinavir, norfloxacin, ritonavir, telithromycin, troleandomycin, verapamil, voriconazole
Inducers:	Carbamazepine, efavirenz, glucocorticoids, macrolide antibiotics, nevirapine, phenytoin, phenobarbital, rifabutin, rifapentine, rifampin, St. John's wort

[a]Increased or decreased (primarily hepatic cytochrome P-450) metabolism of medications may influence the effectiveness of drugs or result in significant drug-drug interactions. Understanding the common cytochrome P-450 isoforms (eg, CYP2C9, CYP2D9, CYP2C19, CYP3A4) and common drugs that are metabolized by (aka "substrates"), inhibit, or induce activity of the isoform helps minimize significant drug interactions. CYP3A is involved in the metabolism of >50% of drugs metabolized by the liver.

Based on data from Katzung B (ed): *Basic and Clinical Pharmacology*, 9th ed. McGraw-Hill, New York, 2004; *The Medical Letter*, Volume 47, July 4, 2004; http://www.fda.gov/cder/drug/drugreactions (accessed September 16, 2006).

TABLE 14
Serotonin syndrome as a result of combined use of selective serotonin reuptake inhibitors (SSRI) and triptans

Serotonin syndrome is a life-threatening condition that can develop when SSRIs and 5-hydroxytryptamine receptor agonists (triptans) are used together. Serotonin syndrome may be more likely to occur when starting or increasing the dose of an SSRI or a triptan.

Signs and symptoms of serotonin syndrome include the following:

restlessness	fast heartbeat
diarrhea	vomiting
hallucinations	increased body temperature
coma	fast changes in blood pressure
loss of coordination	overactive reflexes
nausea	

TABLE 15
Composition of selected multivitamins and multivitamins with mineral and trace element supplements

| | Vitamins | | | | | | | | | | | | |
| | Fat Soluble | | | | Water Soluble | | | | | | | | |
	A	D	E	K	C	B	B_2	B_3	B_6	Folate	B_{12}	Biotin	B_5
Centrum	70	100	100	31	100	100	100	100	100	100	100	10	100
Centrum Performance	70	100	200	31	200	300	300	200	300	100	300	13	100
Centrum Silver	70	100	150	13	100	100	100	100	150	100	417	10	100
NatureMade Multi	60	100	167	31	200	100	100	100	100	100	100	10	100
NatureMade Complete	60	100	100	NA	100	100	100	100	100	100	100	NA	100
NatureMade Multi Daily	60	100	500	50	500	3333	2941	250	2500	100	833	17	500
NatureMade Multi Max	60	100	500	50	500	200	200	100	200	100	417	10	100
NatureMade Multi 50+	100	100	200	13	200	300	200	100	300	100	417	10	100
One-A-Day 50 Plus	50	100	110	25	200	300	200	100	300	100	417	10	150
One-A-Day Essential	100	100	100	NA	100	100	100	100	100	100	100	NA	100

233

TABLE 15
Composition of selected multivitamins and multivitamins with mineral and trace element supplements (continued)

| | Vitamins | | | | | | | | | | | | |
| | Fat Soluble | | | | Water Soluble | | | | | | | | |
	A	D	E	K	C	B_1	B_2	B_3	B_6	Folate	B_{12}	Biotin	B_5
One-A-Day Maximum	50	100	100	31	100	100	100	100	100	100	100	10	100
Therapeutic Vitamin	100	100	100	NA	150	200	200	100	150	100	150	10	100
Theragran-M Advanced Formula High Potency	100	100	200	35	150	200	200	100	300	100	200	10	100
Theragran-M Premier High Potency	70	100	200	31	200	267	235	125	200	100	150	10	100
Theragran-M Premier 50 Plus High Potency	70	100	200	13	125	200	176	125	300	100	500	12	150

234

	Minerals								Trace Elements				
	Ca	P	Mg	Fe	Zn	I	Se	K	Mn	Cu	Cr	Mo	Other
Therapeutic Vitamin + Minerals Enhanced	100	100	200	NA	150	200	200	100	300	100	200	10	100
Unicap M	100	100	100	NA	100	100	100	100	100	100	100	NA	100
Unicap Senior	100	50	50	NA	100	80	82	80	110	100	50	NA	100
Unicap T	100	100	100	NA	833	667	588	500	300	100	300	NA	250
Centrum	16	11	25	100	100	100	29	2	100	100	100	100	
Centrum Performance	10	5	10	100	100	100	100	2	200	100	100	100	lyco-pene
Centrum Silver	20	5	25	NA	100	100	29	2	100	100	125	100	
NatureMade Multi Complete	10	8	25	50	100	100	35	1	100	100	100	33	Ginseng Ginkgo
NatureMade Multi Daily	45	NA	NA	100	100	NA	NA	NA	NA	NA	NA	NA	lycopene
NatureMade Multi Max	10	4	6	50	100	100	100	1	100	100	100	NA	lyco-pene Lutein

TABLE 15
Composition of selected multivitamins and multivitamins with mineral and trace element supplements (continued)

	Minerals								Trace Elements				
	Ca	P	Mg	Fe	Zn	I	Se	K	Mn	Cu	Cr	Mo	Other
NatureMade Multi 50+	20	5	25		100	100	71	2	100	100	100	33	
One-A-Day 50 Plus	12	NA	25	NA	150	100	150	1	200	100	150	120	Lutein
One-A-Day Essential	NA	NA	NA	NA	NA	100	NA	NA	NA	NA	NA	NA	
One-A-Day Maximum	16	11	25	100	100	100	29	2	175	100	54	213	
Therapeutic 7 Vitamin	NA	NA	NA	NA	NA	NA	NA	NA	NA	NA	NA	NA	
Theragran-M Advanced Formula High Potency	4	3	26	50	100	100	100	1	100	100	42	100	
Theragran-M Premier High Potency	17	11	25	100	100	100	286	2	100	175	100	107	Lutein
Theragran-M Premier 50 Plus High Potency	20	5	25	0	113	100	286	2	175	100	125	100	Lutein

Therapeutic Vitamin + Minerals Enhanced	4	3	25	50	100	100	<1	100	100	42	100
Unicap M	6	5	NA	100	100	NA	<1	50	NA	NA	NA
Unicap Senior	10	8	8	56	100	100	<1	50	50	NA	NA
Unicap T	NA	NA	NA	100	100	14	<1	50	50	NA	NA

Common multivitamins available without a prescription are listed. Most chain stores have generic versions of many of the multivitamin supplements listed above; thus, specific generic brands are not listed. Many specialty vitamin combinations are available, but not included in this list. [Examples are B vitamins plus C, supplements for a specific condition or organ, pediatric and infant formulations, and prenatal vitamins.)

Values are listed as percentages of the Daily Value based on Recommended Dietary Allowances or Dietary Reference Intakes (Food and Nutrition Board, Institute of Medicine, National Academy of Science).

[1] Common generic brands (when other than the store name itself) are: Osco Drug Central-Vite (Albertson's); Spectravite (CVS); Kirkland Signature Daily Multivitamin (Costco); Whole Source, PharmAssure (Rite Aid); CentroVite (Safeway); Member's Mark (Sam's Club); Vitasmart (Kmart); Century (Target); A thru Z Select, Super Avitinol, Ultra Choice (Walgreens) Equate Complete or Spring Valley, Sentury-Vite (Wal-Mart).

Vitamins: B₁ = Thiamine; B₂ = Riboflavin; B₆ = Niacin; B₆ = Pyridoxine; B₁₂ = Cyanocobalamin. Elements: Ca = calcium; Cr = chromium; Cu = copper; Fe = iron; Fl = fluoride; I = iodine; K = potassium; Mg = magnesium; Mn = manganese; Mo = Molybdenum; P = phosphorus; Se = selenium; Zn = zinc; NA = not applicable or not available.

Index